ENDOCRINOLOGY RESEARCH AND CLINICAL DEVELOPMENTS

LEPTIN

BIOSYNTHESIS, FUNCTIONS AND CLINICAL SIGNIFICANCE

ENDOCRINOLOGY RESEARCH AND CLINICAL DEVELOPMENTS

Additional books in this series can be found on Nova's website
under the Series tab.

Additional e-books in this series can be found on Nova's website
under the e-book tab.

ENDOCRINOLOGY RESEARCH AND CLINICAL DEVELOPMENTS

LEPTIN

BIOSYNTHESIS, FUNCTIONS AND CLINICAL SIGNIFICANCE

EDWARD L. BLUM
EDITOR

NOVA BIOMEDICAL

New York

For permission to use material from this book please contact us:
Telephone 631-231-7269; Fax 631-231-8175
Web Site: http://www.novapublishers.com

Library of Congress Cataloging-in-Publication Data

Library of Congress Control Number: 2013956183

ISBN: 978-1-62948-801-1

Published by Nova Science Publishers, Inc. † New York

CONTENTS

Preface **vii**

Chapter 1 Leptin in Alzheimer's Disease and other Cognitive Disorders and its Association with Underlying Lipid Abnormalities **1**
Jane M. Johnston, George Perry, J. Wesson Ashford and Nikolaos Tezapsidis

Chapter 2 Fat, Salt and Blood Pressure: The Leptin-Renal Axis **17**
Cristian Del Carpio Tenorio, Pramesh Dhakal, Garry P. Reams, Ronald H. Freeman, Robert Spear, Kan Liu and Daniel Villarreal

Chapter 3 Melanoma and Leptin **33**
Arash Sabetisoofyani

Chapter 4 Inhibition of Oncogenic Effects of Leptin by cAMP Elevation in Triple Negative Breast Cancer Cells **39**
Annamaria Spina, Francesca Di Maiolo, Luigi Sapio, Luca Sorvillo and Silvio Naviglio

Chapter 5 Leptin: From Energy Balance to Inflammatory Process in Obesity **45**
Flávia Campos Corgosinho, Andrea Frontini, Antonio Giordano, Saverio Cinti and Ana Raimunda Dâmaso

Chapter 6 Leptin Regulation of Intestinal Nutrients Absorption **61**
Jaione Barrenetxe, Carmen Fanjul and María Pilar Lostao

Chapter 7 Implications of Leptin in Male Reproductive Function **83**
Luc J. Martin

Chapter 8 Role of Leptin in Early Life Increases the Metabolic Vulnerability in Adults: Physiological, Pathological and Potential Therapeutic Implications **111**
L. Manuel Apolinar and E. de la Chesnaye Caraveo

Chapter 9 The Skeletal Effects of Leptin **129**
Natalie K. Y. Wee and Paul A. Baldock

Chapter 10 The Physiological Roles of Leptin in the Oral and Maxillofacial Region: Promotive Effects on Mucosal Wound Healing and Tooth Development **141**
Reiko Tokuyama and Kazuhito Satomura

Chapter 11 Respiratory Responses to Microinjections of Leptin into the Pre-Bötzinger Complex of the Rat **157**
Alexey N. Inyushkin and Elena M. Inyushkina

Chapter 12 Leptin as a Reproductive Modulator: An Eco-Physiological Approach **173**
Elena Bukovetzky and Abraham Haim

Index **189**

PREFACE

Leptin was originally described for its role in obesity and energy homeostasis. This book focuses on the biosynthesis, functions and overall clinical significance of leptin. Leptin's association to Alzheimer's diseases and other cognitive disorders is discussed along with the leptin-renal axis; the relationship of leptin and melanoma; the inhibition of oncogenic effects of leptin by cAMP elevation in triple negative breast cancer cells; the leptin regulation of intestinal nutrients absorption; the implications of leptin in male reproductive function; the role of leptin in early life metabolism and its physiological, pathological, and potential therapeutic implications; the skeletal effects of leptin; the physiological roles of leptin in oral and maxillofacial region; the respiratory responses to microinjectons of leptin; and leptin as a reproductive modulator.

Chapter 1 - Leptin was originally described for its role in obesity and energy homeostasis. These properties are centrally mediated through leptin receptors (ObR) in the arcuate nucleus of the hypothalamus. However, neuromodulatory properties of leptin in neuroanatomically diverse regions of the brain may play significant roles in other physiological functions. For example, the high density of functional leptin receptors found in the hippocampus and cortical regions of the brain may underline its involvement in memory and cognition. *In vitro* studies support a role of leptin in synaptic function and plasticity along with amyloidogenesis, amyloid removal and tau-phosphorylation. *In vivo* studies have confirmed a role in Alzheimer's disease (AD)-related pathology and a beneficial effect on cognitive deterioration of AD-transgenic animals. Epidemiological studies show that low levels of circulating plasma leptin are associated with dementia and depression, conditions often observed in patients presenting with various disorders including AD, Parkinson's dementia, Huntington's and prion diseases. Herein, the authors review the role of leptin in brain, cognitive impairment and underlying lipid abnormalities and discuss the benefits of leptin replacement therapy.

Chapter 2 - Leptin is a 16-kDa-peptide hormone that is primarily synthesized and secreted by adipose tissue. One of the major actions of this hormone is the control of energy balance by binding to receptors in the hypothalamus, leading to reduction in food intake, elevation in temperature and energy expenditure. In addition, available evidence suggests that leptin, through both direct and indirect mechanisms, plays an important role in cardiovascular and renal regulation. While the relevance of endogenous leptin needs further clarification, it appears to function as a pressure and volume-regulating factor under conditions of health. However, in abnormal situations characterized by chronic hyperleptinemia such as obesity, it may function pathophysiologically for the development of hypertension and for direct renal and vascular damage.

Chapter 3 - Epidemiological studies suggest that obesity increases the risk of developing several cancers, including melanoma. Obesity increases the expression of angiogenic factors, such as leptin, that may contribute to tumor growth. However, a direct cause and effect relationship between obesity and tumor growth has not been clearly established and the role of leptin in accelerating tumor growth is unclear. The role of diet in melanoma has been explored in several studies but the findings have been inconsistent. Specifically, high intake of specific agents, such as antioxidants and retinoid-rich food has been linked to a protective effect against melanoma development. Similar associations have been found with higher blood levels of a-tocopherol , b-carotene and retinol, as well as with greater dietary intakes of vitamin E and b-carotene in several case–control studies. Anthropometrical measures, such as height, weight and body mass index (BMI); have been associated with an increased risk of several malignancies, including melanoma. Leptin, a hormone secreted by adipose tissue, controls food intake and energy balance by providing signals to the hypothalamus. Serum levels of leptin are positively related with body composition and insulin levels, female sex and alcohol consumption and inversely related to cigarette smoking.

Chapter 4 - Triple-negative breast cancers (TNBC) are characterised by an aggressive phenotype and have been associated with poor prognosis. Triple-negative breast cancer patients are unresponsive to current targeted therapies and other treatment options are only partially effective. Therefore, new pharmacological approaches are needed.

Given the relevant role of leptin in breast cancer growth and metastasis, leptin system has emerged as a new and promising therapeutic target for breast cancer. Importantly, recent studies provide initial evidence of cAMP elevation as a simple way to neutralize leptin-induced biological effects in TNBC cells, including proliferation and migration.

The underlying molecular mechanisms, the potential clinical significance and therapeutic applications by these studies will be presented.

Chapter 5 - Obesity is a public health problem worldwide, resulting from a positive energy balance. Body weight is regulated by a complex circuitry involving central and peripheral factors, mainly by adipose organ-brain crosstalk. Leptin is a 16-kDa polypeptide that is primarily produced by adipose tissue, thus, circulation levels are in proportion of body mass, serving as a key adiposity signal. Leptin plays an important role in energy balance, acting as a major signaling in anorexigenic pathway. In human obesity, central and peripheral leptin resistance are proposed in association with state of hyperleptinemia. Studies suggest that an extended period of exposure to high levels of leptin, especially in the hypothalamus, may result in the development of central leptin resistance. Hyperleptinemia is also associated with the chronic subclinical inflammatory state, being involved in the development of many other diseases such as insulin resistance, cardiovascular disease and metabolic syndrome. Furthermore, recent studies have suggested the importance of this adipokine in weight loss process. This review focuses on the structure, role and effects of Leptin on obesity, metabolic syndrome development, and weight loss process.

Chapter 6 - Leptin is a hormone implicated in the control of food intake and energy balance. Although leptin was first thought to be only expressed in the adipose tissue, today we know that it is also produced in different organs such as skeletal muscle, pituitary gland, placenta and stomach, which secretes the hormone to the gastric juice.

In this chapter, the authors present different findings in rodents and Caco-2 cells, which contribute to the vision of leptin as an important hormonal signal for the regulation of intestinal absorption of nutrients and therefore, describe another important function for the hormone, apart from its well-known action on appetite control and obesity.

Luminal leptin inhibits intestinal sugar transport in a short-term manner, by reducing the density of the Na^+/glucose co-transporter SGLT1 at the brush border membrane of the enterocytes. Likewise, leptin inhibits glutamine uptake by decreasing both ASCT2 and B^oAT1 transporters trafficking to the apical membrane. In contrast, luminal leptin increases GLUT2 and GLUT5 insertion in the brush border membrane enhancing galactose and fructose absorption respectively. Similarly, intestinal transport of peptides and butyrate is increased by leptin, through the regulation of the expression in the membrane of the proton-coupled co-transporter PEPT1 and the monocarboxylate transporter MCT1, respectively. Leptin regulation of nutrients absorption has also been observed when leptin is acting from the basolateral membrane. The effect of both apical and basal leptin is rapidly and completely reverted when the hormone is removed. Different kinases seem to be involved in the leptin signaling pathways which regulate these nutrients transporters.

Chapter 7 - Obesity is associated with reduced quality of life, increased subfertility, and increased morbidity for diseases as a result of reduced testosterone production in aging males. Leptin is a metabolic hormone produced by white adipose tissue whose production is directly correlated with the level of obesity. It is well documented that leptin has influences on the physiology of reproduction. Indeed, leptin interacts with its receptor at every levels of the hypothalamus-pituitary-gonads (HPG) axis in males. However, most obese individuals develop a functional leptin resistance, rendering them insensitive to increased endogenous leptin concentrations. Such alterations in leptin signaling can lead to abnormal functioning of the endocrine and reproductive systems. In males, an inability of leptin action may contribute to hypogonadism and male infertility. Indeed, leptin resistance or leptin insufficiency impairs the hypothalamic function and normal physiology of the testis. In this chapter, the authors will do an update on the mechanisms of action of leptin at each components of the HPG axis. Furthermore, the effects of leptin on testosterone production and spermatogenesis in relation to male reproduction will be discussed.

Chapter 8 - Leptin, the protein product of the *obese (ob* or *Lep)* gene, is a hormone synthesized by adipocytes that signals available energy reserves to the brain, thereby influencing development, growth, metabolism and reproduction. In mammals, leptin acts as an adiposity signal: circulating leptin fluctuates in proportion to fat mass, exerting its action on the hypothalamus to suppress food intake. In this manner, central leptin signaling plays a pivotal role in the regulation of ~~the~~ metabolic activity. More importantly, leptin levels during the perinatal period are essential for the development of metabolic systems involved in energy homeostasis. Moreover, maternal nutrition and the hormonal environment during pregnancy and lactation may also modulate the offspring's response to postnatal modifications in leptin levels.

There are several reports showing that hyperleptinemia positively correlates with atherogenic processes including promotion of platelet aggregation and thrombosis, as well as with hypertension, production of inflammatory cytokines and metabolic syndrome. Thereby endothelial dysfunction takes place and underlies metabolic and vascular alterations that contribute to the development of both cardiovascular disease and type 2 diabetes. In fact, it has been demonstrated that an increase of leptin serum levels in humans, are also associated with a higher risk of myocardial infarction and stroke independent of obesity and obesity-related cardiovascular risk factors.

The present study highlights the importance of leptin levels during the perinatal period in the development of metabolic systems that control energy homeostasis and how modifications of these levels may induce long-lasting and potentially irreversible effects on metabolism, which in turn may contribute to the development of different cardio-metabolic diseases.

Chapter 9 - Whole body energy homeostasis is known to influence bone metabolism. Of particular interest in this relationship is the adipokine, leptin. Leptin was first demonstrated to be an instrumental component of bone regulation through studies of the leptin-deficient *ob/ob* and leptin receptor deficient *db/db* mouse models. These mice were found to have a complex bone phenotype with opposing roles in cancellous and cortical bone involving indirect, central, as well as direct local effects on bone cell activity inboth osteoblastic and osteoclastic lineages.

This complexity has led to some confusion regarding the leptin/bone interactions. This chapter focusses on the multiple pathways that leptin regulates to exert its skeletal effects.

Central pathways (fat-brain-bone axis) are important in the regulation of bone metabolism by leptin. Circulating leptin released from peripheral adipocytes regulates neuropeptide expression within several areas of the hypothalamus, which control both osteoblasts and osteoclastsvia efferent sympathetic nervous system pathways. These pathways have been shown to regulate cortical and cancellous bone mass via separate mechanisms.

Interestingly, leptin also has direct effects upon bone cells, promoting bone formation and inhibiting resorption. In addition, leptin is implicated in influencing mesenchymal stem cell differentiation towards osteoblasts and away from adipocytes. These responses are in contrast to the central effects upon cancellous bone, and have also provided conflicting conclusions in the field.

Thus, the study of leptin and its role in bone regulation has highlighted several pathways, both central and peripheral, that reveal important and complex interactions between adipose tissue, brain and bone.

A better understanding of the interactions between leptin and bone are important in this era of rapidly increasing rates of obesity.

Chapter 10 - Leptin, a 16 kDa circulating anti-obesity hormone, is a product of the obese (*ob*) gene. This molecule has been known to exhibit many physiological actions on body weight homeostasis, lipid metabolism, hematopoiesis, thermogenesis, ovarian function, and angiogenesis. Recently, leptin was reported to exist in saliva. However, its function in oral cavity remains to be elucidated. In this chapter, the physiological roles of leptin in oral and maxillofacial region are discussed, especially by focusing on the leptin's effects on wound healing of oral mucosa, and tooth development.

Immunohistochemical analysis revealed leptin receptor (Ob-R) was expressed in spinous cells and granular cells of human and rabbit gingival epithelium. In addition, locally administered leptin induced more rapid healing of chemical burn wounds artificially created in gingiva by enhancing the migration of oral mucosal epithelial cells and stimulating angiogenesis in connective tissue beneath the wounded area.

A topical administration of leptin also promoted the healing of chemical burn wounds created on the back skin of mice accelerating the angiogenesis in the subcutaneous connective tissue beneath the ulcer and the cell migration of skin keratinocytes. These findings strongly suggest that leptin could be a potent and promising medicine to promote the wound healing in mucosa and skin.

On the other hand, another immunohistochemical study revealed that leptin was expressed in two major tooth-forming cells in tooth germs: ameloblasts (enamel-forming cells) and odontoblasts (dentin-forming cells). More interestingly, dental papilla cells in the vicinity of odontoblastic layer expressed much more leptin. In addition, more CD31-positive vascular endothelial cells were distributed in this area. Judging from the previous study that leptin has an angiogenic effect, these findings strongly suggest the possibility that ameloblasts, odontoblasts and some dental papilla cells are recruiting the blood vessels into tooth germs by secreting leptin to ensure the immaculate tooth development.

In summary, leptin, a multi-functional molecule not only as a systemic hormone but also as a local growth factor, plays important physiological roles in oral and maxillofacial region.

Chapter 11 - In recent studies dealing with the central control of respiration, the authors reported that a pleiotropic hormone mainly produced by white adipose tissue, leptin has a substantial dose-dependent excitatory effect on breathing when it is microinjected into the nucleus of the solitary tract. The present study was undertaken to assess the characteristics of the respiratory effects induced by action of leptin in the pre-Bötzinger complex, a region primarily involved in respiratory rhythm generation both *in vitro* and *in vivo*. Therefore, the respiratory responses to unilateral microinjections (200 nl) of 0.1 nM, 10 nM and 1 μM leptin into the pre-Bötzinger complex were investigated in urethane anesthetized, spontaneously breathing Wistar rats. No changes in respiration were induced by 0.1 nM leptin microinjections. At higher (10 nM and 1 μM) concentrations leptin microinjections into the pre-Bötzinger complex elicited a dose-related increase in respiratory minute volume with the highest concentration resulting in an increase from 77.2 ± 3.2 to 95.5 ± 4.9 ml/min ($p<0.001$: Holm-Sidak test). This increase was due primarily to an elevation in respiratory frequency from 64.4 ± 2.7 to 82.3 ± 4.6 breaths/min ($p<0.001$: Holm-Sidak test) without obvious changes in tidal volume or peak amplitude of diaphragm or external intercostal muscles integrated EMG. The elevation in respiratory rate was largely a result of a significant decrease in expiratory duration in a dose-related fashion, whereas inspiratory duration was not significantly altered.

The time course of respiratory facilitatory effect of leptin was characterized by a moderately rapid onset and long duration. Excitation was observed within 3 min after microinjection with a peak effect occurring at approximately 20 min after administration. In general, the effect was over within 50 min.

To the author's knowledge, these results are the first to indicate that leptin causes respiratory stimulation by a direct action on the pre-Bötzinger complex. Taken together with the author's previous data, these results suggest that leptin may be involved in matching ventilation to metabolic requirements to stimulate ventilation. Further studies will require identifying central mechanisms by which activation of leptin receptors alters the respiratory control.

Chapter 12 - The survival of a species in an unpredictable ecosystem as the desert depends among others on the adaptation of its reproductive system, in terms of matching reproductive activity with water and food availability in the habitat, and halting it when these are limited. Integration of the various environmental cues will eventually determine which populations will be able to breed at an appropriate time thus surviving as a species in xeric environments. Osmotic stress was noted as an effective internal signal for reducing reproductive activity in desert-adapted *Acomys* populations.

In the basis of the author's study lies the assumption that a possible mechanism by which dietary salinity causes an osmotic stress, which affects reproduction in desert adapted common spiny mice *Acomys cahirinus* in association with osmoregulatory hormones; vasopressin and aldosterone. As leptin regulates energy intake, it seemed of great interest to assess its role in reproduction of desert adapted rodents, inhabiting an unpredictable environment.

For a long time energy source storage seemed as the only role of WAT, apart from providing thermal and mechanical insulation. For now WAT in the author's understanding is a highly dynamic, endocrine tissue, being involved in a wide range of physiological and metabolic processes far beyond the paradigm of fuel storage.

White adipocytes secrete several major hormones, protein signals and factors, most notably is the peptide hormone leptin. Circulating leptin levels serve as a signal for the state of body energy repletion to body cells most importantly the central nervous system (CNS) where it suppresses food intake and permits energy expenditure. In addition to its metabolic effects, leptin is well known as a modulator of reproduction.

The results of the author's studies show an involvement of leptin in metabolism and regulation of reproductive function in rodents. The authors tested desert and mesic adapted *A. cahirinus* for investigating the role of leptin as a modulator of reproductive pathways in *Acomys* populations from two different ecosystems.

The authors data and those of previous studies including the desert adapted golden spiny mouse, reported on a massive reduction of body mass in salinity treated (ST)-mice, under short and long day photoperiod conditions for males and females, coupled with a colossal reduction of WAT, leading to a complete absence of the tissue in 85% of ST-mice. ST caused a significant ($p < 0.05$) decrease in serum leptin levels in both, LD- and SD-acclimated desert-adapted A. cahirinus females, compared with their control groups.

In general, by using the reverse transcriptase polymerase chain reaction (RT-PCR) method, the authors detected a significant increase in expression levels of mRNA receptor genes for leptin (Ob-RT) in testis and WAT of ST-treated mice. High gene expression levels of leptin (Ob-Rt) mRNA receptors were noted in ovaries of SD-ST desert-adapted females ($p < 0.05$), while in the testes high gene expression levels were noted only in LD-ST desert-adapted individuals ($p < 0.05$), compared with their controls.

The authors results on endocrine and molecular levels are of importance for the proposed idea that, in desert rodents, reproduction is being controlled not only by water availability but, also by the amount of energy resources. Such rodents show that the hormone leptin, which regulates energy storage through its receptors presented on the gonads, or on WAT or hypothalamus, is involved in regulation of desert-adapted rodents' reproduction.

In: Leptin: Biosynthesis, Functions and Clinical Significance
Editor: Edward L. Blum
ISBN: 978-1-62948-801-1

Chapter 1

Leptin in Alzheimer's Disease and Other Cognitive Disorders and Association with Underlying Lipid Abnormalities

***Jane M. Johnston*[1], *George Perry*[2], *J. Wesson Ashford*[3] and *Nikolaos Tezapsidis*[1]**

[1]Neurotez Inc., Bridgewater, NJ, US
[2]University of Texas San Antonio, TX, US
[3]Department of Psychiatry and Behavioral Sciences, Stanford University School of Medicine, Palo Alto, CA, US

Abstract

Leptin was originally described for its role in obesity and energy homeostasis. These properties are centrally mediated through leptin receptors (ObR) in the arcuate nucleus of the hypothalamus. However, neuromodulatory properties of leptin in neuroanatomically diverse regions of the brain may play significant roles in other physiological functions. For example, the high density of functional leptin receptors found in the hippocampus and cortical regions of the brain may underline its involvement in memory and cognition. In vitro studies support a role of leptin in synaptic function and plasticity along with amyloidogenesis, amyloid removal and tau-phosphorylation. In vivo studies have confirmed a role in Alzheimer's disease (AD)-related pathology and a beneficial effect on cognitive deterioration of AD-transgenic animals. Epidemiological studies show that low levels of circulating plasma leptin are associated with dementia and depression, conditions often observed in patients presenting with various disorders including AD, Parkinson's dementia, Huntington's and prion diseases. Herein, we review the role of leptin in brain, cognitive impairment and underlying lipid abnormalities and discuss the benefits of leptin replacement therapy.

LEPTIN PHYSIOLOGY

Leptin, a 167 amino acid secreted by adipocytes, is a pleiotropic hormone that was originally described for its role in obesity and energy homeostasis [1, 2]. The tertiary structure of leptin resembles that of helical cytokines [3] which include leukemia inhibitory factor (LIF), ciliary neurotrophic factor (CNTF) and interleukin-6 (IL-6), IL-11 and IL-12 [4] and has lead to the classification of leptin as an adipokine. However, Leptin would be more accurately put into the larger growing list of adipose-derived hormones that includes adiponectin and resistin. Leptin exerts its effects by binding to specific leptin receptors (ObR), located on a variety of endocrine organs including liver [5] and reproductive organs [6] as well as specific brain regions such as the hypothalamus [7], hippocampus and cortex [8]. Thus, leptin may directly or indirectly modulate a variety of metabolically active tissues as well as the central nervous system and does not directly act on the immune system.

Leptin is secreted from adipose tissue in a pulsatile fashion, with peak levels reached between midnight and early morning in proportions related to both the body mass index (BMI) and the amount of body fat. Circulating plasma leptin are generally higher in females than in males [9] and although there is a post-menopause decline in females, leptin levels are still higher than those of males (Johnston et al., 2013). Leptin circulates bound to serum macromolecules, which may regulate bioavailability, and with a short half-life of approximately three to four hours [10]. Because leptin can target multiple neuroendocrine organs, circulatory disturbances may lead to a variety of disorders [11]. Clinical conditions linked to leptin excess or hyperleptinemia include obesity [12] and diabetes [11]. Prolonged leptin excess may lead to leptin resistance, which has not been clinically well defined and may occur due to saturation of the leptin transporter at the blood-brain-barrier [13]. On the other hand, leptin–related clinical conditions may also occur due to leptin deficiency or hypoleptinemia. These include energy deficient states such as anorexia [14, 15], lipodystrophy [16] or dementia [17, 18] and congenital leptin deficiency, a genetic disorder presenting with obesity [19]. Behavioral changes are associated with a number of these disorders [20, 21], under scoring the significance of leptin on brain function and cognition [22, 23].

LEPTIN SIGNALING

The leptin receptor (ObR) is widely distributed in the peripheral and central systems and is a member of the class 1 cytokine receptor superfamily [4]. At least six isoforms of the ObR (ObRa through ObRf) have been identified [24]. Of these, the long isoform of the leptin receptor (ObRb) is the most well known and complete deletion of this receptor leads to obesity in mice [25]. ObRa and ObRc are believed to function in leptin transport across the blood brain barrier as they are highly expressed in cerebral microvessels [26, 27] and ObRe may be a soluble receptor isoform that buffers free leptin in the circulation [24], common for other receptors of the cytokine family [28]. The ObRb isoform is highly expressed in brain [29], particularly in the hypothalamus, where leptin receptors are involved in the control of energy homeostasis, and also in the hippocampus and neocortex where leptin receptors are involved in memory and cognition [8].

The main signaling cascades activated by ObRb occur through JAKs (Janus kinases) and STATs (signal transducers and activators of transcription) [30]. Leptin binding to the ObRb receptor stimulates JAK2, which subsequently phosphorylates STAT3 to mediate transcription of a number of target genes [4]. Leptin signaling can be suppressed by the suppressor of cytokine signaling (SOC). SOC3 is a cytokine induced signal suppressor which blocks JAK2 activity to inhibit leptin signaling. ObRb can also activate the mitogen-activated protein kinase cascade (MAPK), especially the extracellular signal-related kinases (ERK) through JAK2 activation or independently of phosphorylation. These kinases activate a number of cellular pathways leading to differentiation [31], proliferation [32] or apoptosis [33]. Additionally, leptin can stimulate phosphatidylinositol 3-kinase (PI3K) signaling in a number of tissues including the hypothalamus [34], liver [35] and muscle [36]. Downstream targets of these pathways are diverse including 5'-adenosine monophosphate-activated protein kinase (AMPK) [37], calcium activated potassium channels [38], caspases [39], proinflammatory cytokines [40, 41] and actin filaments [42]. Thus leptin can activate a number of different signaling pathways to influence biological function.

Leptin in Brain and Neuronal Function

Leptin has a significant role in neurodevelopment [23, 29], which was first demonstrated in the brains of the genetically leptin deficient *ob/ob*, obese and diabetic mice [43]. These animals were shown to have reduced brain weights and cortical volumes when compared to control, lean mice [23, 44]. Further, a reduced density of neurons along with altered brain protein expression was observed and these deficits could be corrected by leptin replacement during early life [44]. Recent labeling experiments with 5-bromo-deoxyuridine have shown that leptin maintains the neural lineage of progenitor cells [45] and leptin deficiency during development reduces cortical neurons in embryonic life [46, 47]. Interestingly, human volumetric MRI studies of obese subjects, both genetic and non-genetic, have shown reduced gray matter in several regions compared to normal individuals [48, 49] which could be increased by leptin replacement [48].

The first effects of leptin on neuronal function were shown in hypothalamic slices, from control rats [50], but not Zucker fatty rats with mutated leptin receptors, and demonstrated a role for leptin in feeding behavior in the genetically obese ob/ob mice. However, the distribution of leptin receptors in hippocampal and cortical regions of the brain suggested additional roles, involving neuronal populations known to be important in memory and other cognitive functions, as was also shown originally in the *ob/ob* mice. Specifically, these mice have defects in glial and neuronal proteins and reduced cortical volumes and leptin administration can correct these alterations and improve synaptogenesis as well as memory and learning behavior [23, 44, 51]. Other rodent models of obesity, the *fa/fa* and *db/db* models, that are also leptin insensitive, have impaired hippocampal function and synaptic activity [52], implicating leptin in synaptic function. These rodents have deficits in hippocampal long-term potentiation (LTP) and long-term depression (LTD) [52] which are activity-dependent forms of synaptic plasticity and control synaptic strength to influence both memory and learning. Direct administration of leptin into the hippocampus significantly improves rodent performance in spatial memory and learning tests [51]. Further, treatment of hippocampal slices with leptin *in vitro* results in the conversion of short-term potentiation (STP) to LTP.

At the cellular level, leptin has been shown to increase activity-dependent synaptogenesis by enhancing Ca2+ influx through N-methyl-D-aspartate (NMDA) receptors. Studies in Xenopus oocytes expressing recombinant NMDA receptors have shown that leptin receptor signaling is a prerequisite for the enhancement of NMDA mediated currents. Furthermore, leptin is reported to increase NMDA activity by increasing NMDA receptor trafficking to the cell membrane. NMDA receptors are composed of NR1, NR2 and sometimes an NR3 subunit and the NMDA receptor subunit composition varies during development [53-55] and leptin has been shown to increase NR1/NR2 expression at the cell surface [56, 57]. NMDA receptors are also known to influence the expression of α-amino-3-hydroxy-5-methylisoxazole-4- propionic acid (AMPA) receptors and their subunit composition which is also linked to activity-dependent changes in synaptic function. In addition, AMPA receptor subunit composition may also be variable consisting of GluR1-4 subunits with GluR2 predominately expressed in the hippocampus until increased synaptic activity, or leptin stimulation, leads to a reduction in GluR2 subunits [58]. Thus, leptin can alter AMPA and NMDA receptor function via rapid vesicular trafficking of subunits [56, 58] or modulation of lipid rafts [59] to regulate synaptogenesis in normal brain, and leptin deficiency is clearly associated with disease-related neurodegeneration processes.

BRAIN LIPIDS AND COGNITIVE DYSFUNCTION

Lipid homeostasis is vital to normal brain function and dysregulation has been linked to neurodegenerative disorders [60], including Alzheimer's, Parkinson's and Huntington's diseases, suggesting common features might underlie disease progression [61]. Abnormal lipid inclusions in AD were first described in glial cells in the brain of Auguste Deter in 1906, the first reported AD case, by Alzheimer in his original paper [62]. However, this observation received little attention and the complex pathways of lipid synthesis, metabolism and excretion have made it difficult to decipher pathways and mechanisms relevant to memory and learning. While lipids are a diverse class of dietary substances, cholesterol, omega-3 fatty acids and triglycerides have received the most interest with regard to cognitive effects [63]. Of these, cholesterol and triglycerides may impair cognition and diedocosahexanoic acid (DHA), an omega-3 fatty acid may have beneficial effects. Indeed statins, cholesterol-lowering drugs, have been shown to have beneficial effects on AD and memory function in both human [64] and animal models [65], as well as improve cognitive and motor impairments in Parkinson's disease (PD) models [66] and prevent epileptogenesis in transgenic mice [67].

The brain has a lipoprotein transport system that is independent of the circulation and cholesterol does not cross the blood brain barrier. Instead, astrocytes produce cholesterol and apolipoprotein E (APOE) which transports cholesterol and phospholipids to neurons where they are endocytosed [68]. Interestingly, the stongest genetic risk factor for AD is expression of the apolipoprotein E4 allele (APOE4) [69, 70] which suggests that dysfunctional lipoprotein transport and subsequent uptake may underlie disease progression. Cholesterol balance/transport may also be altered in Huntingtons and Parkinson's disease [68] as well as prion disease [71]. Indeed, plasma membrane microdomains or caveolae, with cholesterol or phospholipids have many functions, including cellular signaling and cytoskeletal arrangement [72], all of which could be influenced by lipid dysfunction as well as lead to the accumulation of toxic proteins, such as hyperposphorylated Tau, in neurons.

The function of leptin in lipid dynamics, membrane processing and cellular transport [73], underscores a role for leptin deficiency as a common mediator in cognitive pathology (Figure 1). Indeed, genetically obese leptin receptor deficient rodents were shown to have altered lipid-raft fatty acid composition [74] and translocator protein expression in muscle [75] and brain tissue [76]. Thus, leptin controls membrane recycling in neurons [73, 77] and alters protein movement within the cell. Leptin has been shown to alter the accumulation of toxic amyloid proteins in cellular models of model of AD, in a process dependent upon the integrity of cholesterol-rich lipid rafts [59, 71]. Vesicular trafficking of AMPA and NMDA subunits, important for synaptogenesis, has also been shown to occur in hippocampal neurons in response to leptin treatment [56, 58]. Furthermore, low plasma leptin levels have been correlated with many aspects of cognition and behavior [78] including suicide, eating disorders and certain neurodegenerative diseases. Taken together, these studies implicate leptin in normal brain function, mediating lipid balance and cognitive function and further suggest that plasma leptin status may function as a common biomarker identifying individuals at risk of cognitive impairment (Figure 1).

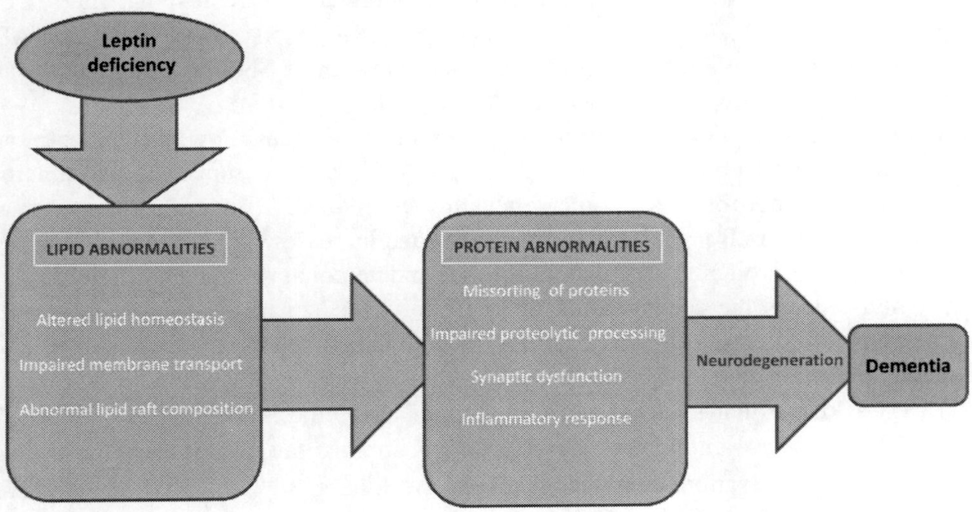

Figure 1. Leptin deficiency can alter lipid processes in neurons, leading to a variety of effects including altered lipid raft composition and membrane transport. Impaired membrane events may lead to the accumulation of cellular proteins such as b-amyloid, tau and a- synuclein as well as modulate synaptic function via NMDA receptors. Thus leptin deficiency underlies a common pathway in neurodegenerative disease and cognitive impairment.

Alzheimer's Disease (AD)

Given the role of leptin in lipid homeostasis and synaptogenesis, it is not surprising that leptin deficiency has been implicated in AD. The pathologic hallmarks of the disease include the accumulation of amyloid (Aβ) plaques in the brain, an extraneuronal protein deposit, and hyperphosphorylation of Tau protein to form intraneuronal deposits and neurofibillary tangles [79]. These events take place silently during aging, often decades before cognitive impairment manifests.

A number of independent studies point to an association of low circulating plasma leptin levels in subjects with or at risk of AD.

The first small study, reported this association in 2001 [80] and was followed by a larger prospective analysis of 2871 subjects [17] that showed individuals with high leptin levels were less likely to develop AD than those with low leptin levels over the four year study period. A third study of 41 patients also correlated low circulating leptin levels with early AD [81]. A fourth study by Leib et al. (2009) followed 785 healthy individuals from the Framingham cohort for 8.3 years and demonstrated that individuals with low leptin had an increased risk of dementia [18]. These authors also noted that high leptin levels were protective among individuals with normal body mass index (BMI) but not obese individuals, whose high leptin levels may contribute to leptin resistance. Finally, we recently analyzed data derived from the Alzheimer's Disease Neuroimaging Initiative (ADNI) program database (Johnston et al., 2013) and have shown that circulating plasma leptin levels in subjects with Mild Cognitive Impairment (MCI) or AD were lower than those with normal cognition (NC). Approximately 70% of both men and women with MCI present with plasma leptin levels lower than the median values of NC. Additionally, cerebrospinal fluid (CSF) leptin measurements reflected the levels of leptin in CSF in all groups (NC/MCI/AD), suggesting that plasma leptin deficiency provides an indication of CNS leptin deficiency and diagnostic information about the presence of MCI and AD.

An important therapeutic possibility is that individuals who have low plasma leptin and MCI may benefit from leptin replacement [22, 78, 82, 83] which is supported by numerous preclinical studies from our, and other, laboratories [84, 85]. Indeed, leptin reduces extracellular Aβ secretion from cultured neurons [85] and increases apolipoprotein E (ApoE)-dependent Aβ uptake through the regulation of lipids and neuronal membrane fluidity [59]. In addition, leptin reduces the accumulation of phosphorylated tau in SH-SY5Y cells and in primary neurons [86]. Leptin can reduce both Aβ accumulation and tau hyperphosphorylation independently and directly, most likely though the activation of AMP-activated kinase (AMPK) [87] a kinase that switches cells from lipid biosynthesis to glucose oxidation to generate ATP and control energy availability. AMPK inhibits tau phosphorylation through AMPK-dependent deactivation of gylycogen synthase kinase 3β (GSK3β) [88, 89] Thus leptin has the potential to modulate AD pathogenesis.

Chronic 8 week leptin treatment of CRND8 transgenic AD mice has shown beneficial effects on AD pathology and cognitive decline *in vivo* [90]. Treated animals showed reduced plaque size, reduced Aβ levels in brain and serum, and reduced tau phosphorylation compared with control animals. In behavioral testing, leptin treated animals showed improved novel object recognition as well as contextual and cued fear conditioning compared with saline treated transgenic controls. Indeed, the direct injection of leptin into rodent hippocampus improves memory processing by modulating LTP and synaptic plasticity [51].

Parkinson's Disease (PD)

Parkinson's disease is a pathologically heterogeneous disorder that can be either degenerative or non degenerative [91, 92]. Non-degenerative parkinsonism is a functional disorder that can be caused by the effects of toxins, drugs or metabolic disturbances. Degenerative parkinsonisms may be familial or sporadic and involve progressive neuropathology. Multiple system atrophy (MSA), progressive supranuclear palsy (PSP) corticobasal degeneration, chronic traumatic encephalopathy and frontotemporal (FTLD) lobar degeneration are parkinsonisms with common symptoms and progressive neuronal loss but with heterogenous pathology [91].

The majority of patients with Parkinson's disease (PD) develop dementia over the course of their disease [93]. Indeed up to 45.5% of patients in the Norwegian ParkWest study that presented with MCI had developed dementia within three years [94]. Cognitive impairment is accompanied by progressive brain changes [92], including a loss of dopamine neurons and the deposition of α-synuclein in the form of protein aggregates or Lewy bodies [95]. α-synuclein is a membrane protein that functions in synaptic plasticity and neurotransmission [96] and mutations of the α-synuclein gene lead to the onset of familial PD [97]. Significant amounts of α-synuclein are also associated with AD [98, 99], and the cognitive changes in AD are believed to be more aggressive when Lewy bodies are present, suggesting that α-synuclein, β-amyloid and tau can promote each other's aggregation Autopsy data analyzed by Kotzbauer et al. [100] suggest that PD patients with β-amyloid deposits and dementia have a lower survival rate than other PD pathologic subgroups. Thus preventing the formation of one or more of these aggregates could improve cognitive changes associated with their accumulation [95].

Surprisingly, little is known regarding the role of leptin in PD patients with and without dementia. Epidemiological studies to date are few [101-103], with conflicting results due to broad groupings of subjects and diverse ongoing treatment therapies [104-107], all of which can influence both BMI and circulating plasma leptin. Future studies will require participants to be stratified according to specific clinical criteria, cognitive profile [108] combined with rigorous biomarker analysis to fully evaluate plasma leptin level and MCI/ incident dementia in PD. In addition, leptin has been shown to have neurotrophic effects on dopaminergic neurons in vitro [109-111] and PD clinical symptoms, bradykinesia, tremor, rigity and postural instability result from the loss of these neurons in the substantia nigra in the brains of the afflicted. The protective actions of leptin are mediated via anti-apoptotic mechanisms [110] and mitogen-activated protein kinase signaling. Thus leptin may have a beneficial effect as a PD therapy in patients with cognitive impairment, alpha-synuclein deposition and degeneration of the substantia nigra, either as a monotherapy or in combination with other pharmaceuticals.

Huntington's Disease (HD)

Huntington's disease (HD) is a neurodegenerative disorder in which a mutant protein, huntingtin, is ubiquitously expressed, leading to motor disturbances, dementia and psychiatric problems. Other abnormalities, including weight loss occur in the afflicted which may reflect a dysregulation of circulating plasma leptin. Surprisingly few studies to date have examined the role of leptin in the disease pathology and clinical studies that have measured circulating leptin report varying results [112, 113], likely due to small patient cohorts as well as a lack of patients stratified for gender, body weight, cognitive status and medication profile. Interestingly, animal studies suggest that HD mutant mice with low leptin have adipose tissue dysfunction that correlates with disease progression [114]. Thus it seems that an investigation on the potential use of leptin therapy in HD is certainly worth exploring.

Prion Disease

Prion diseases are rare, fatal neurodegenerative disorders that result from the accumulation of a misfolded protein and lead to progressive dementia [115]. Most cases of prion disease arise sporadically although Creutzfeldt-Jakob disease (CJD) is a familial prion disease. A variant form of CJD, (vCJD), can be acquired by eating meat contaminated with bovine spongiform encephalopathy (BSE). Familial forms of prion disease are caused by inherited mutations in the prion protein (PrP) gene (PRNP) which is believe to be a copper transporter. The normal protein, PrP^{C} is conveted into mutant protein PrP^{Sc} and which has the capability to convert other normal prion protein, forming clumps in brain tissue.

Previous research suggests a pathogenic link between prion and AD [115]. Indeed, hamsters infected with transmissible prion proteins have suppressed leptin levels [116] and PrP^{c} has been shown to bind to Aβ with high affinity to mediate synaptic toxicity in cultures and mouse models [71, 117] by a mechanism that involves protein misfolding [117, 118] as well as impaired tau and glutamate transmission in the hippocampus.

Depression

Mood and depression have been linked to increase risks for the development of a variety of disorders including cancer, diabetes, stroke, epilepsy and dementia [119]. Pathological changes in depression include decreased hippocampal volumes and changes in neurotrophic support. Leptin has been suggested to exert antidepressant-like effects, possibly through an effect of the hypothalamic-pituitay axis and hippocampus. Indeed low plasma leptin has been associated with depression in patients, as has decreased leptin gene expression and polymorphins in the leptin gene [120].

Epilepsy

Leptin has been suggested to influence hippocampal processes implicated in epileptic seizures and had been implicated as an anticonvulsant agent [121]. Xu et al. [122] showed that administration of intranasal leptin to rodent models prevented seizures by a mechanism involving suppression of glutamate–induced excitatory post synaptic events mediated by AMPA receptors. Additional studies have shown that leptin reduces cellular injury in kainic acid-induced status epilepticus in rodents [123] possibly due to astrocytic leptin receptor upregulation, shown to occur in mouse seizure models [124]. Interestingly, knockout mice lacking astrocyte specific leptin receptors have a higher lethality rate when seizures are induced [124]. It is not know how plasma leptin levels may correlate with epileptic states, given the heterogeneity of the disorder and the available medications, which have complicated interpretation of longitudinal studies.

CONCLUSIONS

Leptin deficiency may lead to disturbed lipid homeostasis in brain which may be a common pathway in a number of neurodegenerative disorders in which protein accumulations occur. Strong links to date suggest that leptin replacement may be beneficial in Alzheimer's disease in patients presenting with low circulating plasma leptin levels. Other neurodegenerative disorders are additional indicators for leptin replacement, but require further confirmatory analysis of plasma leptin in the subgroups based on gender, BMI, medication profile and other parameters as we have shown in the ADNI cohort (Johnston et al., 2013). Clearly, further exploration of leptin deficiencies in patients with the neurodegenerative disorders described is needed, since replacement therapy may produce significant gains in cognition (Figure 1).

REFERENCES

[1] Zhang, Y., et al., Positional cloning of the mouse obese gene and its human homologue. *Nature*, 1994. 372(6505): p. 425-32.

[2] Halaas, J.L., et al., Weight-reducing effects of the plasma protein encoded by the obese gene. *Science*, 1995. 269(5223): p. 543-6.

[3] Zhang, F., et al., Crystal structure of the obese protein leptin-E100. *Nature*, 1997. 387(6629): p. 206-9.

[4] Fruhbeck, G., Intracellular signalling pathways activated by leptin. *Biochem. J.*, 2006. 393(Pt 1): p. 7-20.

[5] Kaplan, L.M., Leptin, obesity, and liver disease. *Gastroenterology*, 1998. 115(4): p. 997-1001.

[6] Mantzoros, C.S., Role of leptin in reproduction. *Ann. N Y Acad. Sci.*, 2000. 900: p. 174-83.

[7] Halaas, J.L. and J.M. Friedman, Leptin and its receptor. *J. Endocrinol.*, 1997. 155(2): p. 215-6.

[8] Williams, L.M., et al., Leptin receptor and neuropeptide Y gene expression in the sheep brain. *J. Neuroendocrinol.*, 1999. 11(3): p. 165-9.

[9] Licinio, J., et al., Sex differences in circulating human leptin pulse amplitude: clinical implications. *J. Clin. Endocrinol. Metab.*, 1998. 83(11): p. 4140-7.

[10] Chan, J.L., et al., Pharmacokinetics of recombinant methionyl human leptin after subcutaneous administration: variation of concentration-dependent parameters according to assay. *J. Clin. Endocrinol. Metab.*, 2007. 92(6): p. 2307-11.

[11] Luchsinger, J.A., Adiposity, hyperinsulinemia, diabetes and Alzheimer's disease: an epidemiological perspective. *Eur. J. Pharmacol.*, 2008. 585(1): p. 119-29.
[12] Sorensen, T.I., S. Echwald, and J.C. Holm, Leptin in obesity. *BMJ,* 1996. 313(7063): p. 953-4.
[13] Caro, J.F., et al., Decreased cerebrospinal-fluid/serum leptin ratio in obesity: a possible mechanism for leptin resistance. *Lancet,* 1996. 348(9021): p. 159-61.
[14] Grinspoon, S., et al., Serum leptin levels in women with anorexia nervosa. *J. Clin. Endocrinol. Metab.*, 1996. 81(11): p. 3861-3.
[15] Eckert, E.D., et al., Leptin in anorexia nervosa. *J. Clin. Endocrinol. Metab.*, 1998. 83(3): p. 791-5.
[16] Oral, E.A., et al., Leptin-replacement therapy for lipodystrophy. *N. Engl. J. Med.*, 2002. 346(8): p. 570-8.
[17] Holden, K.F., et al., Serum leptin level and cognition in the elderly: Findings from the Health ABC Study. *Neurobiol Aging*, 2009. 30(9): p. 1483-9.
[18] Lieb, W., et al., Association of plasma leptin levels with incident Alzheimer disease and MRI measures of brain aging. *JAMA,* 2009. 302(23): p. 2565-72.
[19] Montague, C.T., et al., Congenital leptin deficiency is associated with severe early-onset obesity in humans. *Nature,* 1997. 387(6636): p. 903-8.
[20] Morrison, C.D., Leptin signaling in brain: A link between nutrition and cognition? *Biochim. Biophys. Acta,* 2009. 1792(5): p. 401-8.
[21] Grosshans, M., et al., Association of leptin with food cue-induced activation in human reward pathways. *Arch. Gen. Psychiatry*. 69(5): p. 529-37.
[22] Paz-Filho, G.J., et al., Leptin replacement improves cognitive development. *PLoS One,* 2008. 3(8): p. e3098.
[23] Steppan, C.M. and A.G. Swick, A role for leptin in brain development. *Biochem. Biophys. Res. Commun.*, 1999. 256(3): p. 600-2.
[24] Lee, G.H., et al., Abnormal splicing of the leptin receptor in diabetic mice. *Nature,* 1996. 379(6566): p. 632-5.
[25] Cohen, P., et al., Selective deletion of leptin receptor in neurons leads to obesity. *J. Clin. Invest.,* 2001. 108(8): p. 1113-21.
[26] Bjorbaek, C. and B.B. Kahn, Leptin signaling in the central nervous system and the periphery. *Recent Prog. Horm Res.*, 2004. 59: p. 305-31.
[27] Hileman, S.M., et al., Characterizaton of short isoforms of the leptin receptor in rat cerebral microvessels and of brain uptake of leptin in mouse models of obesity. *Endocrinology*, 2002. 143(3): p. 775-83.
[28] Heaney, M.L. and D.W. Golde, Soluble hormone receptors. *Blood*, 1993. 82(7): p. 1945-8.
[29] Udagawa, J., et al., Expression of the long form of leptin receptor (Ob-Rb) mRNA in the brain of mouse embryos and newborn mice. *Brain Res.*, 2000. 868(2): p. 251-8.
[30] Tartaglia, L.A., The leptin receptor. *J. Biol. Chem.*, 1997. 272(10): p. 6093-6.
[31] Ben-Eliezer, M., M. Phillip, and G. Gat-Yablonski, Leptin regulates chondrogenic differentiation in ATDC5 cell-line through JAK/STAT and MAPK pathways. *Endocrine,* 2007. 32(2): p. 235-44.
[32] Burguera, B., et al., Leptin increases proliferation of human steosarcoma cells through activation of PI(3)-K and MAPK pathways. *Med. Sci. Monit.*, 2006. 12(11): p. BR341-9.

[33] Najib, S. and V. Sanchez-Margalet, Human leptin promotes survival of human circulating blood monocytes prone to apoptosis by activation of p42/44 MAPK pathway. *Cell Immunol.*, 2002. 220(2): p. 143-9.

[34] Won, J.C., et al., Central administration of an endoplasmic reticulum stress inducer inhibits the anorexigenic effects of leptin and insulin. *Obesity* (Silver Spring), 2009. 17(10): p. 1861-5.

[35] Kunjara, S., et al., Insight into the role of inositol phosphoglycans in insulin response and the regulation of glucose and lipid metabolism illustrated by the response of adipocytes from two strains of rats. *Mol. Genet Meta.b*, 2008. 94(2): p. 263-6.

[36] Kunjara, S., et al., Inositol phosphoglycans and the regulation of the secretion of leptin: in vitro effects on leptin release from adipocytes and the relationship to obesity. *Mol. Genet Metab.*, 2000. 70(1): p. 61-8.

[37] Steinberg, G.R., J.W. Rush, and D.J. Dyck, AMPK expression and phosphorylation are increased in rodent muscle after chronic leptin treatment. *Am. J. Physiol. Endocrinol. Metab.*, 2003. 284(3): p. E648-54.

[38] Harvey, J., et al., Essential role of phosphoinositide 3-kinase in leptin-induced K(ATP) channel activation in the rat CRI-G1 insulinoma cell line. *J. Biol. Chem.*, 2000. 275(7): p. 4660-9.

[39] Dineva, J., et al., Expression of atrial natriuretic peptide, progesterone, apoptosis-related proteins and caspase-3 in in vitro luteinized and leptin-treated porcine granulosa cells. *Endocr. Regul*, 2007. 41(1): p. 11-8.

[40] Ahmed, M., et al., Induction of proinflammatory cytokines and caspase-1 by leptin in monocyte/macrophages from holstein cows. *J. Vet. Med. Sci.,* 2007. 69(5): p. 509-14.

[41] Pinteaux, E., et al., Leptin induces interleukin-1beta release from rat microglial cells through a caspase 1 independent mechanism. *J. Neurochem.*, 2007. 102(3): p. 826-33.

[42] O'Malley, D., A.J. Irving, and J. Harvey, Leptin-induced dynamic alterations in the actin cytoskeleton mediate the activation and synaptic clustering of BK channels. *FASEB J.,* 2005. 19(13): p. 1917-9.

[43] Bereiter, D.A. and B. Jeanrenaud, Altered neuroanatomical organization in the central nervous system of the genetically obese (ob/ob) mouse. *Brain Res.*, 1979. 165(2): p. 249-60.

[44] Ahima, R.S., et al., Regulation of neuronal and glial proteins by leptin: implications for brain development. *Endocrinology*, 1999. 140(6): p. 2755-62.

[45] Udagawa, J., et al., Leptin and its intracellular signaling pathway maintains the neurosphere. *Neuroreport*. 21(18): p. 1140-5.

[46] Harris, R.B., et al., A leptin dose-response study in obese (ob/ob) and lean (+/?) mice. *Endocrinology,* 1998. 139(1): p. 8-19.

[47] Udagawa, J., et al., The role of leptin in the development of the cerebral cortex in mouse embryos. *Endocrinology*, 2006. 147(2): p. 647-58.

[48] Matochik, J.A., et al., Effect of leptin replacement on brain structure in genetically leptin-deficient adults. *J. Clin. Endocrinol. Metab.*, 2005. 90(5): p. 2851-4.

[49] Pannacciulli, N., et al., Relationships between plasma leptin concentrations and human brain structure: a voxel-based morphometric study. *Neurosci. Lett.*, 2007. 412(3): p. 248-53.

[50] Glaum, S.R., et al., Leptin, the obese gene product, rapidly modulates synaptic transmission in the hypothalamus. *Mol. Pharmacol.*, 1996. 50(2): p. 230-5.

[51] Farr, S.A., W.A. Banks, and J.E. Morley, Effects of leptin on memory processing. *Peptides,* 2006. 27(6): p. 1420-5.
[52] Li, X.L., et al., Impairment of long-term potentiation and spatial memory in leptin receptor-deficient rodents. *Neuroscience,* 2002. 113(3): p. 607-15.
[53] Liu, L., et al., Role of NMDA receptor subtypes in governing the direction of hippocampal synaptic plasticity. *Science,* 2004. 304(5673): p. 1021-4.
[54] Bartlett, T.E., et al., Differential roles of NR2A and NR2B-containing NMDA receptors in LTP and LTD in the CA1 region of two-week old rat hippocampus. *Neuropharmacology*, 2007. 52(1): p. 60-70.
[55] Moult, P.R. and J. Harvey, NMDA receptor subunit composition determines the polarity of leptin-induced synaptic plasticity. *Neuropharmacology*. 61(5-6): p. 924-36.
[56] Shanley, L.J., A.J. Irving, and J. Harvey, Leptin enhances NMDA receptor function and modulates hippocampal synaptic plasticity. *J. Neurosci.*, 2001. 21(24): p. RC186.
[57] O'Malley, D., et al., Leptin promotes rapid dynamic changes in hippocampal dendritic morphology. *Mol Cell Neurosci*, 2007. 35(4): p. 559-72.
[58] Moult, P.R., et al., Leptin regulates AMPA receptor trafficking via PTEN inhibition. *J. Neurosci.*. 30(11): p. 4088-101.
[59] Fewlass, D.C., et al., Obesity-related leptin regulates Alzheimer's Abeta. *FASEB J,* 2004. 18(15): p. 1870-8.
[60] Schreurs, B.G., The effects of cholesterol on learning and memory. *Neurosci. Biobehav. Rev*. 34(8): p. 1366-79.
[61] Golde, T.E., et al., Thinking laterally about neurodegenerative proteinopathies. *J. Clin. Invest.* 123(5): p. 1847-55.
[62] Foley, P., Lipids in Alzheimer's disease: A century-old story. *Biochim. Biophys. Acta.* 1801(8): p. 750-3.
[63] Morley, J.E. and W.A. Banks, Lipids and cognition. *J. Alzheimers Dis*. 20(3): p. 737-47.
[64] Rockwood, K., et al., Use of lipid-lowering agents, indication bias, and the risk of dementia in community-dwelling elderly people. *Arch Neurol*, 2002. 59(2): p. 223-7.
[65] Zhang, Y.Y., et al., Atorvastatin attenuates the production of IL-1beta, IL-6, and TNF-alpha in the hippocampus of an amyloid beta1-42-induced rat model of Alzheimer's disease. *Clin. Interv. Aging*. 8: p. 103-10.
[66] Castro, A.A., et al., Atorvastatin improves cognitive, emotional and motor impairments induced by intranasal 1-methyl-4-phenyl-1,2,3,6-tetrahydropyridine (MPTP) administration in rats, an experimental model of Parkinson's disease. *Brain Res*. 1513: p. 103-16.
[67] Osterweil, E.K., et al., Lovastatin corrects excess protein synthesis and prevents epileptogenesis in a mouse model of fragile X syndrome. *Neuron*. 77(2): p. 243-50.
[68] Vance, J.E., Dysregulation of cholesterol balance in the brain: contribution to neurodegenerative diseases. *Dis. Model Mech*. 5(6): p. 746-55.
[69] Raber, J., Y. Huang, and J.W. Ashford, ApoE genotype accounts for the vast majority of AD risk and AD pathology. *Neurobiol. Aging*, 2004. 25(5): p. 641-50.
[70] Strittmatter, W.J., et al., Apolipoprotein E: high-avidity binding to beta-amyloid and increased frequency of type 4 allele in late-onset familial Alzheimer disease. *Proc. Natl. Acad. Sci. USA,* 1993. 90(5): p. 1977-81.

[71] Rushworth, J.V., et al., Prion protein-mediated toxicity of amyloid-beta oligomers requires lipid rafts and the transmembrane LRP1. *J. Biol. Chem.*. 288(13): p. 8935-51.

[72] Head, B.P., H.H. Patel, and P.A. Insel, Interaction of membrane/lipid rafts with the cytoskeleton: Impact on signaling and function: Membrane/lipid rafts, mediators of cytoskeletal arrangement and cell signaling. *Biochim Biophys Acta*.

[73] Fanjul, C., et al., Leptin regulates sugar and amino acids transport in the human intestinal cell line Caco-2. *Acta Physiol.* (Oxf). 205(1): p. 82-91.

[74] Ruth, M.R., S.D. Proctor, and C.J. Field, Feeding long-chain n-3 polyunsaturated fatty acids to obese leptin receptor-deficient JCR:LA- cp rats modifies immune function and lipid-raft fatty acid composition. *Br. J. Nutr.*, 2009. 101(9): p. 1341-50.

[75] Sainz, N., et al., Leptin reduces the expression and increases the phosphorylation of the negative regulators of GLUT4 traffic TBC1D1 and TBC1D4 in muscle of ob/ob mice. *PLoS One*. 7(1): p. e29389.

[76] Giannaccini, G., et al., Serotonin transporter (SERT) and translocator protein (TSPO) expression in the obese ob/ob mouse. *BMC Neurosci.* 12: p. 18.

[77] Benomar, Y., et al., Insulin and leptin induce Glut4 plasma membrane translocation and glucose uptake in a human neuronal cell line by a phosphatidylinositol 3-kinase-dependent mechanism. *Endocrinology*, 2006. 147(5): p. 2550-6.

[78] Johnston, J.M., et al., Repositioning leptin as a therapy for Alzheimer's disease. *Therapy*. 8(5): p. 481-490.

[79] Selkoe, D.J., Alzheimer's disease: genes, proteins, and therapy. *Physiol. Rev.*, 2001. 81(2): p. 741-66.

[80] Power, D.A., et al., Circulating leptin levels and weight loss in Alzheimer's disease patients. *Dement Geriatr Cogn Disord*, 2001. 12(2): p. 167-70.

[81] Bigalke, B., et al., Adipocytokines and CD34 progenitor cells in Alzheimer's disease. *PLoS O*ne. 6(5): p. e20286.

[82] Tezapsidis, N., et al., Leptin: a novel therapeutic strategy for Alzheimer's disease. *J. Alzheimers Dis.*, 2009. 16(4): p. 731-40.

[83] Harvey, J., Leptin: the missing link in Alzheimer disease? *Clin. Chem.* 56(5): p. 696-7.

[84] Marwarha, G. and O. Ghribi, Leptin signaling and Alzheimer's disease. *Am. J. Neurodegener Dis.* 1(3): p. 245-65.

[85] Doherty, G.H., et al., Leptin prevents hippocampal synaptic disruption and neuronal cell death induced by amyloid beta. *Neurobiol. Aging*. 34(1): p. 226-37.

[86] Greco, S.J., et al., Leptin reduces Alzheimer's disease-related tau phosphorylation in neuronal cells. *Biochem. Biophys. Res. Commun.*, 2008. 376(3): p. 536-41.

[87] Greco, S.J., et al., Leptin regulates tau phosphorylation and amyloid through AMPK in neuronal cells. *Biochem. Biophys. Res. Commun.*, 2009. 380(1): p. 98-104.

[88] Greco, S.J., et al., Leptin inhibits glycogen synthase kinase-3beta to prevent tau phosphorylation in neuronal cells. *Neurosci. Lett.,* 2009. 455(3): p. 191-4.

[89] Marwarha, G., et al., Leptin reduces the accumulation of Abeta and phosphorylated tau induced by 27-hydroxycholesterol in rabbit organotypic slices. *J. Alzheimers Dis.* 19(3): p. 1007-19.

[90] Greco, S.J., et al., Leptin reduces pathology and improves memory in a transgenic mouse model of Alzheimer's disease. *J. Alzheimers Dis*. 19(4): p. 1155-67.

[91] Dickson, D.W., Parkinson's disease and parkinsonism: neuropathology. *Cold Spring Harb Perspect Med*. 2(8).

[92] Dexter, D.T. and P. Jenner, Parkinson disease: from pathology to molecular disease mechanisms. *Free Radic Biol. Med.* 62: p. 132-44.

[93] Hely, M.A., et al., The Sydney multicenter study of Parkinson's disease: the inevitability of dementia at 20 years. *Mov. Disord.*, 2008. 23(6): p. 837-44.

[94] Pedersen, K.F., et al., Prognosis of mild cognitive impairment in early Parkinson disease: the Norwegian ParkWest study. *JAMA Neurol.* 70(5): p. 580-6.

[95] Bellucci, A., et al., alpha-Synuclein synaptic pathology and its implications in the development of novel therapeutic approaches to cure Parkinson's disease. *Brain Res.* 1432: p. 95-113.

[96] Burre, J., M. Sharma, and T.C. Sudhof, Systematic mutagenesis of alpha-synuclein reveals distinct sequence requirements for physiological and pathological activities. *J. Neurosci.*. 32(43): p. 15227-42.

[97] Houlden, H. and A.B. Singleton, The genetics and neuropathology of Parkinson's disease. *Acta Neuropathol.* 124(3): p. 325-38.

[98] Jellinger, K.A., Alpha-synuclein pathology in Parkinson's and Alzheimer's disease brain: incidence and topographic distribution--a pilot study. *Acta Neuropathol*, 2003. 106(3): p. 191-201.

[99] Marsh, S.E. and M. Blurton-Jones, Examining the mechanisms that link beta-amyloid and alpha-synuclein pathologies. *Alzheimers Res. Ther.* 4(2): p. 11.

[100] Kotzbauer, P.T., et al., Pathologic accumulation of alpha-synuclein and Abeta in Parkinson disease patients with dementia. *Arch. Neurol.* 69(10): p. 1326-31.

[101] Aziz, N.A., et al., Leptin, adiponectin, and resistin secretion and diurnal rhythmicity are unaltered in Parkinson's disease. *Mov. Disord.* 26(4): p. 760-1.

[102] Fiszer, U., et al., Leptin and ghrelin concentrations and weight loss in Parkinson's disease. *Acta Neurol. Scand.* 121(4): p. 230-6.

[103] Evidente, V.G., et al., Serum leptin concentrations and satiety in Parkinson's disease patients with and without weight loss. *Mov. Disord*, 2001. 16(5): p. 924-7.

[104] Markaki, E., et al., The role of ghrelin, neuropeptide Y and leptin peptides in weight gain after deep brain stimulation for Parkinson's disease. *Stereotact Funct. Neurosurg.* 90(2): p. 104-12.

[105] Novakova, L., et al., Hormonal regulators of food intake and weight gain in Parkinson's disease after subthalamic nucleus stimulation. *Neuro. Endocrinol. Lett.* 32(4): p. 437-41.

[106] Escamilla-Sevilla, F., et al., Change of the melanocortin system caused by bilateral subthalamic nucleus stimulation in Parkinson's disease. *Acta Neurol. Scand.* 124(4): p. 275-81.

[107] Rustembegovic, A., E. Sofic, and I. Wichart, Serum prolactin, leptin, lipids and lipoproteins levels during antipsychotics treatment in Parkinson's disease and related psychosis. *Med. Arh,* 2006. 60(4): p. 211-2.

[108] Hildebrandt, H., et al., Cognitive profiles of patients with mild cognitive impairment or dementia in Alzheimer's or Parkinson's disease. *Dement Geriatr Cogn Dis Extra.* 3(1): p. 102-12.

[109] Guo, Z., et al., Leptin-mediated cell survival signaling in hippocampal neurons mediated by JAK STAT3 and mitochondrial stabilization. *J. Biol. Chem.*, 2008. 283(3): p. 1754-63.

[110] Doherty, G.H., C. Oldreive, and J. Harvey, Neuroprotective actions of leptin on central and peripheral neurons in vitro. *Neuroscience*, 2008. 154(4): p. 1297-307.
[111] Weng, Z., et al., Leptin protects against 6-hydroxydopamine-induced dopaminergic cell death via mitogen-activated protein kinase signaling. *J. Biol. Chem.*, 2007. 282(47): p. 34479-91.
[112] Popovic, V., et al., Circulating and cerebrospinal fluid ghrelin and leptin: potential role in altered body weight in Huntington's disease. *Eur. J. Endocrinol.*, 2004. 151(4): p. 451-5.
[113] Aziz, N.A., et al., Leptin secretion rate increases with higher CAG repeat number in Huntington's disease patients. *Clin. Endocrinol.* (Oxf). 73(2): p. 206-11.
[114] Phan, J., et al., Adipose tissue dysfunction tracks disease progression in two Huntington's disease mouse models. *Hum. Mol. Genet*, 2009. 18(6): p. 1006-16.
[115] Lauren, J., Cellular Prion Protein as a Therapeutic Target in Alzheimer's Disease. *J. Alzheimers Dis.*
[116] Bailey, J.D., et al., Prominent pancreatic endocrinopathy and altered control of food intake disrupt energy homeostasis in prion diseases. *J. Endocrinol.*, 2008. 197(2): p. 251-63.
[117] Morales, R., et al., Molecular cross talk between misfolded proteins in animal models of Alzheimer's and prion diseases. *J. Neurosci.*. 30(13): p. 4528-35.
[118] Jeffrey, M., Review: membrane-associated misfolded protein propagation in natural transmissible spongiform encephalopathies (TSEs), synthetic prion diseases and Alzheimer's disease. *Neuropathol. Appl. Neurobiol.* 39(3): p. 196-216.
[119] Lang, U.E. and S. Borgwardt, Molecular mechanisms of depression: perspectives on new treatment strategies. *Cell Physiol. Biochem.* 31(6): p. 761-77.
[120] Kloiber, S., et al., Resistance to antidepressant treatment is associated with polymorphisms in the leptin gene, decreased leptin mRNA expression, and decreased leptin serum levels. *Eur. Neuropsychopharmacol.* 23(7): p. 653-62.
[121] Diano, S. and T.L. Horvath, Anticonvulsant effects of leptin in epilepsy. *J. Clin. Invest.*, 2008. 118(1): p. 26-8.
[122] Xu, L., et al., Leptin inhibits 4-aminopyridine- and pentylenetetrazole-induced seizures and AMPAR-mediated synaptic transmission in rodents. *J. Clin. Invest.*, 2008. 118(1): p. 272-80.
[123] Obeid, M., et al., Neuroprotective effects of leptin following kainic acid-induced status epilepticus. *Epilepsy Behav.* 19(3): p. 278-83.
[124] Jayaram, B., et al., Protective role of astrocytic leptin signaling against excitotoxicity. *J. Mol. Neurosci.* 49(3): p. 523-30.

In: Leptin: Biosynthesis, Functions and Clinical Significance ISBN: 978-1-62948-801-1
Editor: Edward L. Blum

Chapter 2

FAT, SALT AND BLOOD PRESSURE: THE LEPTIN-RENAL AXIS

Cristian Del Carpio Tenorio*[1,2]*, Pramesh Dhakal*[1,2]*,
Garry P. Reams*[3]*, Ronald H. Freeman*[3]*,
Robert Spear*[1]*, Kan Liu*[1,2]*,
and Daniel Villarreal*[1,2,*]*,
[1]Department of Internal Medicine,
SUNY- Upstate Medical University, NY, US
[2]Veterans Affairs Medical Center,
Syracuse, NY, US
[3]Departments of Internal Medicine and Physiology,
University of Missouri-Columbia,
Columbia, MO, US

ABSTRACT

Leptin is a 16-kDa-peptide hormone that is primarily synthesized and secreted by adipose tissue. One of the major actions of this hormone is the control of energy balance by binding to receptors in the hypothalamus, leading to reduction in food intake, elevation in temperature and energy expenditure. In addition, available evidence suggests that leptin, through both direct and indirect mechanisms, plays an important role in cardiovascular and renal regulation. While the relevance of endogenous leptin needs further clarification, it appears to function as a pressure and volume-regulating factor under conditions of health. However, in abnormal situations characterized by chronic hyperleptinemia such as obesity, it may function pathophysiologically for the development of hypertension and for direct renal and vascular damage.

Keywords: Diuresis, Hemodynamics, Natriuresis, Nitric Oxide, Hypertension

---

* Correspondence: Daniel Villarreal, MD, FACC, FAHA, FIACS, Department of Medicine, Division of Cardiology, SUNY Upstate Medical University, Room 6142, 750 East Adams Street, Syracuse, New York 13210 USA. Telephone Number: (315) 464-9578, Fax Number: (315) 464-9571. E-mail: Villarrd@upstate.edu.

INTRODUCTION

The prevalence of obesity in the adult population of the United States has risen markedly in the last three decades, contributing to the increased incidence of diabetes, hypertension and heart disease [1 - 3]. Indeed, epidemiological evidence indicates that 65-75% of the risk for hypertension is attributed to excess weight [4, 5]. In the last decade, an area of research in obesity and hypertension that links these two pathologic conditions is the endocrinology of adipose tissue. It is now recognized that adipose tissue is a prolific organ which secretes several immunomodulators and bioactive molecules [3, 6]. Of these various factors, leptin has emerged as an important hormone with significant pleiotropic actions on several organ-systems [7, 8].

The first described major action of leptin was on the hypothalamus to control body weight and fat deposition through its effects on appetite inhibition, as well as stimulation of the metabolic rate and thermogenesis [9, 10]. However, current evidence suggests that the biology of leptin extends to other organs including the kidney, the heart, the sympathetic nervous system and the systemic vasculature [7, 8, 11- 14].

LEPTIN RECEPTORS: LOCALIZATION AND FUNCTION

The leptin receptor (LR), a product of the lepr gene, is a member of the extended class I cytokine receptor family having at least six splice variants LR (a-f) [15- 19], being LRb the longest, described in most of the signal transduction studies [20 – 21]. Significant expression of the leptin receptor occurs in the lung and adipocytes, while only moderate levels appear in the kidney, with relatively lower levels demonstrated in other tissues like the heart, brain, spleen, liver, and muscle [22]. Although the extracellular domain of the leptin receptor and the short splice variant (LRa) have been detected in many peripheral tissues, the long splice variant (LRb) is expressed in fewer organ systems including the hypothalamus, adrenal gland, kidney and heart [22]. Most biological effects of leptin are mediated by this LRb receptor through the activation of the Janus kinases (a family of tyrosine kinases) to promote transcription via activation of the signal transduction and activator of transcription (STAT-3), phosphoinositol-3 kinase (PI3K) and inhibition of adenosine monophosphate-activated protein kinase (AMPK) [15-19, 22]. The functions of the short-form LR's (a,c,d,f) and the soluble form of LRe are less clear, but their proposed roles include transport of leptin across the blood brain barrier, clearance of leptin from the circulation and the regulation of free leptin. [23] LRa and LRb can also stimulate mitogen activated protein kinase (MAPK) which may be involved in the induction of hypertrophy [24]. Finally, suppression of cytokine signaling protein 3 (SOCS3) and protein tyrosine phosphatase 1b (PTB1b) have been identified as negative regulators of leptin signaling [15-19].

Leptin, Sympathetic Tone and the Regulation of Arterial Blood Pressure

It is well-established that leptin can activate the sympathetic nervous system both by local peripheral actions as well as through centrally mediated effects on the hypothalamus [25]. Studies with direct infusion of leptin into the cerebral ventricles of normal rats have demonstrated a slow increase of mean arterial pressure (MAP) of approximately 10 % [13]. Importantly, a similar hypertensive response has been recently demonstrated with the central administration of leptin in the diet-induced obese rat model [26], which exhibits resistance to the actions of the hormone in other peripheral organs, such as the kidney [14]. To this end, it is pertinent to point out that leptin signaling in the nucleus tracti solitarii increased renal sympathetic flow in normal rats but not in obese Zucker rats, indicating that intact leptin receptors are essential for this vasoactive response [25].

In other investigations conducted both in normotensive as well as hypertensive rats [12, 14, 27], the acute systemic administration of leptin was associated with the peripheral activation of the sympathetic nervous system without elevation in MAP. This raises the possibility of the simultaneous local activation of counter- regulatory vasodilatory mechanisms [14, 28, 29]. In-vitro studies have demonstrated a dose-dependent leptin-induced vasorelaxation in the aortic rings of Wistar-Kyoto rats [28] which is mediated by nitric oxide [NO]. An elevation in plasma NO with intravenous administration of synthetic leptin in normal rats has also been demonstrated [29]. In these studies, blockade of NO led to a leptin-induced enhancement of arterial blood pressure while blockade of the sympathetic nervous system led to leptin-mediated reduction in blood pressure [29]. Thus, leptin's lack of effect on arterial blood pressure in normal subjects may represent a balanced action of vasodilatation primarily mediated by NO, and vasoconstriction primarily mediated by the sympathetic nervous system, with a resultant neutral hemodynamic effect [29, 30]. This concept requires further validation because the vasodilatory actions of leptin in other vascular beds have been found to be inconsistent [31, 32]. In high calorie fed obese rats, however, it has been shown that acutely infused leptin was associated with a hypertensive effect, related, at least in part, to impaired vascular NO production characteristic of obesity [33].

Chronic Hyperleptinemia, Leptin Resistance and Hypertension

In chronic hyperleptinemic conditions such as obesity, the potential neutral effect of leptin on peripheral vascular resistance may no longer prevail. It has been previously demonstrated that the agouti yellow obese mouse model is resistant to the satiety actions of leptin but not to the effects of leptin on the sympathetic nervous system [34, 35], although this stimulation may be attenuated with the progression of obesity [36]. From these findings, the concept of "selective leptin resistance" as a mechanism for the development of hypertension in obesity has emerged [34, 35]. The precise factors behind this selectivity are yet to be fully defined [35, 37], but may involve alterations in the SOCS3 signaling pathway or insulin receptor substrate-1 (IRS-1) serine residue phosphorylation [33, 38, 39, 40]. A recent study by Beltowski et al in rats made hyperleptinemic by administration of leptin for 7 days suggested that resistance to the natriuretic and NO-mimetic effects of leptin may involve, at least in part, a reduced expression of leptin receptor in target tissues. [41] This concept is supported by prior investigations which indicate that hyperleptinemia reduces expression of leptin receptor in the hypothalamus and the kidney [42]. Finally, increased CRP production induced by hyperleptinemia [43] has been implicated as a possible mechanism for leptin resistance, since CRP impairs the effect of leptin on AKT phosphorilation, eNOS phosphorylation as well as cGMP generation by endothelial cells [43].

Independent of the possibility of selective leptin resistance in obesity, studies in normal rats have demonstrated that chronic hyperleptinemia leads to a persistent elevation in MAP and this hypertensive effect is rapidly reversed upon cessation of the hormone administration [44]. Similar increases in systolic blood pressure have been demonstrated in transgenic mice overexpressing leptin where the endogenous level of the hormone was elevated twenty-fold [45]. In this regard, it is relevant to point out that hyperleptinemia may increase vascular smooth muscle cell proliferation [46], an effect that could contribute to the development and/or perpetuation of hypertension. Moreover, mice with leptin deficiency [ob/ob] or with a leptin receptor defect, [db/db] exhibit significant obesity but do not develop hypertension, suggesting that at least in animal models, leptin may play a role in the regulation of systemic hemodynamics [35]. In humans, evidence suggests a direct relationship between hyperleptinemia and hypertension in both men and women [47, 48], and this effect may be independent of body mass index and insulin resistance [49].

Leptin and the Renal Regulation of Sodium-volume Balance

Previous studies have indicated that the LRb leptin receptor is localized in the renal medulla [22, 50] which suggests a functional role of this hormone in renal biology. Indeed, numerous investigations have demonstrated that acute administration of synthetic leptin in the rat produces a significant elevation in urinary sodium and water excretion [14, 50 - 52].

Villarreal et al., [14] demonstrated that in normotensive rats, an intravenous bolus of leptin produced a robust six to seven fold elevation in urinary sodium excretion and fractional excretion of sodium; in contrast, hypertensive rats were refractory to the renal effects of leptin. Interestingly, the natriuretic effect was also attenuated in obese Zucker rats (Figure 1) [14]. MAP and creatinine clearance remained unchanged in all of the rat strains with the acute infusion of the hormone. Collectively, these findings were interpreted to suggest that leptin might be a natriuretic hormone primarily acting at the tubular level for promotion of sodium and water excretion in normal rats, and that leptin may function pathophysiologically in obesity and hypertension, where chronic hyperleptinemia may contribute to a preferential stimulation of the sympathetic nervous system and a blunted natriuresis and diuresis [2, 7, 53]. Moreover, in a rat model of diet-induced obesity, studies by Patel et al. have shown markedly attenuated natriuretic and diuretic effects of synthetic leptin as well as reduced urinary excretion of NO (Figure 2) [54]. These findings suggest that in obesity, alterations in leptin-induced renal NO production and/or metabolism may account, at least in part, for the blunted natriuretic effects.

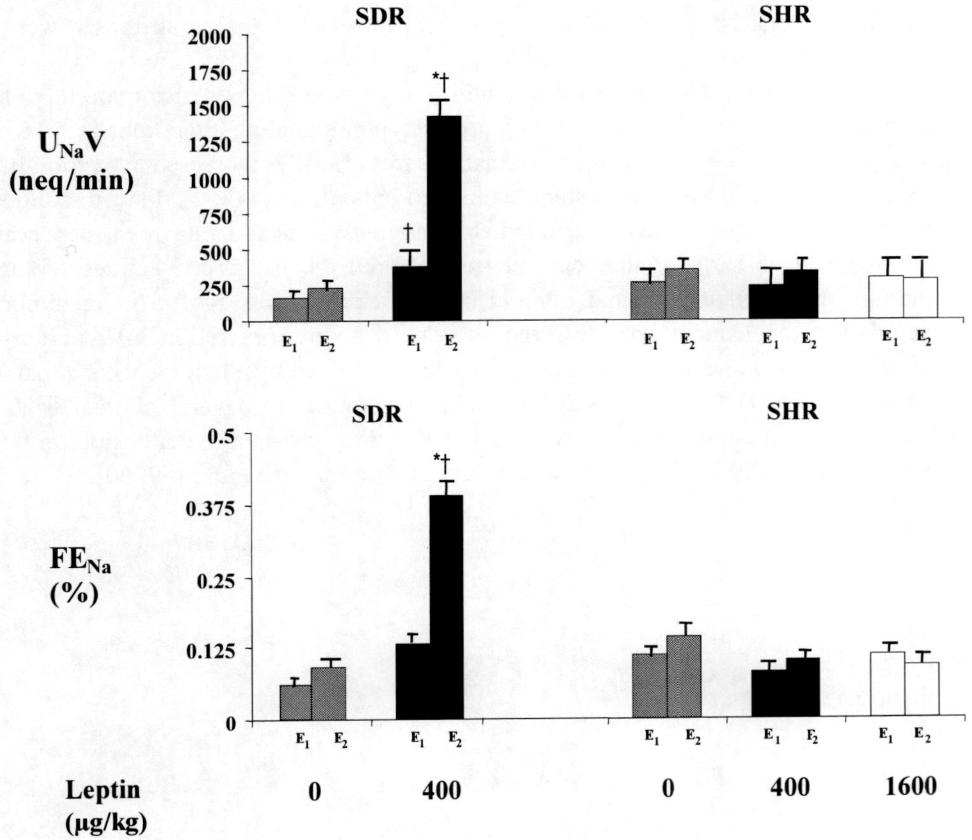

Figure 1. Renal effects of leptin in Sprague Dawley Rats (SDR) and Spontaneously Hypertensive Rats (SHR). *Top*: Urinary sodium excretion (UNaV). *Bottom*: Fractional excretion of sodium (FENa). Control (0 dose, $n = 8$); leptin 400 μg/kg ($n = 8$); leptin 1,600 μg/kg ($n = 8$). Values are means ± SE. E1 and E2, experimental periods (45 min each). * $P < 0.05$ vs E1. † $P < 0.05$ vs control of corresponding experimental period. From Villarreal, D., Reams, G., Freeman, R.H., Taraben, A. Am J. Physiol 1998; 275: R2056-R2060 (Reproduced with permission from The American Physiological Society).

However, additional observations in diet-induced obese rats indicate that caloric restriction was associated with the restoration of the natriuretic actions of leptin as well as with the renal generation of NO (Figure 3) [54]. In the aggregate, these studies are consistent with the concept that obesity is associated with renal leptin resistance [14, 55], and this resistance, at least in part, is reversible with caloric restriction and weight loss [54].

The significance of NO in the direct modulation of leptin-induced sodium excretion has been investigated in rats chronically treated with L-NG-Nitroarginine Methyl Ester (L-NAME) to inhibit NO production [56]. In this study by Villarreal et al, L-NAME-treated rats failed to produce significant natriuresis. However, there was a two to threefold elevation in sodium excretion induced by leptin with the restoration of NO by sodium nitroprusside [56], indicating that NO may play an important role in mediating or modulating the tubular natriuretic effects of leptin. These observations are supported by the investigations of Beltowski et al., [55] which demonstrated that leptin produces a time- and dose-dependent reduction of renal medullary Na-K-ATPase, which may in part be regulated by NO [56, 57]. Furthermore, Beltowski et al. [55] reported that in diet-induced obese rats, leptin-mediated stimulation of plasma NO, reduction of renal Na-K-ATPase, and natriuresis were all significantly impaired.

The mechanisms for renal resistance to leptin in obesity and hypertension are thought to include receptor down regulation [12, 42, 54], post-receptor signaling alterations [12, 16, 17], excessive degradation of NO produced by oxidative stress [58], or increased activation of the efferent renal sympathetic nervous system leading to antinatriuresis [52]. Indeed, studies in hypertensive rats [52] which have examined this latter hypothesis using renal denervation (RD) indicated that ablation of the renal nerves restored the natriuretic actions of leptin. These findings suggest that the renal efferent sympathetic nervous system is an important counter-regulatory mechanism impeding leptin-induced sodium excretion in hypertension, and perhaps also during obesity, which is similarly characterized by a heightened sympathetic nervous tone (Figure 4) [2, 7]. This information is germane to several clinical trials on bilateral renal sympathetic denervation for treatment of drug resistant hypertension, in which a significant reduction in blood pressure was observed after the procedure [59, 60].

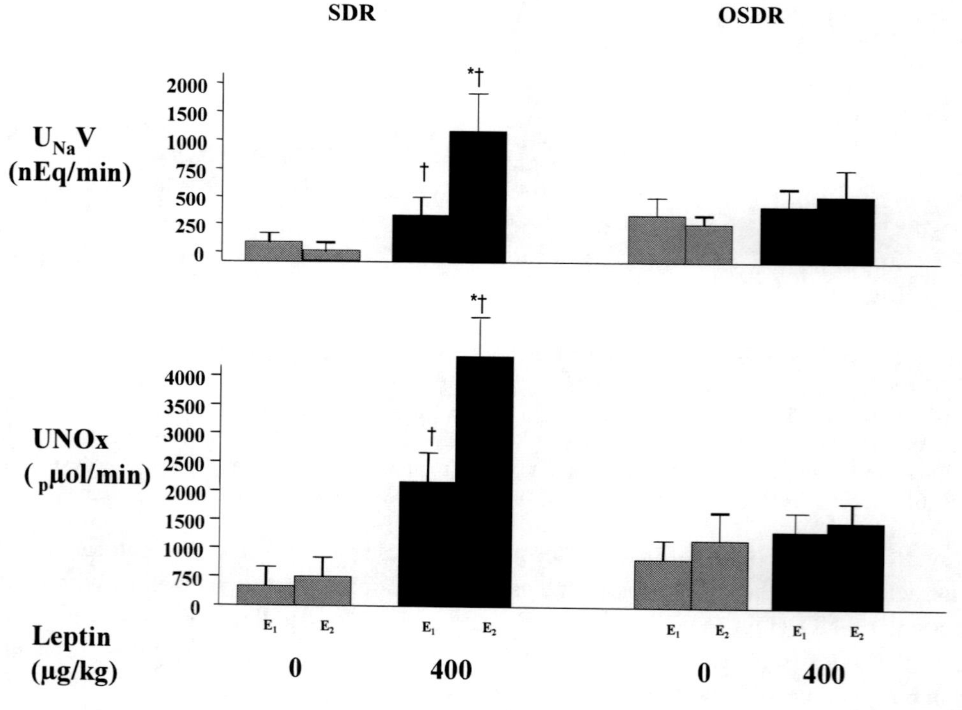

Figure 2. Renal effects of intravenous bolus of leptin in normal Sprague Dawley Rats (SDR) and in Sprague Dawley Rats with diet-induced obesity fed high caloric/fat diet for 12 weeks (OSDR). Top: Urinary sodium excretion (UNaV). Bottom: Urinary nitric oxide excretion (UNOx). Control rats (0 dose, $n = 4$), leptin rats (400 µg/kg $n = 4$). Values are means ± SE. E1 and E2, experimental periods (45 min each). * $P < 0.05$ vs E1. †$P < 0.05$ vs control of corresponding experimental period. From Patel, S.B., Villarreal, D., Kundra, A., et al. Cardiac Hormone2008: 111-127. (Reproduced with permission from Transworld Research Network.).

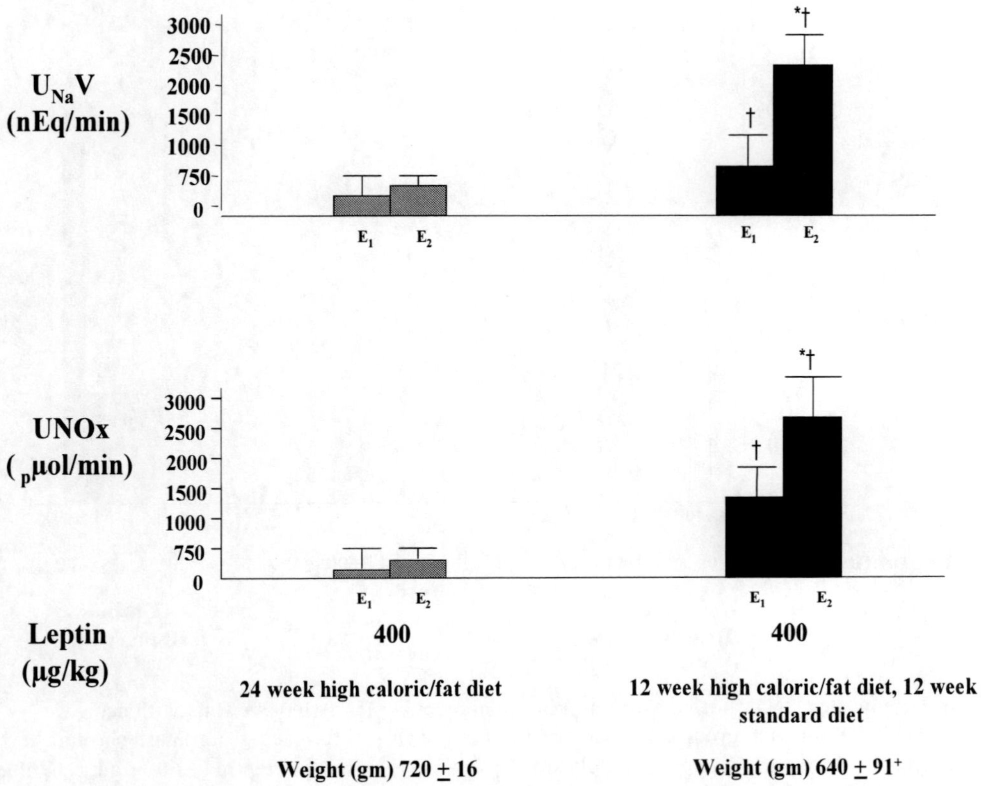

Figure 3. Renal effects of intravenous bolus of leptin in Sprague Dawley Rats with diet-induced obesity (OSDR) fed high caloric/fat diet for 24 weeks ($n = 4$) [left panel] and in OSDR fed high caloric/fat diet for this initial 12 weeks and switched to standard rat chow for additional 12 weeks ($n = 4$) [right panel]. Abbreviations as in figure 2. Values are means ± SE. E1 and E2 , experimental periods (45 min each). * $P < 0.05$ vs E1. †$P < 0.05$ vs corresponding experimental period between groups. From Patel, S.B., Villarreal, D., Kundra, A., et al. Cardiac Hormone2008: 111-127. (Reproduced with permission from Transworld Research Network.).

The relevance and importance of endogenous leptin as a distinct sodium-volume regulatory hormone has been examined in normal Sprague Dawley rats that were in a state of mild sodium/volume expansion [61]. Urinary sodium and volume excretion were reduced by approximately 20-25% after blockade of leptin with a polyclonal antibody, indicating a significant physiologic role for this hormone in the daily renal control of salt and water balance. The importance of leptin as a regulator of sodium and volume is further supported by recent investigations [62, 63] which have demonstrated that leptin expression in adipose tissue is directly proportional to dietary sodium, a response that would be expected for mechanisms regulating sodium balance.

Thus, the available information to date suggests that leptin's net effect on renal sodium metabolism may reflect both direct natriuretic and indirect anti-natriuretic actions. The responsiveness to leptin at various sites which regulate natriuresis may differ under diverse physiological and pathophysiological conditions, and this in turn, will be a determinant for the overall magnitude of leptin-induced urinary sodium excretion.

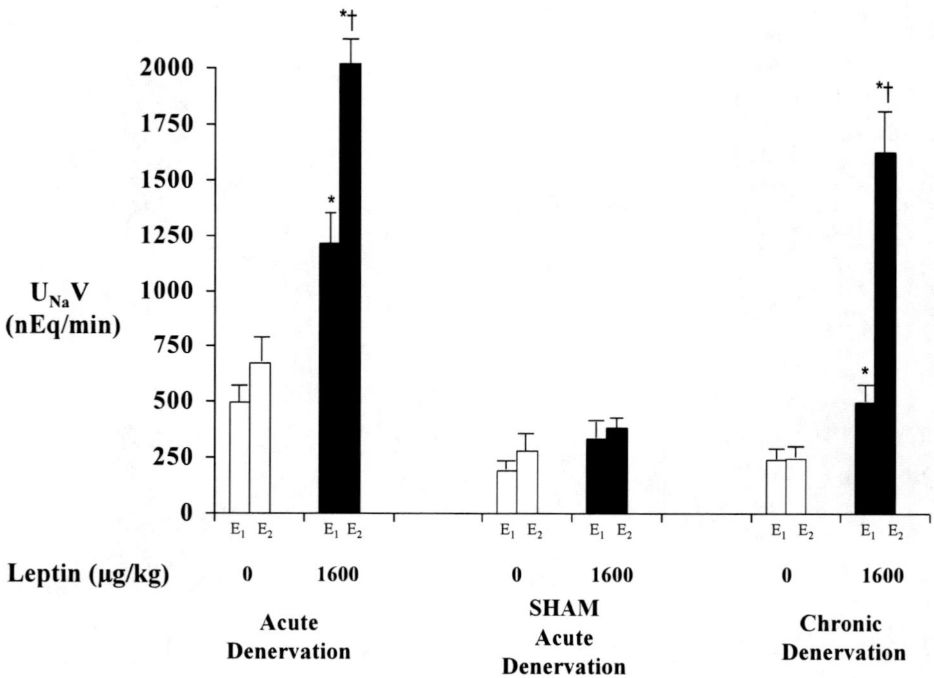

Figure 4. Natriuretic (UNaV) effects of leptin in Spontaneously Hypertensive Rats with acute denervation ($N = 8$ for each group), sham acute denervation ($N = 6$ for each group), and chronic denervation ($N = 8$ for each group). Symbols are [□] vehicle (0 dose); [■] leptin (1,600 µg/kg). Values are means ± SEM. E1-2 are the experimental periods of 45 minutes each. * $P < 0.05$ vs. the corresponding period at 0 dose within each experimental series; †$P < 0.05$ vs. E1. From Villarreal, D., Reams, G., Freeman, R.H. Kidney Int 2000; 58: 989-994. (Reproduced with permission from Blackwell Science LTD).

Leptin and Chronic Kidney Disease

Leptin's role in renal physiology and pathophysiology is complex. As indicated earlier, leptin may play a significant role in the regulation of sodium and water balance in normal situations. However, in conditions of chronic hyperleptinemia, the hormone has been linked to renal structural changes that specifically have been associated with obesity [64]. Elegant studies by Wolf et al. have determined that in glomerular endothelial cells, leptin can stimulate cellular proliferation, expression of TGF-β1 and type IV collagen synthesis leading to fibrosis [64]. Indeed, long term infusion of leptin in normal rats promoted the development of glomerulosclerosis and proteinuria [65]. It is of interest that similar renal abnormalities have been found in mice with chronic high fat diet and the metabolic syndrome [66], which is characterized by sustained elevations of circulating leptin [67].

Inappropriate elevation in serum leptin levels has been demonstrated in patients with chronic kidney disease [68-70]. The origin and significance of hyperleptinemia in these patients is not completely defined, but it must be emphasized that the marked elevation of leptin is out of proportion to obesity and persists after correction for body mass index [71]. Since the kidney is involved in clearance of leptin, its elevated levels in renal insufficiency are primarily due to reduced renal filtration and metabolism [68, 72]. It remains to be determined whether an increased rate of leptin production also contributes to the high serum leptin levels in renal insufficiency.

It has been previously demonstrated that leptin induces the synthesis of type I collagen in mesangial cells as well as type IV collagen in glomerular endothelial cells contributing to extracellular matrix deposition, glomerulosclerosis, and proteinuria [65, 73]. Based on this information, a link has been described between the increased incidence of glomerulosclerosis in patients with severe obesity and serum leptin concentration [74], supporting the studies by Wolf et al. in hyperleptinemic rats [65].

Leptin levels appear to be higher in patients undergoing peritoneal dialysis [PD] compared to hemodialysis [HD] [75]. The reasons for this phenomenon are multifactorial. It is likely that the elevated body fat mass in patients with PD contributes to the increase in serum leptin [76]. However, other factors are probably involved. For instance, the continuous glucose load in PD results in chronic hyperinsulinemia, an important finding considering that insulin upregulates lepr gene expression [69]. In this regard, it is of interest that even higher leptin levels are observed in patients with renal insufficiency with elevated insulin levels compared to patients with low insulin levels [69, 76].

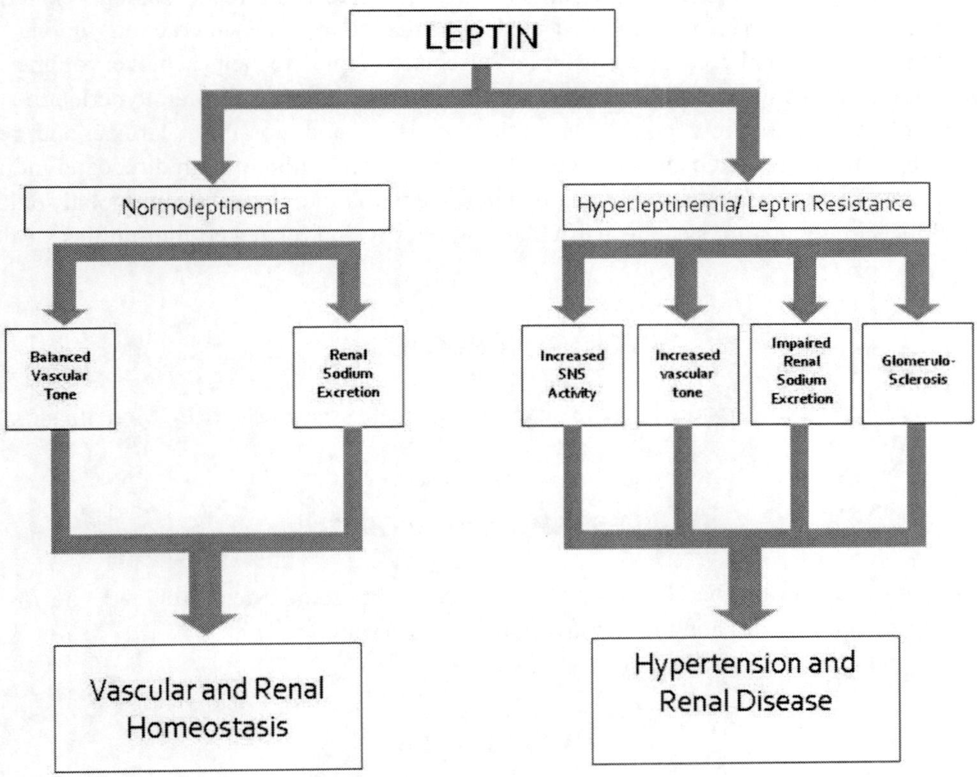

Figure 5. Vascular and Renal Action of Leptin. *SNS* sympathetic nervous system. Modified from Kshatriya S., Reams G., Spear RM. et al. Curr Opin Nephrol Hypertens. 2010; 19(1):72-8. Reproduced with permission from Wolters Kluwer/Lippincott, Williams and Wilkins).

The pathophysiological significance of hyperleptinemia in renal insufficiency is not completely understood. High levels of leptin have been associated with weight loss in dialysis patients [71, 77-79], and therefore it has been suggested that hyperleptinemia may be a contributing factor in uremic-induced cachexia [70, 77-83]. Other suggested actions in patients with end-stage renal disease include leptin-induced reduction in erythropoiesis [84, 85], promotion of renal osteodystrophy [86, 87], chronic inflammation [82] and glomerulosclerosis [73, 74]. Clearly additional research is necessary for the better definition of the potential reversibility of these abnormalities, particularly in the context of the blockade of leptin effects with receptor antagonists.

Summary and Conclusion

It is well established that cardiovascular and renal functions require the activation of multiple neuro-hormonal mechanisms designed to maintain homeostasis. The hormone leptin has multiple actions in physiological and pathophysiological cardiovascular and renal regulation (Figure 5). Potentially prominent are its effects on renal sodium excretion, sympathetic nervous system activation and vascular tone. The interaction among the vasoconstricting, vasodilatory and natriuretic effects of leptin to help achieve volume and pressure homeostasis in normal conditions may be disrupted during chronic hyperleptinemia, and this effect could likely contribute to hypertension and possibly, cardiac and renal dysfunction. Further research awaits the additional characterization of both direct and indirect mechanisms of action of leptin, including its interface with other important hormonal sodium-volume-pressure regulatory systems particularly in obesity and related co-morbidities.

Acknowledgment

The authors wish to acknowledge the expert technical assistance Jeffrey Montalbano.

Research Support

Supported in part by the Veteran Affairs Research Program [Merit Review], the Joseph C. Georg Research Award and the Hendricks Research Award.

References

[1] Ogden, CL; Carroll, MD; Curtin; et al. Prevalence of overweight and obesity in the United States, *JAMA*, 2006 295, 1549-1555.

[2] Hall, JE; Crook, ED; Jones DW; et al. Mechanisms of obesity associated cardiovascular and renal disease. *Am. J. Med. Sci.* 2002 324, 27-37.

[3] Hajer, GR; Van Haeften, TW; Visseren, FLJ. Adipose tissue dysfunction in obesity, diabetes and vascular diseases. *Eur. Heart J.,* 2008 9, 2959-2971.

[4] Garrison, RJ; Kannel, B; Stokes J 3rd; et al. Incidence and precursors of hypertension in young adults: The Framingham Offspring Study. *Prev. Med.,* 1987 16, 235-251.

[5] Wofford, MR; Hall, JE. Pathophysiology and Treatment of Obesity Hypertension. *Curr. Pharmaceutical Design*, 2004 10, 3621-3637.

[6] Hutley, L; Prins, J. Fat as an Endocrine Organ: Relationship to the Metabolic Syndrome. *Am. J. Med. Sci.*, 2005 330, 280-289.

[7] Guha, PK; Villarreal, D; Reams, GP; et al. Role of leptin in the regulation of body fluid volume and pressures. *Am. J. Ther.*, 2003 10, 211-218.

[8] Sharma, V; McNeill, J. The Emerging Roles of Leptin and Ghrelin in Cardiovascular Physiology and Pathophysiology. *Curr. Vasc. Pharmacol.*, 2005 3, 169-180.

[9] Misra, A; Garg, A. Leptin: Its receptor and obesity. *J. Invest. Med.,* 1996 44, 540-548.

[10] Lonnqvist, F. The obese (ob) gene and its product leptin: A new route towards obesity treatment in man? *QJM,* 1996 89, 327-332.

[11] Beltowski, J. (x) Role of leptin in blood pressure regulation and arterial hypertension. *J. Hypertens.,* 1996 24, 789-801.

[12] Haynes, WG; Morgan, DA; Walsh, S.A; et al. Receptor-mediated regional sympathetic nerve activation by leptin. *J. Clin. Invest.,* 1997 100, 270-278.

[13] Dunbar, JC; Hu, Y; Lu, H. Intracerebroventricular leptin increases lumbar and renal sympathetic nerve activity and blood pressure in normal rats. *Diabetes*, 1997 46, 2040-2043.

[14] Villarreal, D; Reams, G; Freeman, RH; et al. Renal effects of leptin in normotensive. hypertensive and obese rats. *Am. J. Physiol.* 1998 275: R2056-R2060.

[15] Chen, H; Charlat, O; Tartaglia, LA, et al. Evidence that diabetes gene encodes leptin receptor: Identification of a mutation in the leptin receptor gene in db/db mice. *Cell,* 1996 84, 491-495.

[16] Banks, AS; Davis, SM; Bates, SH; et al. Activation of downstream signals by the long form of the leptin receptor. *J. Biol. Chem.*, 2000 275, 14563-14572.

[17] Munzberg, H; Myers, MG Jr. Molecular and anatomical determinants of central leptin resistance. *Nature*, 2005 8, 566-570.

[18] Tartaglia, LA; Dembski, M; Weng, X; et al. Identification and expression of cloning of a leptin receptor. OB-R. *Cell*, 1995 83: 1263-1271.

[19] Wang, M-Y; Zhou, YT; Neward, CB; et al. A novel leptin receptor isoform in rat. *FEBS Let.*, 1996 392: 87-90.

[20] Zoccali, C; Mallamaci, F; Tripepi, G. Adipose tissue as a source of inflammatory cytokines in health and disease: Focus on end-stage renal disease. *Kidney Int.*, 2003 63, S65–S66.

[21] Chen, H; Charlat, O; Tartaglia, LA; et al. Evidence that the diabetes gene encodes the leptin receptor: identification of a mutation in the leptin receptor gene in db/db mice. *Cell,* 1996 84, 491-495.

[22] Hoggard, N; Mercer, JG; Rayner, DV; et al. Localization of leptin receptor mRNA splice variants in murine peripheral tissues by RT-PCR and in situ hybridization. *Biochem. Biophys. Res. Commun.*, 1997 232, 383-387.

[23] Lee, GH; Proenca, R; Montez, JM; et al. Abnormal splicing of the leptin receptor in diabetic mice. *Nature,* 1996 379, 632-635.

[24] Anubhuti; Arora, S. Leptin and its metabolic interactions – an update. *Diabetes Obes. Metab.*, 2008 10, 973-993.

[25] Mark, AL; Agassandian, K; Morgan; et al. Leptin signaling in the nucleus tractus solitarii increases sympathetic nerve activity to the kidney. *Hypertension*, 2009 53, 375-380.

[26] Dubinion, JH; Da Silva, AA; Hall, JE. Chronic blood pressure and appetite responses to central leptin infusion in rats fed a high fat diet. *J. Hypertens.,* 2011 29, 758-762.

[27] Beltowski, J; Jochem, J; Wojcicka, G; et al. Influence of intravenously administered leptin on nitric oxide production. renal hemodynamics and renal function in the rat. *Regul. Pept.,* 2004 *1*20, 59–67.

[28] Lembo L; Vecchione C; Fratta, L; Leptin induces direct vasodilation through distinct endothelial mechanisms. *Diabetes*, 2000 49, 293-297.

[29] Fruhbeck, G. Pivotal role of nitric oxide in the control of blood pressure after leptin administration. *Diabetes*, 1999 48, 903-908.

[30] Brook, RD; Bard, RL; Bodary, PF; et al. Blood Pressure and Vascular Effects of Leptin in Humans. *Metab. Syndr. Relat. Disord.*, 2007 5, 270-274.

[31] Mitchell, JL; Morgan, DA; Correia, MLG; et al. Does leptin stimulate nitric oxide to oppose the effects of sympathetic activation? *Hypertension*, 2001 38, 1081-1086.

[32] Gardiner, SM; Kemp, PA; March, JE; et al. Regional hemodynamic effects of recombinant murine or human leptin in conscious rats. *Br. J. Pharmacol.*, 2000 130, 805-810.

[33] Beltowski, J; Wojcicka, G; Jamroz-Wisniewska, A; et al. Resistance to acute NO-mimetic and EDHF-mimetic effects of leptin in the metabolic syndrome. *Life Sciences*, 2009 85, 557-567.

[34] Mark, AL; Shaffer, RA; Correia, ML. Contrasting blood pressure effects of obesity in leptin-deficient ob/ob mice and agouti yellow obese mice. *J. Hypertension*, 1999 17, 1949-1953.

[35] Correia, MI; Haynes, WG; Rahmouni K. The concept of selective leptin resistance: evidence from agouti yellow obese mice. *Diabetes*, 2002 51, 439-442.

[36] Morgan, DA; Thedens, DR; Weiss, R; et al. Mechanisms mediating renal sympathetic activation to leptin in obesity. *Am. J. Physiol. Regul. Integr. Comp. Physiol.*, **2008** 295: R1730-R1736.

[37] Rahmouni, K; Correia, LG; Haynes, WG; et al. Obesity-Associated Hypertension. new insights into mechanisms. *Hypertension*, 2005 45, 9-14.

[38] Tune, JD; Consodine, R. Effects of leptin on cardiovascular physiology. *J. Am. Soc. Hypertens.*, 2007 14, 231-241.

[39] Bjorbaek, C; Elmquist, JK; Frantz, JD; et al. Identification of SOCS-3 as a potential mediator of central leptin resistance. *Mol. Cell,* 1998 191, 619–625.

[40] Nava, E; Wiklund, NP; Salazar, FJ. Changes in nitric oxide release in vivo in response to vasoactive substances. *Br. J. Pharmacol.,* 1996 119, 1211–1216.

[41] Bełtowski, J; Jamroz-Wiśniewska, A; Borkowska, E; et al. Up-regulation of renal Na+, K+-ATPase: the possible novel mechanism of leptin-induced hypertension. *Pol. J. Pharmacol.*, Mar-Apr 2004 56(2), 213-222.

[42] Zhang, Y; Scarpace, PJ. The role of leptin in leptin resistance and obesity. *Physiol. Behav.,* 2006 88, 249–256.

[43] De Rosa, S; Cirillo, P; Pacileo, M; et al. Leptin stimulated C-reactive protein production by human coronary artery endothelial cells. *J. Vasc. Res.*, 2009 46, 609–617.

[44] Shek, EW; Brands, MW; Hall, JE. Chronic leptin infusion increases arterial pressure. *Hypertension*, 1998 31, 409-414.

[45] Aizawa-Abe, M; Ogawa, Y; Masuzaki H; et al. Pathophysiological role of leptin in obesity-related hypertension. *J. Clin. Invest.*, 2000 105, 1243-1252.

[46] Huang, F; Xiong, X; Wang, H; et al. Leptin-induced vascular smooth muscle cell proliferation via regulating cell cycle. activating ERK ½ and NF-KB. *Acta Biochim. Biophys. Sin.*, 2010 42, 325-331.

[47] Galletti, F; D'Elia, L; Barba, G; et al. High-Circulating leptin Levels are associated with a greater risk of hypertension in men independently of body mass and insulin resistance: Results of an eight-year follow-up study. *J. Clin. Endocrinol. Metab.*, 2008 93, 3922-3926.

[48] Ma, D; Feitosa, MF; Wilk, JB; et al. Leptin is associated with blood pressure and hypertension in women from the National Heart. Lung. and Blood Institute Family Heart Study. *Hypertension*, 2009 5, 473-479.

[49] Mak, RH; Cheung, W; Cone, RD; et al. Leptin and inflammation-associated cachexia in chronic kidney disease. *Kidney Int.*, 2009 69, 794–797.

[50] Serradeil-Le, G; Raufaste, D; Brossard, G; et al. Characterization and localization of leptin receptors in the rat kidney. *FEBS Lett.*, 1997 404, 185-191.

[51] Jackson, EK; Li, P. Human leptin has natriuretic activity in the rat. *Am. J. of Physiol.*, 1997 272, F333-F338.

[52] Villarreal, D; Reams, G; Freeman, RH. Effects of renal denervation on the sodium excretory action of leptin in hypertensive rats. *Kidney Int.*, 2000 58, 989-994.

[53] DiBona, GF. The kidney in the pathogenesis of hypertension: The role of renal nerves. *Am. J. Kidney Dis.*, 1985 5: A27-A31.

[54] Patel, S; Villarreal; D; Kundra, A; et al. Cardiovascular and renal actions of leptin. In Vesely D. L. Ed. *Cardiac Hormones. Transworld Research Network, Kerala, India.* 2008, 111-127.

[55] Beltowski, J; Wojcicka, G. Human leptin administered intraperitoneally stimulates natriuresis and decreases renal medullary Na+. K+-ATPase activity in the rat-impaired effect in dietary-induced obesity. *Med. Sci. Monit.,* 2002 *8.* BR221-BR229.

[56] Villarreal, D; Reams, G; Samar, H; et al. Effects of Chronic Nitric Oxide Inhibition on the Renal Excretory Response to Leptin. *Obes. Res.*, 2004 12, 1006-10.

[57] Lin, L; Martin, R; Schaffenhauier, AO; et al. Acute changes in the response to peripheral leptin with alteration in the diet composition. *Am. J. Physiol.*, 2001 280, R504-R509.

[58] Bouloumine, A; Marumo, T; Lofanton, M. Leptin induces oxidative stress in human endothelial cells. *FASEB J.*, 1999 13, 1231-1238.

[59] Krum, H; Schlaich, M; Whitbourn, R; et al. Catheter-based renal sympathetic denervation for resistant hypertension: a multicentre safety and proof-of-principle cohort study. *Lancet*, 2009 373, 1275-1281.

[60] A, Sobotka; Murray, D; Esler, Henry Krum; et al. One-Year Results From the Symplicity HTN-2 RCT: Renal Sympathetic Denervation for Treatment of Drug-Resistant Hypertension *Circulation,* 2012 126, 2976-2982.

[61] Villarreal, D; Reams, G; Samar, H. Leptin blockade attenuates sodium excretion in saline-loaded normotensive rats. *Mol. Cell Biochem.*, 2006 283, 153-157.

[62] Dobrian, AD; Schriver, SD; Lynch, T; et al. Effect of salt on hypertension and oxidative stress in rat model on diet-induced obesity. *Am. J. Physiol.*, 2003 285, F619-F628.

[63] Adomczak, M; Koleot, F; Chutek, J; et al. Effect of renin angiotensin system activation by dietary sodium restriction and upright position on plasma leptin concentration in patients with essential hypertension. *Med. Sci. Monit.*, 2002 8, CR473-CR477.

[64] Wolf, G; Ziyadeh, FN. Leptin and renal fibrosis. *Contrib. Nephrol.*, 2006 151, 175–183.

[65] Wolf, G; Chen, S; Han, DC; et al. Leptin and renal disease. *Am. J. Kidney Dis.*, 2002 39, 1-11.

[66] Deji, N; Kume, S; Araki, S-I; et al. Structural and functional changes in the kidneys of high-fat diet-induced mice. *Am. J. Physiol. Renal Physiol.*, 2008 296, F118-F126.

[67] Gannagé-Yared, M-H; Khalife, S; Semaan, M; et al. Serum adiponectin and leptin levels in relation to the metabolic syndrome. androgenic profile and somatotropic axis in healthy non-diabetic elderly men. *Eur. J. Endocrinol.*, 2006 155, 167-176.

[68] Sharma, K; Considine, RV; Michael, B; et al. Plasma leptin is partly cleared by the kidney and is elevated in hemodialysis patients. *Kidney Int.*, 1997 51, 1980–1985.

[69] Nordfors, L; Lönnqvist, F; Heimbürger, O; et al. Low leptin gene expression and hyperleptinemia in chronic renal failure. *Kidney Int.*, 1998 54, 1267–1275.

[70] Stenvinkel, P; Lönnqvist, F; Schalling, M. Molecular basis of renal disease. Molecular studies of leptin: implications for renal disease. *Nephrol. Dial. Transplant.*, 1999 4, 1103-1112.

[71] Heimburger, O; Lönnqvist, F; Danielsson, A; et al. Serum immunoreactive leptin concentration and its relation to the body fat content in chronic renal failure. *J. Am. Soc. Nephrol.,* 1997 8, 1423-1430.

[72] Cumin, F; Baum, HP; de Gasparo M; et al. Removal of endogenous leptin from the circulation by the kidney. *Int. J. Obes. Relat. Metab. Disord.*, 1997 21, 495-504.

[73] Ballermann, BJ. A role for leptin in glomerulosclerosis? *Kidney International*, 1999 56 3, 1154–1155.

[74] M, Tesauro; A, Mascali; O, Franzese; et al. Chronic Kidney Disease, Obesity, and Hypertension: The Role of Leptin and Adiponectin. *Intl. J. of Hypertension,* vol. 2012, Article ID 943605, 7 pages, 2012. doi:10.1155/2012/943605.

[75] Johansen, KL; Mulligan, K; Tai, V; et al. Leptin. body composition. and indices of malnutrition in patients on dialysis. *J. Am. Soc. Nephrol.*, 1998 9, 1080-1084.

[76] Stenvinkel, P; Heimbürger, O; Lönnqvist, **F.** Serum leptin concentrations correlate to plasma insulin concentrations independent of body fat content in chronic renal failure. *Nephrol. Dial. Transplant.*, 1997 12, 1321-1325.

[77] Fontan, PM; Rodriguez-Carmona, R; Cordido, F; et al. Hyperleptinemia in uremic patients undergoing conservative management. peritoneal dialysis. and hemodialysis: A comparative analysis. *Am. J. Kidney Dis.*, 1999 34, 824-831.

[78] Bossola, M; Tazza, L; Giungi, S; et al. Anorexia in hemodialysis patients: an update. *Kidney Int.*, 2006 70, 417-22.

[79] Stenvinkel, P; Lindholm, B; Lönnqvist, F; et al. Increases in serum leptin levels during peritoneal dialysis are associated with inflammation and a decrease in lean body mass. *J. Am. Soc. Nephrol.,* 2000 **11,** 1303–1309.

[80] Odamaki, M; Furuya, R; Yoneyama, T. Association of the serum leptin concentration with weight loss in chronic hemodialysis patients. *Am. J. Kidney Dis.,* 1999 **33,** 361–368.

[81] Kshatriya, S; Liu, K; Salah, A; et al. Obesity Hypertension: The Regulatory Role of Leptin. *Int. J. Hypertens.*, vol. 2011, Article ID 270624, 8 pages, 2011. doi:10.4061/2011/270624.

[82] Mak, RH; Cheung, W; Cone, RD; et al. Leptin and inflammation-associated cachexia in chronic kidney disease. *Kidney Int.*, 2006 69, 794–797.

[83] Cheung, W; Yu, PX; Little, BM; et al. Role of leptin and melanocortin signaling in uremia-associated cachexia. *J. Clin. Invest.,* 2005 115**,** 1659–1665.

[84] Axelsson, J; Qureshi, A; Heimbürger; et al. Body Fat Mass and Serum Leptin Levels Influence Epoetin Sensitivity in Patients With ESRD. *Am. J. Kidney Dis.*, 2005 46, 628-634.

[85] Hung, S-C; Tung, T-Y; Yang, C-S; et al. High-calorie supplementation increases serum leptin levels and improves response to rHuEPO in long-term hemodialysis patients. *Am J. Kidney Dis.*, 2005 45, 1073-1083.

[86] Coen, G; Ballanti, P; Fischer, M; et al. Serum leptin in dialysis renal osteodystrophy. *Am. J. Kidney Dis.*, 2003 42, 1036-1042.

[87] Mallamaci, F; Tripepi, G; Zoccali, C. Leptin in end stage renal disease (ESRD): a link between fat mass. bone and the cardiovascular system. *J. Nephrol.*, 2005 18, 464-468.

In: Leptin: Biosynthesis, Functions and Clinical Significance ISBN: 978-1-62948-801-1
Editor: Edward L. Blum

Chapter 3

MELANOMA AND LEPTIN

Arash Sabetisoofyani*
University of Arizona, AZ, US

ABSTRACT

Epidemiological studies suggest that obesity increases the risk of developing several cancers, including melanoma. Obesity increases the expression of angiogenic factors, such as leptin, that may contribute to tumor growth. However, a direct cause and effect relationship between obesity and tumor growth has not been clearly established and the role of leptin in accelerating tumor growth is unclear. The role of diet in melanoma has been explored in several studies but the findings have been inconsistent. Specifically, high intake of specific agents, such as antioxidants and retinoid-rich food has been linked to a protective effect against melanoma development. Similar associations have been found with higher blood levels of a-tocopherol , b-carotene and retinol, as well as with greater dietary intakes of vitamin E and b-carotene in several case–control studies [1-3]. Anthropometrical measures, such as height, weight and body mass index (BMI); have been associated with an increased risk of several malignancies, including melanoma [4-6]. Leptin, a hormone secreted by adipose tissue, controls food intake and energy balance by providing signals to the hypothalamus [7]. Serum levels of leptin are positively related with body composition and insulin levels, female sex and alcohol consumption and inversely related to cigarette smoking [8-10].

Keywords: Melanoma, Obesity, Leptin

INTRODUCTION

Obesity has increased dramatically in the United States in the past three decades; approximately32% of adults are obese with a body mass index greater than 30 kg/m2 [11]. Epidemiological studies have shown that there is a strong, positive correlation between BMI

* Corresponding author: Arash Sabetisoofyani M.D., University of Arizona, Phone #520-301-5658; Email:arash@ email.arizona.edu, 3993 N. Campbell Ave #4204.

and the incidence of several types of cancer, such as colon, breast, ovarian, prostate, renal cell carcinoma and melanoma. Calle et al. concluded that obesity may account for 50% of cancer deaths in women aged 50 y or older [12]. However, there have been few studies that have demonstrated a direct cause and effect relationship between obesity and cancer. Moreover, the epidemiological evidence suggests that the response to obesity is not the same for all tumors. Consequently, the mechanisms by which obesity may influence carcinogenesis are poorly understood. Adipose tissue secretes several cytokines (i.e., adipokines) that are believed to promote inflammation, cell proliferation and angiogenesis. Leptin, an adipokine that is produced inproportion to the mass of adipose tissue and which circulates in the blood, has been suggested to link obesity with tumor growth [13-15]. Leptin stimulates cell proliferation in several tumor cell lines, enhances endothelial cell migration in vitro, and has been suggested to be an angiogenicfactor [16, 17]. Thus, leptin has several effects that could contribute to tumor growth. However, most of the studies supporting leptin's role in promoting cell proliferation and angiogenesis have been conducted in vitro and have involved the use of large, pharmacological concentrations of leptin to demonstrate the effects.

STRUCTURE

Leptin is an adipocyte-derived hormone that acts as a major regulator for food intake and energy homeostasis. Leptin deficiency or resistance can result in profound obesity, diabetes, and infertility in humans. Since its discovery, our understanding of leptin's biological functions has expanded from antiobesity to broad effects on reproduction, hematopoiesis, angiogenesis, blood pressure, bone mass, lymphoid organ homeostasis, and T lymphocyte systems. Leptin receptor belongs to the class I cytokine receptor superfamily. At least five isoforms of leptin receptor exist, primarily because of alternate splicing. The longest form is capable of full signal transduction. The short forms may serve as leptin binding proteins and play a role in leptin transporting across the blood–brain barrier.

BACKGROUND

The few published animal studies attempting to determine whether leptin and obesity promote tumor growth have produced mixed results. Some studies support the hypothesis that the absence of leptin signaling attenuates mammary tumor growth in mice [18-20]. For example, Gonzalez et al. demonstrated that mouse mammary tumor growth was dramatically reduced when mice were treated with a leptin receptor antagonist [21], suggesting that leptin signaling may be necessary for certain types of breast tumor growth. In apparent contradiction to these studies, obese Zucker rats, which have a mutation in the leptin receptor, developed more mammary tumors at an earlier age than lean Zucker rats after exposure to the carcinogen [22]. Until recently, there had been no studies that have examined the relationship between obesity and the incidence of melanoma. One mechanism by which obesity has been suggested to contribute to enhanced tumor growth is by promoting angiogenesis. The mechanisms that mediate the effects of food restriction on tumor growth are unclear but likely involve numerous metabolic pathways, including those involved in angiogenesis. The mechanisms for leptin's effects on tumor growth are still uncertain, although a role for leptin in promoting angiogensis has been previously suggested. There is indirect evidence from clinical studies that leptin may enhance tumor growth by stimulating angiogenesis. For example, leptin expression correlated well with VEGF expression in human gastric cancers and both factors were associated with poor patient prognosis [23]. Results from a recent study in mice showed that mammary tumor VEGF and tumor growth were significantly reduced when mice were treated with the leptin receptor antagonist. Leptin has been identified in several types of human cancers and may also be linked to poor prognosis. In two studies, leptin and leptin receptor expression were significantly increased in primary and metastatic breast cancer relative to noncancerous tissues in women [24, 25]. In a clinical study of colorectal cancer, leptin expression was positively correlated with tumor grade [26]. Serum leptin and leptin receptor expression in renal cell carcinomas was well correlated with progression-free survival, venous invasion and lymph node metastasis [27]. Leptin has also been shown to be expressed in uterine and endometrial cancers [28]. There is very little previous information on the relationship between leptin and melanoma. One epidemiological study reported that high serum leptin was positively correlated with melanoma risk [29].

Conclusion

Epidemiological studies suggest that hyperglycemia and hyperinsulinemia are associated with increased risk for development of cancer. However, further studies are needed for testing the hypothesis that hyperinsulinemia increases tumor growth in this model of melanoma. The mechanisms by which obesity promotes melanoma growth likely involve increased angiogenesis, since tumors from the obese mice have more VEGF. Leptin deficiency attenuates but does not abolish melanoma tumor growth. A key factor in obesity induced angiogenesis that may be involved in promoting melanoma growth is inflammation. Obesity is often described as a low level inflammatory state and the literature is replete with studies supporting a central role for macrophages in tumor angiogenesis. During weight gain, adipocytes increase in size, preadipocytes differentiate into mature adipocytes and there is a sudden increase in the metabolic demand of the tissue. Adipocytes respond by secreting inflammatory cytokines that recruit macrophages. Macrophages, in turn, initiate angiogenesis by secreting matrix metalloproteinases to break down the extracellular matrix and basement membranes of nearby blood vessels. Together with adipocytes, macrophages secrete angiogenic factors that promote the proliferation and migration of endothelial cells. Once the new blood vessel is formed, macrophages secrete different cytokines that remodel the stroma to support their growth. The similarities between angiogenesis in obesity and cancer suggest that macrophages are central to both scenarios. Future studies should examine whether inhibition of inflammation in obesity reduces tumor growth.

References

[1] Bain C, Green A, Siskind V et al. Diet and melanoma. An exploratory case-control study. *Ann. Epidemiol.,* 1993; 3: 235–238.

[2] Millen AE, Tucker MA, Hartge P et al. Diet and melanoma in a case-control study. *Cancer Epidemiol Biomarkers Prev.,* 2004; 13: 1042–1051.

[3] Naldi L, Gallus S, Tavani A et al. Risk of melanoma and vitamin A, coffee and alcohol: a case-control study from Italy. *Eur. J. Cancer Prev.,* 2004; 13: 503–508.

[4] Gallus S, Naldi L, Martin L et al. Anthropometrical measures and risk of cutaneous malignant melanoma: a case-control study from Italy. *Melanoma Res.,* 2006; 16: 83–87.

[5] Thune I, Olsen A, Albrektsen G, Tretli S. Cutaneous malignant melanoma: association with height, weight and body-surface area. a prospective study in Norway. *Int. J. Cancer,* 1993; 55: 555–561.

[6] Odenbro A, Gillgren P, Bellocco R et al. The risk for cutaneous malignant melanoma, melanoma in situ and intraocular malignant melanoma in relation to tobacco use and body mass index. *Br. J. Dermatol.,* 2007; 156: 99–105.

[7] Wauters M, Considenie RV, Van Gaal LF. Human Leptin: from an adipocyte hormone to an endocrine mediator. *Eur. J. Endocrinol.,* 2000; 143: 293–311.

[8] Thomas T, Burguera B, Melton LJ III et al. Relationship of serum leptin levels with body composition and sex steroid and insulin levels in men and women. *Metabolism,* 2000; 49: 1278–1284.

[9] Havel PJ, Kasim-Karakas S, Dubuc GR et al. Gender differences in plasma leptin concentration. *Nat. Med.,* 1996; 2: 949–950.

[10] Mantzoros CS, Liolios AD, Tritos NA et al. Circulating insulin concentrations, smoking, and alcohol intake are important independent predictors of leptin in young healthy men. *Obes. Res.,* 1998; 6: 179–186.

[11] Flegal KM, Carroll MD, Ogden CL, Johnson CCL. Prevalence and trends in obesity among US adults 1999–2000. *JAMA,* 2002; 288:1723–7.

[12] Calle EE, Rodriguez C, Walker-Thurmond K, Thun MJ. Overweight, obesity and mortality from cancer in a prospectively studied cohort of U.S. adults. *N. Engl. J. Med.,* 2003;348:1625–38.

[13] Stattin P, Lukanova A, Biessy C, Soderberg S, Palmqvist R, Kaaks R, et al. Obesity and colon cancer: does leptin provide a link? *International Journal of Cancer,* 2004;109: 149–52.

[14] Chang S, Hursting SD, Contois JH, Strom SS, Yamamura Y, Babaian RJ, et al. Leptin and prostate cancer. *The Prostate,* 2001;46:62–7.

[15] Saglam K, Aydur E, Yilmaz M, Goktas K. Leptin influences cellular differentiation and progression in prostate cancer. *J. Urol.,* 2003;169:1308–11.

[16] Fenton JI, Hord NG, Lavigne JA, Perkins SN, Hursting SD. Leptin, insulin-like growth factor-1, and insulin-like growth factor-2 are mitogens in ApcMin/+ but not Apc+/+ colonic epithelial cell lines. *Cancer Epidemiol. Biomarkers Prev.,* 2005;14:1646–52.

[17] Bouloumie A, Drexler HC, Lafontan M, Busse R. Leptin, the product of Ob gene, promotes angiogenesis. *Circulation,* 1998;83:1059–66.

[18] Cleary MP, Phillips FC, Getzin SC, Jacobson TL, Jacobson MK, Christensen TA, et al. Genetically obese MMTV-TGFalpha/Lep (ob) Lep (ob) female mice do not develop mammary tumors. *Breast Cancer Res. Treat.,* 2003;77:205–15.

[19] Cleary MP, Grande JP, Maihle NJ. Effect of high fat diet on body weight and mammary tumor latency in MMTV-TGFα mice. *Int. J. Obes. Relat. Metab. Disord.,* 2004;28:956–62.

[20] Gonzalez RR, Cherfils S, Escobar M, Yoo JH, Carino C, Styer AK, et al. Leptin signaling promotes the growth of mammary tumors and increases the expression of vascular endothelial growth factor (VEGF) and its receptor type two (VEGF-R2). *J. Biol. Chem.,* 2006;281:26320–8.

[21] Hakkak R, Holley AW, Macleod SL, Simpsom PM, Fuchs GJ, Jo CH, et al. Obesity promotes 7,12 dimethylbenz (a) anthracene-induced mammary tumor development in female zucker rats. *Breast Cancer Res.,* 2005;7:627–33.

[22] Sierra-Honigmann MR, Nath AK, Murakami C, Garcia-Cardena G, Papapetropoulos A, Sessa WC, et al. Biological action of leptin as an angiogenic factor. *Science,* 1998;281: 1683–6.

[23] Garofalo C, Koda M, Cascio S, Sulkowska M, Kanczuga-Koda L, Golaszewka J, et al. Increasedexpr ession of leptin and the leptin receptor as a marker of breast cancer progression: possible role of obesity-related stimuli. *Clin. Cancer Res.,* 2006;12:447–53.

[24] Ishikawa M, Kitayama J, Nagawa H. Enhanced expression of leptin and leptin receptor (OB-R) in human breast cancer. *Clin. Cancer Res.,* 2004;10:4325–31.

[25] Koda M, Sulkowska M, Kanczuga-Koda L, Surmacz E, Sulkowski S. Overexpression of the obesity hormone leptin in human colorectal cancer. *J. Clin. Pathol.,* 2007;60:902–6.

[26] Horiguchi A, Sumitomo M, Asakuma J, Asano A, Zheng R, Nanus DM, et al. Leptin promotes invasiveness of murine renal cancer cells via extracellular signal-regulated kinases and rho dependent pathway. *J. Urol.,* 2006;176:1636–41.

[27] Koda M, Sulkowska M, Wincewicz A, Kanczuga-Koda L, Musiatowicz B, Szymanska M, et al. Expression of leptin, leptin receptor and hypoxia-inducible factor 1alpha in human endometrial cancer. *Ann. N Y Acad. Sci.,* 2007;1095:90–8.

[28] Gogas H, Trakatelli M, Dessypris N, Terzidis A, Katsambas A, Chrousos GP, et al. Melanoma risk in association with serum leptin levels and lifestyle parameters: a case-control study. *Ann. Oncol.,* 2008;19:384–9.

[29] Ablamunits V, Cohen Y, Brazee IB, Gaetz HP, Vinson C, Klebanov S. Susceptibility to induced and spontaneous carcinogenesis is increased in fatless A-ZIP/F-1 but not in obese ob/ob mice. *Cancer Res.,* 2006;66:8897–902.

In: Leptin: Biosynthesis, Functions and Clinical Significance ISBN: 978-1-62948-801-1
Editor: Edward L. Blum

Chapter 4

INHIBITION OF ONCOGENIC EFFECTS OF LEPTIN BY cAMP ELEVATION IN TRIPLE NEGATIVE BREAST CANCER CELLS

Annamaria Spina, Francesca Di Maiolo, Luigi Sapio, Luca Sorvillo and Silvio Naviglio*

Department of Biochemistry, Biophysics and General Pathology,
Second University of Naples, Medical School, Naples, Italy

ABSTRACT

Triple-negative breast cancers (TNBC) are characterised by an aggressive phenotype and have been associated with poor prognosis. Triple-negative breast cancer patients are unresponsive to current targeted therapies and other treatment options are only partially effective. Therefore, new pharmacological approaches are needed.

Given the relevant role of leptin in breast cancer growth and metastasis, leptin system has emerged as a new and promising therapeutic target for breast cancer. Importantly, recent studies provide initial evidence of cAMP elevation as a simple way to neutralize leptin-induced biological effects in TNBC cells, including proliferation and migration.

The underlying molecular mechanisms, the potential clinical significance and therapeutic applications by these studies will be presented.

Breast cancer is a common disease and a major cause of death with high incidence among female worldwide [1]. Breast cancer is a heterogeneous disease with varied morphological appearance, molecular features, behaviour and response to therapy [2].

Triple-negative breast cancer (TNBC) represents 10–20 % of all mammary tumors and is defined as tumors that are negative for estrogen receptor (ER), progesterone receptor (PR) and human epidermal growth factor receptor 2 (HER2) [3]. TNBC has several characteristic aggressive clinicopathological features, including young age at onset and large tumour size.

* Correspondence to: Silvio Naviglio, e-mail: silvio.naviglio@unina2.it.

Its histological hallmarks include high grade, high proliferative activity, focal areas of necrosis, absence of infiltrative margin, absence of gland formation, presence of central scar/fibrotic foci and prominent lymphoplasmacytic inflammatory infiltrate [3, 4]. TNBC patients have a poor prognosis in terms of disease-free and overall survival and currently there is a lack of targeted therapies for this group of patients [5, 6].

Because of its expression profile, TNBC is not amenable to treatment with hormone therapy or the anti-HER2 monoclonal antibody trastuzumab, and systemic treatment options are currently limited to cytotoxic chemotherapy. Overall survival, whether in early-stage or advanced disease, is poor compared with that in patients who have other phenotypes.

A number of targeted approaches to TNBC are undergoing clinical evaluation, including the use of agents with poly-(ADP-ribose) polymerase inhibitory properties such as iniparib (the United States Adopted Name for the investigational agent BSI-201), olaparib (AZD2281), and veliparib (ABT-888), antiangiogenic agents such as bevacizumab and sunitinib, and epidermal growth factor receptor blockers such as cetuximab and erlotinib. Encouraging results with some of these agents have been reported, thereby offering the promise for improved outcomes in patients with TNBC [4-7]. However, optimal conditions for the therapeutic assessment of women with triple-negative breast tumours and for the management of their disease have yet to be validated in prospective investigations and new pharmacological approaches for TNBC patients are warranted.

In recent years, interests have grown in the relationship between obesity and cancer. For breast cancer, a clear association between obesity and disease risk has been established [8, 9], and new studies confirming this observation and investigating explanatory hypotheses for the relationship continue to appear regularly. Obesity increases the risk of TNBC [10], too, and this is greatly due to the influence of adipokine leptin [11, 12].

Leptin is one of the most important adipose-derived hormones and it is manufactured mainly by adipose tissue, but can also be synthesized in secondary sources like placenta, stomach, and skeletal muscle as well as in normal or malignant breast tissue [13].

Remarkably, both leptin and its receptors are overexpressed in breast cancer, especially in high-grade tumors including triple-negative cancers and leptin acts as a mitogen/survival factor in breast cancer cells [14-17].

Overall, leptin is strongly proposed as cytokine link between obesity and breast cancer, including TNBC [9-12]. Importantly, given the relevant role of leptin in breast cancer growth and metastasis, leptin system has emerged as a new and promising therapeutic target for breast cancer [11, 18, 19].

Actually, agents able to block leptin activity, including soluble leptin receptors that bind free circulating leptin, leptin antagonists that bind to, but do not activate leptin receptors, and either specific anti-leptin receptors monoclonal antibodies that bind to the receptor preventing leptin signaling or anti-leptin antibodies, are in initial stages of development [18, 19]. However, novel strategies to suppress leptin signalling and counteract its biological effects are warranted.

Elevation of cAMP inhibits the proliferation and expression of transformed phenotype in a wide variety of cancer models, including breast cancer, through the induction of apoptosis and/or cell cycle arrest [20, 21].

Unfortunately, despite their potent antitumor effects in many cancer cells, substances that increase intracellular cAMP levels are not recommended to be used as anti-cancer drugs because of their high cytotoxicity. Therefore, it would be interesting to study new strategies able to potentiate the antitumor activity of these agents in order to reduce the dosage of cAMP elevating compounds required to obtain antiproliferative effects while limiting the potential toxicity [22].

Recently, we demonstrated that in MDA-MB-231 triple-negative breast cancer cells, intracellular cAMP elevation, irrespective of cAMP elevating agent used, completely abrogates both ERK1/2 and STAT3 phosphorylation in response to leptin and, very surprisingly, provided evidence that leptin, when cAMP levels are increased, drives cells towards apoptosis accompanied by a marked down-regulation of Bcl2 protein levels in a Protein Kinase A (PKA) dependent manner [23, 24]

Interestingly, we found a positive pharmacological interaction between leptin and cAMP elevating compounds that allowed a reduction in the effective doses of cAMP elevating drugs in vitro, thus potentially decreasing their undesirable side-effects in vivo.

More recently, we reported that cAMP elevation acts as a potent inhibitor of some leptin-induced metastatic properties of MDA-MB-231 highly aggressive breast cancer cells. Particularly, we found that cAMP increase strongly inhibits leptin-induced migration of MDA-MB-231 cells and that this phenomenom is accompanied by a strong decrease of levels of β3 integrin subunit and Focal Adhesion Kinase pro-metastatic proteins and preceded by an inhibition of pro-proliferative and pro-metastatic ERK1/2 and STAT3 signalling pathways [25].

To the best of our knowledge, above data represent the first evidence indicating a neutralization of leptin-induced oncogenic effects simply by raising intracellular cAMP levels [22, 26].

Triple-negative breast cancers (TNBC) are characterised by an aggressive phenotype and have been associated with poor prognosis. Triple-negative breast cancer patients are unresponsive to current targeted therapies and other treatment options are only partially effective [27]. Therefore, new pharmacological approaches are needed.

Importantly, the costs of therapies and their economic impact are increasingly becoming more relevant for National Health Services [28].

Due to the heterogeneity of triple-negative tumours and the complexity of the molecular pathways involved in their development and progression, it is postulated that the optimal therapeutic concept for TNBC will eventually comprise a combination approach of cytotoxic and targeted agents in an individual tailored pattern [4, 5, 27].

In this context, further positive results from in vivo studies could indicate that the integration between leptin and cAMP signalling pathways might provide the rationale for the development of a simple, innovative and cheap way for therapeutic intervention in triple negative breast cancer, and potentially in other tumors, implying the use of cAMP elevating drugs at lower and more tolerable doses.

REFERENCES

[1] American Cancer Society: Cancer Facts and Figures 2011. Atlanta, Ga: American Cancer Society, (2011)

[2] K Polyak: Heterogeneity in breast cancer. *J Clin Invest* 121(10), 3786-3788 (2011)

[3] Rakha EA, Chan S. Metastatic Triple-negative Breast Cancer. *Clinical Oncology*. 2011 587-600.

[4] Pal SK, Childs BH, Pegram M. Triple negative breast cancer: unmet medical needs. *Breast Cancer Res Treat*. 2011 125(3):627-636.

[5] Reddy KB. Triple-negative breast cancers: an updated review on treatment options. *Curr Oncol*. 2011 18(4):173-179.

[6] SM Domchek, G Mitchell, GJ Lindeman, NM Tung, J Balmaña, SJ Isakoff, R Schmutzler, MW Audeh, N Loman, C Scott, M Friedlander, B Kaufman, JE Garber, A Tutt, ME Robson: Challenges to the Development of New Agents for Molecularly Defined Patient Subsets: Lessons From BRCA1/2-Associated Breast Cancer. *J Clin Oncol*. 29(32), 4224-4226 (2011)

[7] Alvarez RH, Valero V, Hortobagyi GN. Emerging targeted therapies for breast cancer. *J Clin Oncol*. 2010 28(20):3366-3379.

[8] Ray A, Cleary MP. Obesity and breast cancer: a clinical biochemistry perspective. *Clin Biochem*. 2012 Feb;45(3):189-97.

[9] CM Perks, JM Holly: Hormonal mechanisms underlying the relationship between obesity and breast cancer. *Endocrinol Metab Clin North Am*. 40(3), 485-507 (2011)

[10] Davis AA, Kaklamani VG. Metabolic syndrome and triple-negative breast cancer: a new paradigm. *Int J Breast Cancer*. 2012; 2012:809291.

[11] Guo S, Liu M, Wang G, Torroella-Kouri M, Gonzalez-Perez RR. Oncogenic role and therapeutic target of leptin signaling in breast cancer and cancer stem cells. *Biochim Biophys Acta*. 2012 1825(2):207-22.

[12] García-Robles MJ, Segura-Ortega JE, Fafutis-Morris M. The Biology of Leptin and Its Implications in Breast Cancer: A General View. *J Interferon Cytokine Res*. 2013 Jul 19. [Epub ahead of print]

[13] Yin N, Wang D, Zhang H, Yi X, Sun X, Shi B, et al. Molecular mechanisms involved in the growth stimulation of breast cancer cells by leptin. *Cancer Res*. 2004 64(16):5870-5875.

[14] Ishikawa M, Kitayama J, Nagawa H. Enhanced expression of leptin and leptin receptor (OB-R) in human breast cancer. *Clin Cancer Res*. 2004 10(13):4325–4331.

[15] Jardé T, Caldefie-Chezet F, Damez M, et al. Leptin and leptin receptor involvement in cancer development: a study on human primary breast carcinoma. *Oncol Rep*. 2008 19(4):905–911.

[16] Revillion F, Charlier M, Lhotellier V, et al. Messenger RNA expression of leptin and leptin receptors and their prognostic value in 322 human primary breast cancers. *Clin Cancer Res*. 2006 12(7 Pt 1):2088–2094.

[17] Frankenberry KA, Skinner H, Somasundar P, McFadden DW, Vona-Davis LC. Leptin receptor expression and cell signaling in breast cancer. *Int J Oncol*. 2006 28(4):985-993.

[18] Ray A, Cleary MP. Leptin as a potential therapeutic target for breast cancer prevention and treatment. *Expert Opin Ther Targets*. 2010 14(4):443-451.

[19] Otvos L Jr, Surmacz E. Targeting the leptin receptor: a potential new mode of treatment for breast cancer. *Expert Rev Anticancer Ther*. 2011 11(8):1147-50.

[20] Schwede F, Maronde E, Genieser H, Jastorff B. Cyclic nucleotide analogs as biochemical tools and prospective drugs. *Pharmacol Ther*. 2000 87(2-3):199-226.

[21] Ligumsky H, Wolf I, Israeli S, Haimsohn M, Ferber S, Karasik A, Kaufman B, Rubinek T. The peptide-hormone glucagon-like peptide-1 activates cAMP and inhibits growth of breast cancer cells. *Breast Cancer Res Treat*. 2012 Apr;132(2):449-61.

[22] Vitale G, Dicitore A, Mari D, Cavagnini F. A new therapeutic strategy against cancer: cAMP elevating drugs and leptin. *Cancer Biol Ther*. 2009 8(12):1190-1196.

[23] Naviglio S, Di Gesto D, Romano M, Sorrentino A, Illiano F, Sorvillo L, Abbruzzese A, Marra M, Caraglia M, Chiosi E, Spina A, Illiano G. Leptin enhances growth inhibition by cAMP elevating agents through apoptosis of MDA-MB-231 breast cancer cells. *Cancer Biol Ther* 2009 8(12):1183-90.

[24] Naviglio S, Di Gesto D, Illiano F, Chiosi E, Giordano A, Illiano G, Spina A. Leptin potentiates antiproliferative action of cAMP elevation via protein kinase A down-regulation in breast cancer cells. *J Cell Physiol* 2010 225(3):801-9.

[25] Spina A, Di Maiolo F, Esposito A, Sapio L, Chiosi E, Sorvillo L, Naviglio S. cAMP Elevation Down-Regulates β3 Integrin and Focal Adhesion Kinase and Inhibits Leptin-Induced Migration of MDA-MB-231 Breast Cancer Cells. *Biores Open Access*. 2012 Dec;1(6):324-32.

[26] Spina A, Di Maiolo F, Esposito A, D'Auria R, Di Gesto D, Chiosi E, Sorvillo L, Naviglio S. Integrating leptin and cAMP signalling pathways in triple-negative breast cancer cells. *Front Biosci*. 2013 18:133-44.

[27] Mahamodhossen YA, Liu W, Rong-Rong Z. Triple-negative breast cancer: new perspectives for novel therapies. *Med Oncol*. 2013 30(3):653.

[28] Sullivan R, Peppercorn J, Sikora K, et al: Delivering affordable cancer care in high-income countries. *Lancet Oncol*.12, 933-80 (2011).

In: Leptin: Biosynthesis, Functions and Clinical Significance ISBN: 978-1-62948-801-1
Editor: Edward L. Blum

Chapter 5

LEPTIN: FROM ENERGY BALANCE TO INFLAMMATORY PROCESS IN OBESITY

Flávia Campos Corgosinho[1], Andrea Frontini[2], Antonio Giordano[2], Saverio Cinti[2] and Ana Raimunda Dâmaso[1]

[1]Universidade Federal de São Paulo,
Departamento de Pós-Graduação em Nutrição– UNIFESP, Brazil
[2]Università Politecnica delle Marche,
Department of Experimental and Clinical Medicine, UNIVPM, Italy

ABSTRACT

Obesity is a public health problem worldwide, resulting from a positive energy balance. Body weight is regulated by a complex circuitry involving central and peripheral factors, mainly by adipose organ-brain crosstalk. Leptin is a 16-kDa polypeptide that is primarily produced by adipose tissue, thus, circulation levels are in proportion of body mass, serving as a key adiposity signal. Leptin plays an important role in energy balance, acting as a major signaling in anorexigenic pathway. In human obesity, central and peripheral leptin resistance are proposed in association with state of hyperleptinemia. Studies suggest that an extended period of exposure to high levels of leptin, especially in the hypothalamus, may result in the development of central leptin resistance. Hyperleptinemia is also associated with the chronic subclinical inflammatory state, being involved in the development of many other diseases such as insulin resistance, cardiovascular disease and metabolic syndrome. Furthermore, recent studies have suggested the importance of this adipokine in weight loss process. This review focuses on the structure, role and effects of Leptin on obesity, metabolic syndrome development, and weight loss process.

Keywords: Leptin, Leptin receptors, Hyperleptinemia, Energy balance, Inflamation, Obesity

INTRODUCTION

Leptin is a key component of the physiological systems that regulate food intake. This adipokine coordinates central and peripheral signals, acting as a negative feedback loop in which its anti-obesity actions tend to counteract any increase in fat mass in order to maintain a constant body weight. [1,2] In normal weight individuals, leptin circulates at levels proportional to body fat, showing its ability to respond to weight gain and energy status. Leptin also enters the Central Nervous System (CNS) in proportion to its plasma concentration. [3]

Nevertheless, our group recently demonstrated that hyperleptinemia state (HL) is a commonly altered metabolic condition in obese individuals, both adolescents and adults, which may impair the control of energy balance. This condition hampers weight loss process and seems to be reversed only after big losses of weight. [4-7]

Leptin plays an important role in the chronic proinflammatory state that is observed in obesity, metabolic syndrome, and their complications, such as atherosclerosis. [8] It regulates the production of pro-inflammatory cytokines such as tumor necrosis factor alpha (TNF-α), interleukin1 (IL-1), and interleukin (IL-6). These cytokines in turn regulate the expression of leptin, which sustains a chronic pro-inflammatory state. [1,9]

Interestingly, recently it has been shown a strong negative correlation between the hiperleptinemia state with an anti-inflammatory biomarker adiponectin/leptin ratio and the positive correlation with a pro-inflammatory risk leptin/adiponectin ratio. [7] Together, these results reinforce the role of this adipokine as a powerful biomarker of inflammation in obese adults, according to obesity degree. Therefore, in the present review, we outline the role of leptin in: i) the control of energy homeostasis and ii) pro-inflammatory processes related to obesity.

LEPTIN AND MOLECULAR STRUCTURE

Well known as a potent food intake regulator, this 16-kDa adipocyte-derived hormone orchestrates complex biological effects through both central and peripheral receptors. Leptin is an elongated molecule and consists of four antiparallel a-helices, connected by two long crossover links and one short loop, arranged in a left-hand twisted helical bundle. The structure of leptin reveals numerous exposed hydrophobic residues, which appear to serve an important role in receptor binding. Indeed, the surface hydrophobicity increases the tendency for self-association and aggregation of the molecule. [10,11]

Leptin receptors are expressed in the central nervous system, as well as in peripheral tissues, including the hematopoietic and immune systems. [12-16] Structurally, the leptin receptors belong to the class I cytokine receptor family, containing a so-called Cytokine Receptor Homology (CRH) domain in its extracellular sphere. [17] These structural characteristics of leptin and its receptor help characterize the combined activities of leptin, which includes those of an endocrine hormone and an immune-mediating cytokine. [11]

Up to the present time, six isoforms of leptin receptor (LEPR) were identified from "a" to "f", mainly because of gene alternate splicing. [18,19] Interestingly, LEPR have high similarity with receptors for interleukin-6 (IL-6), leukemia inhibitory factor (LIF), granulocyte-colony stimulating factor (GCSF) and oncostatin. [17] The isoforms have a similar extracellular ligand-binding domain at the amino terminus, but they diverge at the intracellular carboxy-terminal domain. [20]The longest form (LEPRb) has intracellular designs necessary for activation of the JAK-STAT signaling pathways, being capable of full signal transduction and appearing to account for almost all leptin action. Although LEPRb is mainly expressed in the hypothalamus, among important central areas of energy balance regulation, it can also activate signal transduction in a diversity of peripheral tissues, including adipose tissue, T cells, endothelial cells, and pancreatic β-cells, suggesting a wide spectrum of peripheral functions. [11,13,21-23]

Even whether the LEPRb isoform possesses clear signaling capability, the short receptor isoforms may nevertheless be necessary for leptin to exert its full spectrum in vivo functions. High expression levels of the short forms (LEPRa and LEPRc) can be found in choroid plexus and brain microvessels, suggesting that they may serve as leptin binding proteins and play a role in leptin transport across the blood–brain and blood-cerebrospinal fluid barriers. [11,16,20,24,25] Researches have proposed that a secreted isoform (LEPRe) may be an important factor regulating leptin's bioavailability, modulating leptin activity on central and peripheral targets. [23,26] Figure 1 illustrates leptin receptors and their supposed functions, however more studies are needed to better understand their specific role in leptin network.

The Role of Leptin in the Neuroendocrine Regulation of Energy Balance

Energy balance is the result of coordinated metabolic process between energy intake and expenditure. [27,28] Evidences suggest that leptin strongly acts as a key hormone in the regulation of energy balance. In addition, leptin is the primary adipose hormone that conveys an adiposity signal to the brain. Particularly in the hypothalamus, leptin integrates to various other metabolic signals, such as NPY, pro-opiomelanocortin (POMC), Cocaine and amphetamine regulated transcript (CART), α-melanocyte-stimulating hormone (α-MSH) and Melanin-concentrating hormone (MCH) to regulate energy homeostasis and body weight by controlling both behavior and metabolic responses. [21] Leptin decreases body weight both by suppressing appetite and by increasing energy expenditure,[29] as shown in Figure 2.

The neural circuitries that integrate leptin and other metabolic signals to control energy homeostasis and body weight remain largely undefined and are extremely complex. However, the literature has indicated that leptin acts on multiple key sites in the neural circuits involved in the control of energy intake and expenditure. [30,31]

Leptin acts through a complex cascade of reactions by binding to the longest isoform receptor LEPRb and activating Janus-family tyrosine kinase 2 (JAK2) via auto- or cross-phosphorylation. JAK2 then phosphorylates tyrosine residues (Tyr985, Tyr1077, Tyr1138), which will act as sites for the binding of intracellular signaling molecules. JAK2 also generates a substrate called Signal Transducer and Activator of Transcription 3 (STAT-3) that subsequently binds to the phosphorylated Tyr1138. STAT-3 then acts as a promoter for gene transcription of the SOCS family into the cell nucleus. SOCS1 and SOCS3 suppress the leptin action by binding to tyrosine residues and JACK2, stopping signalling (Figure 3). [32,33,34].

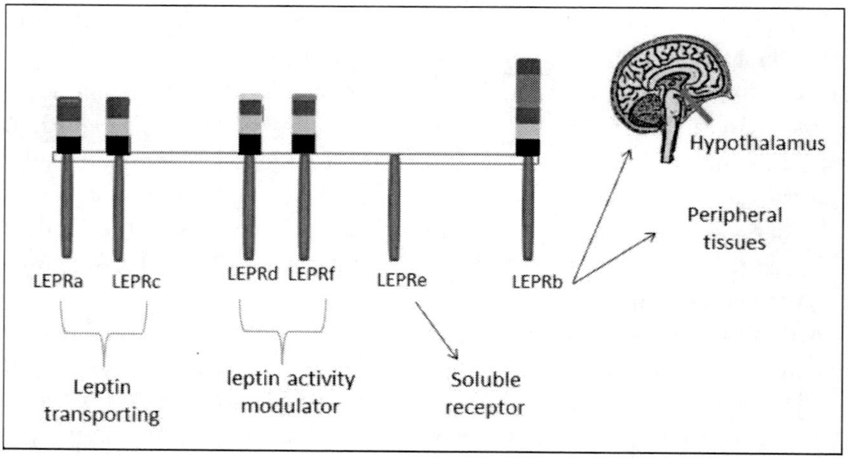

Figure 1. Leptin isoform receptors and their respectively functions.

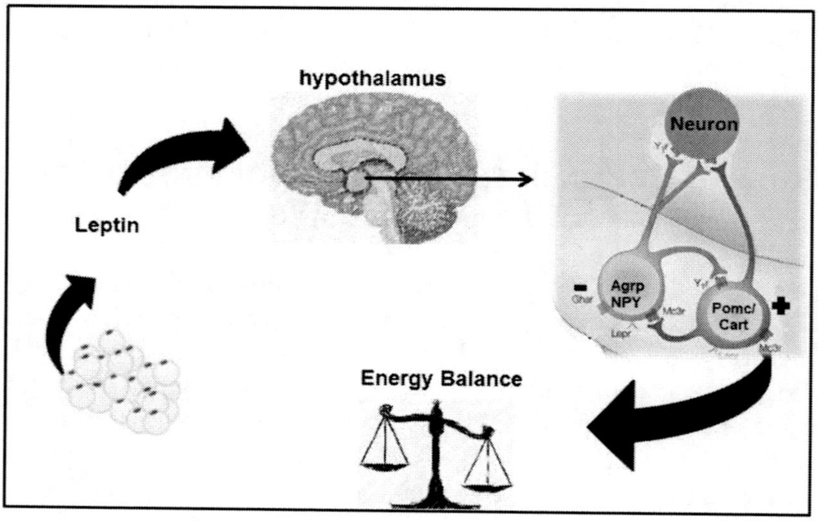

Figure 2. Leptin is secreted by adipose tissue , acting as a marker of adiposity. In the hypothalamus leptin inhibits orexigenic (AgRP/NPY) and stimulate anorexigenic pathways (POMC/CART), hence controlling energy balance. Adapted from Morris & Rui, 2009.

At hypothalamic level, leptin stimulates POMC and CART neurons, and consequently the expression of α-MSH, anorexigenic citokines; simultaneously it inhibits the expression of neuropeptide Y/agouti-related protein (NPY/AgRP). In the other hand, leptin inhibits MCH, an orexigenic marker, reducing hyperphagia, body weight and adiposity. [35,36]

In addition, leptin inhibits GABA release from AgRP neurons, which contributes to increased energy expenditure and decreased adiposity. Therefore, these distinct leptin-responsive neurons may act redundantly, in parallel, and/or synergistically to fully mediate the physiological responses to leptin. [29]

Finally, leptin acts directly on multiple peripheral tissues, including adipose tissue, skeletal muscle, pancreatic islets, and liver. In the adipose tissue, leptin stimulates lipolysis and inhibits lipogenesis; in skeletal muscle it acts improving insulin sensitivity; while it suppresses insulin secretion from pancreatic islets and inhibits stearoyl CoA desaturase in liver. [37,38] Therefore, under normal conditions, leptin controls energy balance, body weight, and systemic metabolism primarily by activating LEPRb in the brain.

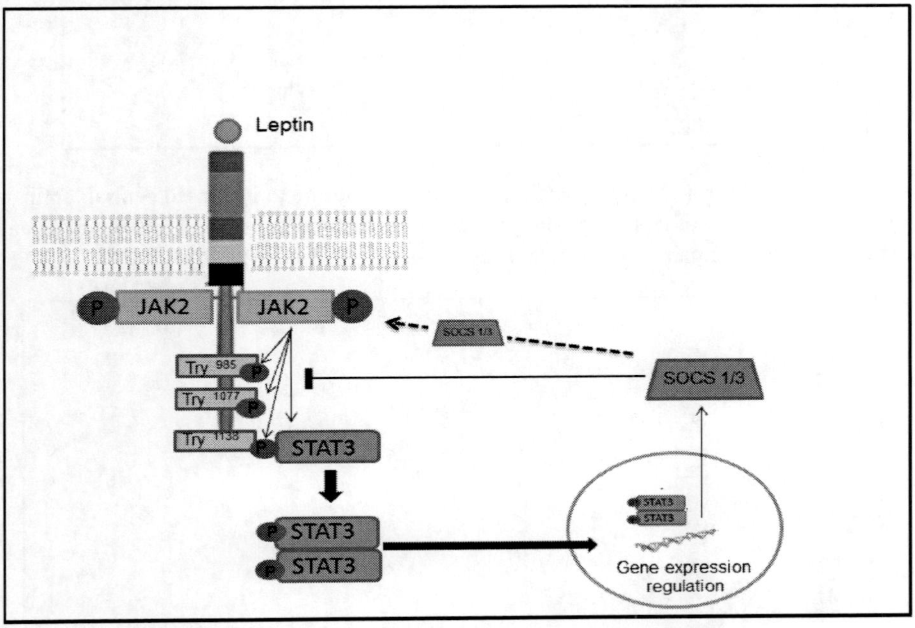

Figure 3. Leptin acts binding to LEPRb and activating Janus-family tyrosine kinase 2 (JAK2) via phosphorylation. JAK2 then phosphorylates tyrosine residues, which will act as sites for the binding of intracellular signaling molecules. A JAK2 substrate called Signal Transducer and Activator of Transcription 3 (STAT-3) binds to the phosphorylated Tyr1138, then acts as a promoter for gene transcription of the SOCS family , that suppress leptin action. JAK2= Janus-family tyrosine kinase 2; P= phosphorylation; Try= tyrosine residues. Adapted from Paz-Filho et al.,2012.

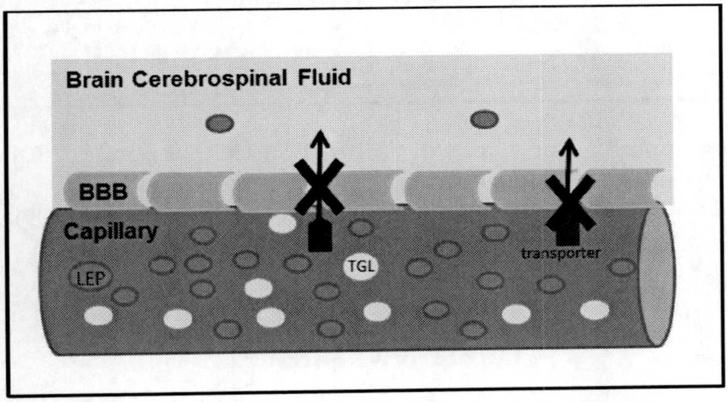

Figure 4-a. Defects in leptin trasporting through blood–brain barriers, which could be due an high concentration of TGL from high fat diet, promoting an interaction with the transporter, altering its affinity with leptin or interaction with leptin altering its affinity with the transporter (Banks, 2008). LEP= leptin; BBB= blood-brain barriers; TGL = tryglicerides.

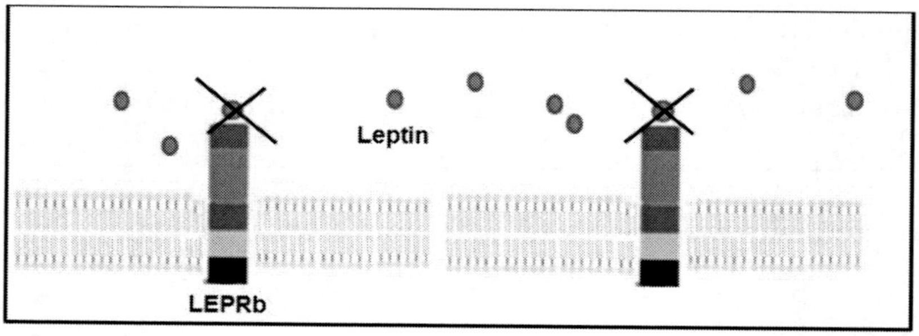

Figure 4-b. Diminished neuronal leptin signaling. Extended exposure to increased central leptin steadily triggers a sub-maximal level of leptin signaling while concurrently desensitizing maximum signaling capacity, which may lead impaired leptin responses (Zhang & Scarpace, 2006).

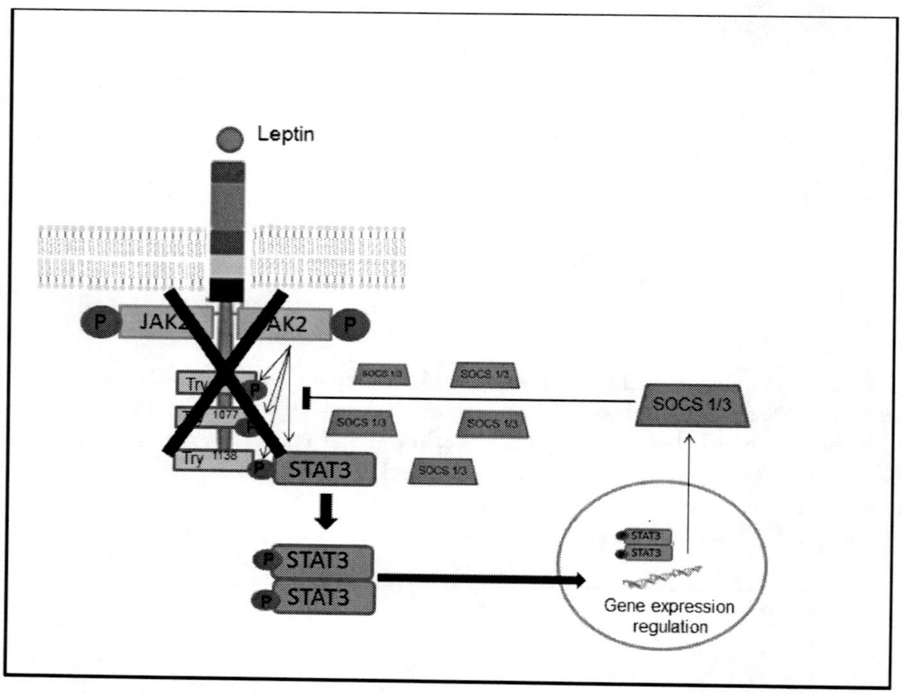

Figure 4-c. Increased expressions of proteins are believed to block leptin signaling. SOCS-3 binds to JAK2 in a leptin-dependent manner, proposing that SOCS-3 weakens leptin receptor signaling, thus increased levels of SOCS-3 might play a part in leptin resistance (Bjørbæk et al., 2009). JAK2= Janus-family tyrosine kinase 2; P= phosphorylation; Try= tyrosine residues.

Leptin in Obesity

Obesity is a chronic disease world-wide, affecting all ages and both genders. An imbalance in energy equilibrium, caused by both sedentary and wrong eating behaviours, leads to a massive increase in adipose tissue. Adipose tissue is the main determinant of leptin gene expression and release. [39,40] Alteration in plasma leptin levels and/or leptin signaling has a profound pathological influence on body weight control. The most common cause of obesity is not genetic defects of leptin, or its receptors, but rather depends on overeating or high fat diet consumption, which may rapidly increase plasma leptin levels and impairs its function. [41]

Although leptin is considered to be involved in neuroendocrine control of energy balance, in human obesity, states of leptin resistance are observed. Furthermore, studies suggest that extended period of exposure of the brain, especially the hypothalamus, to a high level of leptin may result in the development of central leptin resistance. [42,43] In a previous work, we demonstrated that 66% of obese adolescents presented (HL). The study showed that even after weight loss, some of these obese adolescents remained in a hyperleptinemic state. [4]

The central resistance of leptin can be explained by some mechanisms, including 1) defects in leptin transport across the blood–brain barrier, 2) diminished neuronal leptin signaling in target neurons or changes in signaling in downstream target cells and neuro-circuits, 3) increased expression of proteins that block leptin signaling such as the suppressor of cytokine signaling (SOCS)-3 (Figure 4c). [44,45,46,47] The proposed mechanisms are presented in Figure 4.

Defects in Leptin Transport

Although the molecular mechanism behind apparent defect in leptin transport to the hypothalamus is not clearly understood, it is thought to be one of the many defects in obesity. The evidence in support of this theory has come from different but joining findings: (a) the leptin plasma ratio of the cerebrospinal fluid is lower in obese individuals compared to lean controls[45,48]; (b) central injection of leptin is effective in decreasing food intake and body weight in hyperleptinemic diet-induced obese mice (DIO mice), while peripheral leptin administration to does not have any effect on food consumption or body weight of these mice [49]; (c) even though peripheral injection of leptin to DIO mice does not stimulate STAT3 in the hypothalamus, intracerebroventricular administration induces STAT3 activation, however the extent of this induction is 75% lower than that in mice fed the low-fat diet [50]; (d) leptin transport through blood–brain barriers is diminished in numerous models of obesity including the DIO. [51,52]

Further studies are necessary to determine whether a decrease in brain uptake of leptin is the cause or consequence of obesity. Banks and collegues (2006) have hypothesized, that high levels of triglycerides (TGL) may impair leptin transport, since TGL are regulators of the rate at which leptin is transported, being inversely related. During fasting adipose tissue is mobilized and TGL levels are increased, which acts as a starvation signaling to the body. Thus, hypertriglyceridemia caused by high fat diet may be mistaken as a starvation signal by the BBB inducing leptin resistance. [53] The possible two mechanisms suggested are: interaction with the transporter, altering its affinity with leptin or interaction with leptin altering its affinity with the transporter. [54]

Diminished Neuronal Leptin Signaling in Target Neurons

Studies have suggested that obesity due to high fat diet induces central leptin resistance. [42] Widdowson et al. first demonstrated this hypothesis using Wistar rats. [43] They showed that while leptin injection into the lateral cerebroventricle resulted in a dose dependent reduction in food consumption in the animals that were in standard laboratory diet, the anorectic effect of leptin was diminished in the diet-induced obese rats. [55] Interestingly, it was discovered that mice fed on high fat developed leptin resistance only in the arcuate nucleus whereas other hypothalamic regions remain leptin sensitive. [46] It could be mechanistically that high plasma leptin levels associated with obesity may result in a decrease in the number or affinity of the CNS leptin receptors. [56] Furthermore, it is possible, that the extended exposure to increased central leptin steadily triggers a sub-maximal level of leptin signaling while concurrently desensitizing maximum signaling capacity, which may lead impaired leptin responses. [32]

Blockers of Leptin Signaling

Increased expression of proteins, such as protein–tyrosine phosphatase 1B (PTP-1B) and suppressor of cytokine signaling (SOCS)-3 are believed to block leptin signaling. Hyperleptinemia itself may cause leptin resistance by increasing SOCS-3 and PTP-1B expression. [43] Studies in vitro have demonstrated that SOCS-3 protein expression is induced by leptin and that SOCS-3 is a negative regulator of proximal leptin signaling. Furthermore, the data show that SOCS-3 binds to JAK2 in a leptin-dependent manner and propose that SOCS-3 weakens leptin receptor signaling by inhibiting JAK-induced tyrosine phosphorylation of the receptor and of JAK itself, however the mechanisms still not clear and requires further studies. Thus, increased levels of SOCS-3 in central or peripheral leptin-responsive cells might play a part in leptin resistance. [47]

Another study suggests that leptin induces the expression of PTP-1B in SH-SY5Y cells in mouse hypothalamic arcuate nucleus. Furthermore, they showed that overexpression of PTP-1B cDNA in human neuronal cells dramatically affects leptin and insulin. [57] This phosphatase acts by dephosphorylating JAK2 and, thus, it inhibits JAK2-induced phosphorylation of the leptin receptor. [58] In addition, Bence et al. (2006) showed that neuronal deletion of PTP-1B increased leptin and insulin sensitivity, preventing body weight gain in a diet-induced obesity animal model. [59]

Leptin as an Inflammatory Adipokine

Leptin plays role also in the immune system, including inflammation, mainly due to structural similarities with pro-inflammatory citokines. [60] Obesity is considered a chronic sub-inflammatory disease, in which leptin plays an important role in the pro-inflammatory state, by acting on LEPRb, which is expressed by different immune cells, thus activating inflammatory reactions. Leptin modulates the production of cytokines derived from T-cells and increases expression of the activation markers CD25 and CD71 in CD4+ and CD8+ cells. In addition, in monocytes it acts increasing the expression of activation markers and up regulates phagocytosis and cytokine production. Furthermore, in endothelial cells leptin up regulates the expression of adhesion molecules and induces oxidative stress. [61,62]

Concurrently, some inflammatory markers such as IL-1, LPS and TNF-α can increase leptin levels, correlating with inflammation level. Thus, the interfaces between leptin and inflammation are bidirectional: perpetuating the loop of chronic inflammation in obesity. [9,34] The mechanism of leptin- resistance and development of inflammation remains unclear, but it has been reported an imbalance between pro- and anti-inflammatory cytokines, reinforcing the hypothesis that leptin is able to modify the pattern of monocytes/macrophages cytokine secretion through a STAT-3 activated pathway. [63,64]

Moreover, it has been demonstrated that leptin administration, in non-obese diabetic mice, increases both inflammatory infiltrates and IFN-gamma production in peripheral T cells, which speeds-up the destruction of pancreatic beta-cells, anticipating the onset of the disease[34]. Indeed, a recent study from our group suggests that a hyperleptinemic state impairs the attenuation of inflammation and thus leads to a decrease in vascular protection in obese adolescents. The results showed that the influence of interdisciplinary weight loss therapy on the inflammatory response and vascular protection was negatively influenced by HL, mediated by low concentrations of adiponectin. [8]

Moraes et al. (2013) investigated the role of leptinemia, adjusted by tertiles, on inflammatory state in obese adults according to obesity degree. They showed a negative correlation between leptin concentration with adiponectin/leptin ratio (anti-inflammatory marker), and a positive correlation with leptin/adiponectin ratio (pro-inflammatory marker). Indeed, they demonstrated that both ratios were decreased and increased, respectively, according to the obesity degree, reinforcing the role of leptinemia state as a mediator of inflammation in obese adults. [7]

LEPTIN IN METABOLIC SYNDROME

Leptin is a crucial factor for metabolic syndrome, which is characterized by a constellation of risk factors that together are predictors of cardiovascular disease and type 2 diabetes mellitus. [65,66] In fact, studies have implicated leptin as an independent risk factor for cardiovascular disease, suggesting that leptin may be an important link in the development of cardiovascular risk with obesity. [67,68,69]

Esteghamati et al. (2011) studied 3,045 adults, obese and non-obese, and showed that subjects with MetS had significantly higher leptin concentrations, and the significance persisted after adjustment for body mass index. Moreover, though not all components of MetS are independently associated with leptin, its concentrations increased steadily with an increment in the number of MetS components. In addition, after separating subjects into obese and non-obese, leptin concentrations were again significantly higher in subjects with MetS in both groups. [70] In agreement with these results, another study demonstrated, in a sample of the adult Korean population, that leptin was a significant predictor of MetS, independent of BMI.

Recently, Sanches et al. (2013) showed that the HL state in obese human may promote atherosclerosis, since was found correlation between an increased Carotid Intima Media Thickness (cIMT) in these patients compared to a non-hyperleptinemic (NHL) obese group. Also, the hyperleptinemic obese group had higher pro-inflammatory leptin/adiponectin ratio when compared with an obese non-hyperleptinemic group. Moreover, In the NHL group, leptin concentrations were positively correlated with adiponectin and inversely correlated with PAI-1. Together our findings reinforce that a hyperleptinemic state impairs the attenuation of inflammation in obese adolescents undergoing interdisciplinary weight loss therapy, particularly by impeding the increase in adiponectin concentration, which is directly involved in vascular protection in atherosclerosis and other chronic diseases, including metabolic syndrome. [8]

Leptin in the Weight Loss Process

As mentioned above, leptin acts in both CNS and in the peripheral tissues, promoting a reduction in the energy intake and increasing energy expenditure. Unfortunately, in obesity the HL may impair weight loss therapy. In fact, it was showed that NPY, a potent orexigenic neuropeptide down regulated by leptin was increased in the first step of weight loss; however it was returned to basal levels in the subsequent phase of weight loss intervention (after 12 months of therapy). [5] Moreover, it was showed that leptin responses occur as dependent manner to the magnitude effects of weight loss, being recently demonstrated that only after a massive weight loss (> 15.90 kg) this hormone return to reference values in obese adolescents. In addition, the increase in the adiponectin was observed concomitantly and changes in Adiponectin/Leptin ratio were independent predictors of cIMT alterations. [6] Thus, the findings suggest that only after a substantially reduction in the body mass (i.e 10%) the leptin restart its anorexigenic effects, by counteracting the rebound of NPY and decreased α-MSH levels. On the same line, another study demonstrated that a-MSH levels increased as a response to aerobic exercise after one year in association to nutritional counseling. [71]

Additionally, both leptin and exercise may activate UCP1, increasing synergic thermogenesis effects in the brown adipose tissue, promoting a negative energy balance and subsequent weight loss. Uncoupling Protein 1 (UCP1), a key molecule for brown adipose tissue (BAT) thermogenesis, was reported to contribute to the stimulatory effect of leptin on energy expenditure. These results indicate that UCP1 enhances leptin action at hypothalamic level, suggesting UCP1 contributes to the control of energy balance not only through the regulation of energy expenditure but also through appetite control by modulating leptin action. [72,73]

Finally, our group showed that aerobic plus resistance training was more effective than aerobic exercise alone to control HL and to increase adiponectin concentration after one year of interdisciplinary therapy in obese, including clinical, psychological and nutritional counselling. [74]

Conclusion and Future Directions

Leptin regulates sympathetic, metabolic and cardiovascular function under physiological and pathophysiological conditions. Hyperleptinemia is associated with the chronic subclinical inflammatory state, being involved in the development of many other diseases such as insulin resistance, cardiovascular disease and metabolic syndrome. Studies have suggested the importance of this adipokine in weight loss process and that HL can be reversible after substantial weight loss. Leptin is a key role for obesity and should be considered in the clinical practices. However more studies must be done to better understand the mechanisms involved in leptin resistance and its connections with chronic inflammation and obesity related diseases.

REFERENCES

[1] Spiegelman, B. M. & Flier, J. S. (1996). Adipogenesis and obesity: rounding out the big picture. *Cell.*, *87*(3), 377-89

[2] Ahima, R. S. & Flier, J. S. (2000). Adipose tissue as an endocrine organ. *Trends Endocrinol Metab.*, *11*, 327 – 332.

[3] Harrold, J. A., Dovey, T. M., Blundell, J. E. & Halford, J. C. (2012). CNS regulation of appetite. *Neuropharmacology.*, *63*(1), 3-17.

[4] Dâmaso, A. R., de Piano, A., Sanches, P. L., Corgosinho, F., Tock, L., Oyama, L. M., Tock, L., do Nascimento, C. M., Tufik, S. & de Mello, M. T. (2011). Hyperleptinemia in obese adolescents deregulates neuropeptides during weight loss. *Peptides.*, *32*(7), 1384-91.

[5] Oyama, L. M., do Nascimento, C. M., Carnier, J., de Piano, A., Tock, L., Sanches, Pde L., Gomes, F. A., Tufik, S., de Mello, M. T., Dâmaso, AR. (2010). The role of anorexigenic and orexigenic neuropeptides and peripheral signals on quartiles of weight loss in obese adolescents. *Neuropeptides*. 44(6), 467-74.

[6] Masquio, DC., de Piano, A., Sanches, P. L., Corgosinho, F. C., Campos, R. M., Carnier, J., da Silva, P. L., Caranti, D. A., Tock, L., Oyama, L. M., Oller, do Nascimento, C. M., de Mello, M. T., Tufik, S. & Dâmaso, A. R. (2013). The effect of weight loss magnitude on pro-/anti-inflammatory adipokines and carotid intima-media thickness in obese adolescents engaged in interdisciplinary weight loss therapy. *Clin Endocrinol. 79*(1), 55-64.

[7] Moraes, Ados S., Pisani, L. P., Corgosinho, F. C., Carvalho, L. O., Masquio, D. C., Jamar, G., Sanches, R. B., Oyama, L. M., Dâmaso, A. R., Belote, C. & Caranti, D. A. (2013). The role of leptinemia state as a mediator of inflammation in obese adults. *Horm Metab Res.*, *45*(8), 605-10

[8] Sanches, P. L., de Mello, M. T., Elias, N., Fonseca, F. A., Campos, R. M., Carnier, J., de Piano, A., Masquio, D. C., Silva, P. L., Oyama, L. M., Corgosinho, F. C., Nascimento, C. M., Tock, L., D'Elia, C. A., Tufik, S. & Dâmaso, AR. (2013). Hyperleptinemia: Implications on the Inflammatory State and Vascular Protection in Obese Adolescents Submitted to an Interdisciplinary Therapy. *Inflammation*. 2013

[9] Maury, E. & Brichard, S. M. (2010). Adipokine dysregulation, adipose tissue inflammation and metabolic syndrome. *Mol Cell Endocrinol.*, *314*, 1-16.

[10] Zhang, F., Basinski, M. B., Beals, J. M., Briggs, S. L., Churgay, L. M., Clawson, D. K., DiMarchi, R. D., Furman, T. C., Hale, J. E., Hsiung, H. M., Schoner, B. E., Smith, D. P., Zhang, X. Y, Wery, J. P. & Schevitz, R. W. (1997). Crystal structure of the obese protein leptin-E100. *Nature.*, *387*(6629), 206–209.

[11] Zhang, F., Chen, Y., Heiman, M. & DiMarchi, R. (2005). Leptin: Structure, Function and Biology. *Vitamins and Hormones.*, *71*, 345-72.

[12] Covey, S. D., Wideman, R. D., McDonald, C., Unniappan, S., Huynh, F., Asadi, A., Speck, M., Webber, T., Chua, S. C. & Kieffer, T. J. (2006). The pancreatic beta cell is a key site for mediating the effects of leptin on glucose homeostasis. *Cell Metab.*, *4*, 291–302.

[13] Lord, G. M., Matarese, G., Howard, J. K., Baker, R. J., Bloom, S. R. & Lechler, R. I. (1998). Leptin modulates the T-cell immune response and reverses starvation-induced immunosuppression. *Nature.*, *394*(6696), 897-901.

[14] Cohen, P., Zhao, C., Cai, X., Montez, J. M., Rohani, S. C., Feinstein, P., Mombaerts, P. & Friedman, J. M. (2001). Selective deletion of leptin receptor in neurons leads to obesity. *J Clin Invest.*, *108*, 1113–21.

[15] Morioka, T., Asilmaz, E., Hu, J., Dishinger, J. F., Kurpad, A. J., Elias, C. F., Li, H., Elmquist, J. K., Kennedy, R. T. & Kulkarni, R. N. (2007). Disruption of leptin receptor expression in the pancreas directly affects beta cell growth and function in mice. *J Clin Invest.*, *117*, 2860–68.

[16] De Matteis, R., Lucertini, F., Guescini, M., Polidori, E., Zeppa, S., Stocchi, V., Cinti, S. & Cuppini, R. (2013). Exercise as a new physiological stimulus for brown adipose tissue activity. *Nutr Metab Cardiovasc Dis.*, *23*(6), 582-90.

[17] Zabeau, L., Lavens, D., Peelman, F., Eyckerman, S., Vandekerckhove, J. & Tavernier, J. (2003). The ins and outs of leptin receptor activation. *FEBS Lett.*, *546*(1), 45-50.

[18] Ahima, R. S. & Osei, S. Y. (2004). Leptin signaling. *Physiol Behav.*, *81*(2), 223-41.

[19] Lee, G. H., Proenca, R., Montez, J. M., Carroll, K. M., Darvishzadeh, J. G., Lee, J. I., & Friedman, J. M. (1996). Abnormal splicing of the leptin receptor in diabetic mice. *Nature*, *379*, 632–635.

[20] Tartaglia, L. A. (1997). The leptin receptor. *J Biol Chem.*, *272*, 6093–96.

[21] Elmquist, J. K., Maratos-Flier, E., Saper, C. B. & Flier, J. S. (1998). Unraveling the central nervous system pathways underlying responses to leptin. *Nat Neurosci.*, *1*(6), 445-50.

[22] Kim, Y. B., Uotani, S., Pierroz, D. D., Flier, J. S. & Kahn, B. B. (2000). In vivo administration of leptin activates signal transduction directly in insulin-sensitive tissues: overlapping but distinct pathways from insulin. *Endocrinology.*, *141*(7), 2328-39.

[23] Ge, H., Huang, L., Pourbahrami, T. & Li, C. (2002). Generation of soluble leptin receptor by ectodomain shedding of membrane-spanning receptors in vitro and in vivo. *J Biol Chem.*, *277*(48), 45898-903.

[24] Tartaglia, L. A., Dembski, M., Weng, X., Deng, N., Culpepper, J., Devos, R., Richards, G. J., Campfield, L. A., Clark, F. T., Deeds, J., Muir, C., Sanker, S., Moriarty, A., Moore, K. J., Smutko, J. S., Mays, G. G., Wool, E. A., Monroe, C. A. & Tepper, R. I. (1995). Identification and expression cloning of a leptin receptor, OB-R. *Cell*, *83*, 1263-1271.

[25] De Matteis, R. & Cinti, S. (1998). Ultrastructural immunolocalization of leptin receptor in mouse brain. *Neuroendocrinology.*, *68*(6), 412-9.

[26] Lammert, A., Kiess, W., Bottner, A., Glasow, A. & Kratzsch, J. (2001). Soluble leptin receptor represents the main leptin binding activity in human blood. *Biochem Biophys Res Commun.*, *283*(4), 982-8.

[27] Pénicaud, L., Meillon, S. & Brondel, L. (2012). Leptin and the central control of feeding behavior. *Biochimie.*, *94*(10), 2069-74.

[28] Guyenet, S. J. & Schwartz, M. W. (2012). Clinical review: Regulation of food intake, energy balance, and body fat mass: implications for the pathogenesis and treatment of obesity. *J Clin Endocrinol Metab.*, *97*(3), 745-55.
[29] Morris, D. L. & Rui, L. (2009). Recent advances in understanding leptin signaling and leptin resistance. *Am J Physiol Endocrinol Metab.*, *297*(6), E1247-59.
[30] Dubern, B. & Clement, K. (2012). Leptin and leptin receptor-related monogenic obesity. *Biochimie*. *94*(10), 2111-5.
[31] Villanueva, E. C. & Myers, M. G Jr.. (2008). Leptin receptor signaling and the regulation of mammalian physiology. *Int J Obes.*, *32*(7), S8–12
[32] Zhang, Yi. & Scarpace, P. J. (2006). Circumventing central leptin resistance: Lessons from central leptin and POMC gene delivery. *Peptides*. 27350 – 364.
[33] Munzberg, H. (2010). Leptin-signaling pathways and leptin resistance. *Forum Nutr*. *63*, 123-32.
[34] Paz-Filho, G., Mastronardi, C., Franco, C. B., Wang, K. B., Wong, M. L. & Licinio, J. (2012). Leptin: molecular mechanisms, systemic pro-inflammatory effects, and clinical implications. *Arq Bras Endocrinol Metabol.*, *56*(9), 597-607.
[35] Boguszewski, C. L., Paz-Filho, G. & Velloso, L. A. (2010). Neuroendocrine body weight regulation. Integration between fat tissue, gastrointestinal tract, and the brain. *Endokrynologia Polska.*, *61*(2), 194–206.
[36] Diéguez, C., Vazquez, M. J., Romero, A., López, M. & Nogueiras, R. (2011). Hypothalamic control of lipid metabolism: focus on leptin, ghrelin and melanocortins. *Neuroendocrinology.*, *94*(1), 1–11.
[37] Sáinz, N., Rodríguez, A., Catalán, V., Becerril, S., Ramírez, B., Lancha, A., Burgos-Ramos, E., Gómez-Ambrosi, J. & Frühbeck, G. (2012). Leptin Reduces the Expression and Increases the Phosphorylation of the Negative Regulators of GLUT4 Traffic TBC1D1 and TBC1D4 in Muscle of ob/ob Mice. *PLoS One.*, *7*(1), e29389.
[38] Anubhuti, & Arora, S. (2008). Leptin and its metabolic interactions – an update. *Diabetes Obes Metab.,10*, 973–93.
[39] Trayhurn, P., Duncan, J. S., Hoggard, N. & Rayner, D. V. (1998). Regulation of leptin production: a dominant role for the sympathetic nervous system? *Proc Nutr Soc.*, *57*, 413–419.
[40] Blüher, S. & Mantzoros, C. S. (2009). Leptin in humans: lessons from translational research. *Am J Clin Nutr.*, *89*(3), 991S-997S.
[41] Ren, J. (2004). Leptin and hyperleptinemia – from friend to foe for cardiovascular function. *J Endocrinol.*, *181*, 1–10.
[42] Sahu, A. (2004). Leptin signaling in the hypothalamus: emphasis on energy homeostasis and leptin resistance. *Front Neuroendocrinol.*, *24*(4), 225-53.
[43] Leal, V. O. & Mafra, D. (2013). Adipokines in obesity. *Clinica Chimica Acta.*, *419*, 87–94.
[44] Coppari, R. & Bjorbaek, C. (2012). Leptin revisited: its mechanisms of action and potential for treating diabetes. *Nat Rev Drug Discov.*, *11*, 692–708.
[45] Caro, J. F., Kolaczynski, J. W., Nyce, M. R., Ohannesian, J. P., Opentanova, I., Goldman, W. H., Lynn, R. B., Zhang, P. L., Sinha, M. K. & Considine, R. V. (1996). Decreased cerebrospinal-fluid/serum leptin ratio in obesity: a possible mechanism for leptin resistance. *Lancet*, *348*, 159–61.

[46] Munzberg, H., Flier, J. S. & Bjorbaek, C. (2004). Region-specific leptin resistance within the hypothalamus of diet-induced obese mice. *Endocrinology.*, *145*, 4880–9.

[47] Bjorbaek, C., El-Haschimi, K., Frantz, J. D. & Flier, J. S. (1999). The role of SOCS-3 in leptin signaling and leptin resistance. *J Biol Chem.*, *274*, 30059–65.

[48] Schwartz, M. W., Peskind, E., Raskind, M., Boyko, E. J. & Porte, D. Jr. (1996). Cerebrospinal fluid leptin levels: relationship to plasma levels and to adiposity in humans. *Nat. Med.*, 2, 589–93.

[49] Van Heek, M., Compton, D. S., France, C. F., Tedesco, R. P., Fawzi, A. B., Graziano, M. P., Sybertz, E. J., Strader, C. D. & Davis, HR, Jr. (1997). Diet-induced obese mice develop peripheral, but not central, resistance to leptin, *J. Clin. Invest.*, *99*, 385–390.

[50] El-Haschimi, K., Pierroz, D. D., Hileman, S. M., Bjørbaek, C. & Flier, J. S. (2000). Two defects contribute to hypothalamic leptin resistance in mice with diet-induced obesity. *J. Clin. Invest.*, *105*, 1827–32.

[51] Banks, W. A. (2001). Leptin transport across the blood–brain barrier: implications for the cause and treatment of obesity. *Curr. Pharm. Des.*, *7*, 125–33.

[52] Burguera, B., Couce, M. E., Curran, G. L., Jensen, M. D., Lloyd, R. V., Cleary, M. P. & Poduslo, J. F. (2000). Obesity is associated with a decreased leptin transport across the blood–brain barrier in rats. *Diabetes*, *49*, 1219–23.

[53] Banks, W. A., Farr, S. A. & Morley, J. E. (2006). The effects of high fat diets on the blood-brain barrier transport of leptin: failure or adaptation? *Physiol Behav.*, *88*(3), 244-8.

[54] Banks, W. A. (2008). The blood-brain barrier as a cause of obesity. *Curr Pharm Des.*, *14*(16), 1606-14.

[55] Widdowson, P. S., Upton, R., Buckingham, R., Arch, J. & Williams, G. (1997). Inhibition of food response to intracerebroventricular injection of leptin is attenuated in rats with diet-induced obesity. *Diabetes.*, *46*, 1782–1785.

[56] Lu, H., Duanmu, Z., Houck, C., Jen, K. L., Buison, A. & Dunbar, J. C. (1998). Obesity due to high fat diet decreases the sympathetic nervous and cardiovascular responses to intracerebroventricular leptin in rats. *Brain Res., Bull.*, *47*, 331–335.

[57] Benomar, Y., Berthou, F., Vacher, C. M., Bailleux, V., Gertler, A., Djiane, J., & Taouis, M. (2009). Leptin But Not Ciliary Neurotrophic Factor (CNTF) Induces Phosphotyrosine Phosphatase-1B Expression in Human Neuronal Cells (SH-SY5Y): Putative Explanation of CNTF Efficacy in Leptin-Resistant State. *Endocrinology*, *150*, 1182–91.

[58] Myers, M. P., Andersen, J. N., Cheng, A., Tremblay, M. L., Horvath, C. M., Parisien, J. P., Salmeen, A., Barford, D. & Tonks, N. K. (2001). TYK2 and JAK2 are substrates of protein-tyrosine phosphatase 1B. *J Biol Chem.*, *276*, 47771-4.

[59] Bence, K. K., Delibegovic, M., Xue, B., Gorgun, C. Z., Hotamisligil, G. S. & Neel, B. G. et al. (2006). Neuronal PTP1B regulates body weight, adiposity and leptin action. *Nat Med.*, *12*, 917-24.

[60] Kelesidis, T., Kelesidis, I., Chou, S. & Mantzoros, C. S. (2012). Narrative review: the role of leptin in human physiology: emerging clinical applications. *Ann Intern Med.*, *152*, 93-100.

[61] Fantuzzi, G. (2005). Adipose tissue, adipokines, and inflammation. *J Allergy Clin Immunol.*, 115(5), 911-9.

[62] Leon-Cabrera, S., Solís-Lozano, L., Suárez-Álvarez, K., González-Chávez, A., Béjar, Y. L., Robles-Díaz, G. & Escobedo G. (2013). Hyperleptinemia is associated with parameters of low-grade systemic inflammation and metabolic dysfunction in obese human beings. *Front Integr Neurosci.*, *7*, 62.

[63] Faggioni, R., Fantuzzi, G., Gabay, C., Moser, A., Dinarello, C. A., Feingold, K. R., Grunfeld, C. (1999). Leptin deficiency enhances sensitivity to endotoxin-induced lethality, *Am. J. Physiol.*, *276*, 136–142.

[64] Williams, L., Bradley, L., Smith, A. & Foxwell, B. (2004). Signal transducer and activator of transcription 3 is the dominant mediator of the anti-inflammatory effects of IL-10 in human macrophages. *J. Immunol.*, *172*, 567–576

[65] Yun, JE., Kimm, H., Jo, J. & Jee, S. H. (2010). Serum leptin is associated with metabolic syndrome in obese and nonobese Korean populations. *Metabolism.*, *59*, 424e429.

[66] Despres, J. P. & Lemieux, I. (2006). Abdominal obesity and metabolic syndrome. *Nature.*, *444*, 881-87.

[67] Söderberg, S., Ahrén, B., Jansson, J. H., Johnson, O., Hallmans, G., Asplund, K., & Olsson, T. (1999). Leptin is associated with increased risk of myocardial infarction. *J Intern Med.*, *159*, 237–45.

[68] Wallace, A. M., McMahon, A. D., Packard, C. J., Shepherd, J., Gaw, A. & Sattar, N. (2001). Plasma leptin and the risk of cardiovascular disease in the West of Scotland Coronary Prevention Study. *Circulation.*, *104*, 3052–6.

[69] Wannamethee, S. G., Tchernova, J., Whincup, P., Lowe, G. D., Kelly, A., Rumley, A., Wallace, A. M. & Sattar, N. (2007). Plasma leptin: Associations with metabolic, inflammatory and haemostatic risk factors for cardiovascular disease. *Atherosclerosis.*, *191*, 418–426

[70] Esteghamati, A., Noshad, S., Khalilzadeh, O., Morteza, A., Nazeri, A., Meysamie, A., Esteghamati, A. & Nakhjavani, M. (2011). Contribution of serum leptin to metabolic syndrome in obese and nonobese subjects. *Arch Med Res.*, *42*(3), 244-51.

[71] Carnier, J., de Mello, M. T., Ackel-DElia, C., Corgosinho, F. C., Campos, R. M., Sanches, Pde L., Masquio, D. C., Bueno, C. R., Jr., Ganen, Ade P., Martins, A. C., Caranti, D. A., Tock, L., Clemente, A. P., Tufik, S. & Dâmaso, A. R. (2013). Aerobic training (AT) is more effective than aerobic plus resistance training (AT+RT) to improve anorexigenic/orexigenic factors in obese adolescents.

[72] Ringholm, S., Grunnet, Knudsen, J., Leick, L., Lundgaard, A., Munk, Nielsen, M., & Pilegaard, H. (2013). PGC-1α is required for exercise- and exercise training-induced UCP1 up-regulation in mouse white adipose tissue. *PLoS One.*, *8*(5), e64123.

[73] Okamatsu-Ogura, Y., Nio-Kobayashi, J., Iwanaga, T., Terao, A., Kimura, K. & Saito, M. (2011). Possible involvement of uncoupling protein 1 in appetite control by leptin. *Exp Biol Med.*, *236*(11), 1274-81

[74] de Mello, MT., de Piano, A., Carnier, J., Sanches, Pde L., Corrêa, F. A., Tock, L., Ernandes, R. M., Tufik, S. & Dâmaso, A. R. (2011). Long-term effects of aerobic plus resistance training on the metabolic syndrome and adiponectinemia in obese adolescents. *J Clin Hypertens.*, *13*(5), 343-50.

In: Leptin: Biosynthesis, Functions and Clinical Significance ISBN: 978-1-62948-801-1
Editor: Edward L. Blum

Chapter 6

LEPTIN REGULATION OF INTESTINAL NUTRIENTS ABSORPTION

Jaione Barrenetxe, Carmen Fanjul and María Pilar Lostao
Department of Nutrition, Food Science and Physiology,
University of Navarra, Pamplona, Spain

ABSTRACT

Leptin is a hormone implicated in the control of food intake and energy balance. Although leptin was first thought to be only expressed in the adipose tissue, today we know that it is also produced in different organs such as skeletal muscle, pituitary gland, placenta and stomach, which secretes the hormone to the gastric juice.

In this chapter, we present different findings in rodents and Caco-2 cells, which contribute to the vision of leptin as an important hormonal signal for the regulation of intestinal absorption of nutrients and therefore, describe another important function for the hormone, apart from its well-known action on appetite control and obesity.

Luminal leptin inhibits intestinal sugar transport in a short-term manner, by reducing the density of the Na^+/glucose co-transporter SGLT1 at the brush border membrane of the enterocytes. Likewise, leptin inhibits glutamine uptake by decreasing both ASCT2 and B^oAT1 transporters trafficking to the apical membrane. In contrast, luminal leptin increases GLUT2 and GLUT5 insertion in the brush border membrane enhancing galactose and fructose absorption respectively. Similarly, intestinal transport of peptides and butyrate is increased by leptin, through the regulation of the expression in the membrane of the proton-coupled co-transporter PEPT1 and the monocarboxylate transporter MCT1, respectively. Leptin regulation of nutrients absorption has also been observed when leptin is acting from the basolateral membrane. The effect of both apical and basal leptin is rapidly and completely reverted when the hormone is removed. Different kinases seem to be involved in the leptin signaling pathways which regulate these nutrients transporters.

1. Leptin Discovery and Functions

Leptin, the product of the *ob* gene, was identified and cloned from rodent adipose tissue in 1994 (Zhang et al. 1994). Initially, leptin action was restricted to the hypothalamus and it was thought that it was only involved in the regulation of food intake and energy expenditure (Tartaglia et al. 1995). Leptin was then considered as an adipostatic signal implicated in the regulation of the energy balance, as it was demonstrated in leptin deficient obese mice *(ob/ob)*. After leptin treatment, the *ob/ob* mice displayed an increase in energy expenditure and their weight returned to control values (Campfiel et al. 1995; Pelleymounter et al. 1995). Moreover, the impaired immune system and fertility associated with leptin deficiency observed in these mice disappeared, suggesting that the hormone could have different physiological roles in the organism.

Leptin plasma levels are related to the amount of adipose tissue, and are higher in women than in men (Kennedy et al. 1997) and in obese individuals (~ 2- 8 nM) than in lean (normal weight) subjects (0.2- 0.8 nM) (Considine et al. 1996). At present, it is known that leptin is also secreted by other tissues as placenta (Masuzaki et al. 1997), fetal tissues (Shimon et al. 1998), muscle (Wang et al. 1998), ovary (Ryan et al. 2002) and kidney (Martinez-Ansó et al. 1999) among others.

1.1. Physiological Role of Leptin

Leptin reaches the central nervous system by crossing the blood-brain barrier through receptor-mediated endocytosis (Baumann et al. 1996; Banks et al. 1996; Golden et al. 1997), where it regulates the synthesis of different neuropeptides implicated in the control of food intake and energy balance, such as neuropeptide Y (Erickson et al. 1996) and corticotropine releasing hormone (Schwartz et al. 1997) among others (Meister et al. 2000). Leptin also regulates fertility and reproduction by acting on the hypothalamic-pituitary-axis (Gonzalez et al. 2000).

Peripherally, leptin is implicated in a broad range of physiological processes such as angiogenesis (Park et al. 2001), hematopoiesis (Fantuzzi and Fangionni, 2000), immune function (Matarese, 2000), testicular and ovaric function (Caprio et al. 2001), embryonic development (Gonzalez et al. 2000), bone formation (Fleet et al. 2000), wound healing (Frank et al. 2000) and lipid and glucidic metabolism (Hynes and Jones, 2001; Ceddia et al. 2001).

1.2. Leptin and its Receptors

The leptin receptors, Ob-Rs, are members of the class I cytokine receptor family. To date, six alternatively spliced isoforms (Ob-Ra-f) coming from the same gene (*Ob* gene) have been described (Tartaglia, 1997; Frühbeck, 2006). They only differ in the amino acid sequence and the length of their trans-membrane and intracellular domains (Chen et al. 1996; Lee et al. 1996). Ob-Ra, c, d and f possess a relatively short cytoplasmic domain, whereas Ob-Rb, the so-called "long" isoform, has an extended C-terminal region and is the only variant capable of complete intracellular signal transduction (Baumann et al. 1996). Nevertheless, a degree of intracellular signaling has also been demonstrated for the short isoforms (Bjorbaeck et al. 1997; Yamashita et al. 1998; Barrenetxe et al. 2003). Ob-Re, the soluble receptor, is a truncated form of the leptin receptor, which is secreted into the circulation and play a role as a binding protein, regulating leptin bioavailability (Yang et al. 2004) and leptin transport across the blood-brain barrier (Tu et al. 2007).

1.3. Leptin and the Gastrointestinal Tract

Different actions of leptin on the gastrointestinal tract have been described in the literature which support the consideration of leptin as a new gut peptide (Yarandi et al. 2011; Cammisotto and Bendayam, 2012).

1.3.1. Gastric Leptin

It is known that the stomach produces and secretes leptin into the gastric lumen by pepsinogen-containing secretory granules of the chief cells (Bado et al. 1998). These granules also contain the leptin soluble receptor Ob-Re that is released into the gastric lumen together with leptin (Cammisotto et al. 2006). Leptin remains stable in the gastric juice because the binding to its soluble receptor protects it from the acidic pH and proteolytic activity of the gastric lumen (Guilmeau et al. 2003 and 2004). The endocrine cells of the gastric mucosa also secrete leptin to the circulation, in particular after meal consumption, contributing to the plasma leptin levels (Cammisotto et al. 2005; Bado et al. 1998; Cinti et al. 2000).

The nutritional status of the body regulates exocrine secretion of leptin by the gastric mucosa (Coleman and Hermann, 1999). Food intake is also a strong stimulus for gastric leptin secretion together with different neurotransmitters and hormones such as acetylcholine release by the vagus nerve (Sobhani et al. 2002), secretin, CCK (Sobhani et al. 2000), insulin, glucocorticoids and trans-retinoic acids (Goïot et al. 2005). In addition, nutrients as fructose also stimulate leptin production by the gastric mucosa without modifying plasma leptin levels (Sakar et al. 2009).

1.3.2. Leptin in the Intestine

Leptin receptors are present in both the apical and the basolateral membrane of the enterocytes (Barrenetxe et al. 2002). Once secreted into the gastric lumen, leptin reaches the intestine where it can bind to its brush border receptors (Barrenetxe et al. 2002; Aparicio et al. 2004) and regulate different processes of the intestinal wall such as intestinal motility, nutrient absorption, mucus secretion and cell proliferation (El Homsi et al. 2007; Cammisotto et al. 2010 and 2012; Yarandi et al. 2011). Circulating leptin can also act as an endocrine hormone on the enterocytes by binding to the receptors of the basolateral membrane and modify transporters activity (Stan et al. 2001; Fanjul et al. 2013).

2. Intestinal Transport of Nutrients

2.1. Transport Mechanisms across the Intestinal Epithelium

One of the main functions of the small intestine is the absorption of nutrients arising from the diet. Passage of nutrients across the membrane of the enterocytes can be carried out by diffusion or active transport. Diffusion is the net movement of substances along their concentration gradient. In the facilitated diffusion, also called passive transport, the movement of molecules requires the presence of protein channels or carrier proteins. In contrast, active transport is the movement of substances against their concentration gradient. This process needs carrier proteins and chemical energy. In the primary active transport, the energy is obtained from the hydrolysis of ATP, whereas in the secondary active transport the energy source is the electrochemical gradient of Na^+ or H^+.

2.2. Transporters Implicated on Intestinal Nutrients Absorption

2.2.1. Transporters Implicated on Sugars Absorption

Glucose and galactose transport into the enterocytes is an active process that involves co-transport of the sugar with sodium through the SGLT1 transporter. Thus, this transporter is able to concentrate glucose/galactose inside the cells using the sodium electrochemical gradient provided by the Na^+/K^+ ATPase (Wrigth et al. 2007; Wright et al. 2011). SGLT1 is constitutively expressed in the brush-border membrane of the enterocytes, but it can be rapidly mobilized from the apical membrane to the cytoplasm storages and vice versa, after activation of different intracellular signals (Wright et al. 1997). Fructose entry into the enterocytes occurs through the facilitative transporter GLUT5 (Barone et al. 2009). Glucose and fructose transport can also occur through GLUT7, another member of the GLUT facilitative family of transporters (Cheeseman 2008). During post-prandial state, when glucose concentration reaches values over ~30 mM, the low affinity/high capacity glucose transporter GLUT2, constitutively expressed in the basolateral membrane, can be recruited to the brush border membrane from intracellular compartments, providing the small intestine with an absorptive capacity to match dietary glucose uptake during meals (Kellet and Helliwell, 2000; Kellet and Brot-Laroche, 2005). This apical GLUT2 is also able to transport fructose helping the main and fructose specific GLUT5 transporter (Barone et al. 2009). Exit of the three monosaccharides from the enterocytes towards the circulation takes place through GLUT2 (Kellet et al. 2008).

2.2.1. Transporters Implicated on Peptides and Amino Acids Absorption

The proteins partially digested in the stomach and by pancreatic enzymes in the duodenum, are hydrolyzed to peptides and free amino acids through the action of intestinal aminopeptidases, carboxypeptidases and peptidases. The intestinal absorption of di/tri-peptides is exclusively mediated by the proton-dependent transporter PEPT1, whereas multiple transporters are implicated in the intestinal absorption of amino acids. On the other hand, a single amino acid can be transported by more than one transporter.

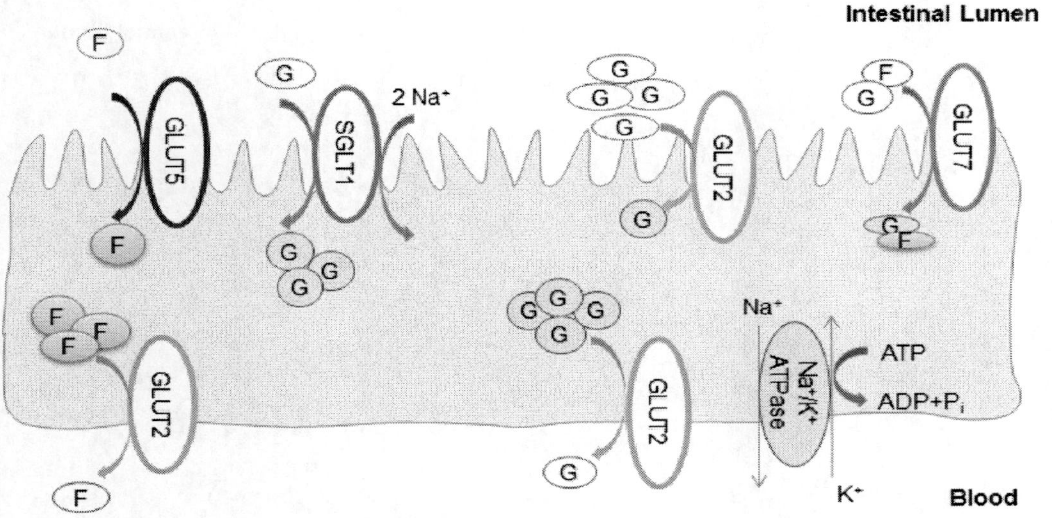

Figure 1. Transporters implicated on intestinal sugars absorption (see text for explanation). F: fructose; G: glucose/galactose.

Glutamine (Gln) is the most abundant amino acid in the plasma, and it is the most important energy source for the enterocytes, lymphocytes and fibroblasts. Gln from the diet is transported into the enterocyte by two sodium-dependent neutral amino acid transporters present in the apical membrane: ASCT2 and B^0AT1 (Broer, 2008). ASCT2 is a neutral amino acid exchanger with high affinity for alanine, cysteine, threonine and glutamine, which can also transport glutamate at low pH (Utsunomiya-Tate et al. 2006). B^0AT1 is a low-affinity transporter, with preference for large neutral amino acids as phenylalanine (Phe), a specific substrate for this transporter (Broer, 2008). Exit of Gln from the enterocyte to the blood occurs through the heterodimeric 4F2hc/LAT2 transporter, a neutral amino acid exchanger located at the basolateral membrane (Segawa et al. 1999; Fraga et al. 2005).

Proline (Pro) is the only protein forming amino acid with a secondary amino group, which is necessary to maintain collagen of the skin, joints, tendons connective tissue and cartilage. In rat intestine, proline transporters include B^0AT1 and PAT1 (Anderson et al. 2004). PAT1 is a sodium-independent but proton-dependent low affinity transporter for small, unbranched, zwitteronic α-, β-, γ- amino and imino acids, such as β-alanine (β-Ala) (Anderson et al. 2004; Iñigo et al. 2006; Thwaites and Anderson 2007a/b). In human Caco-2 cells, PAT1-mediated amino acid influx across the apical membrane leads to an intracellular acidification, which activates the apical Na^+/H^+ exchanger NHE3 (Thwaites et al. 2002). This functional coupling with NHE3 means that in intact epithelia, such as Caco-2 cells or rat intestine, the Na^+-independent PAT1 becomes partially dependent upon extracellular Na^+ (Anderson et al. 2004) as NHE3 cannot function in the absence of Na^+. In rabbit intestine, the transporters that contribute to Pro absorption are B^0AT1 and IMINO, a high affinity Na^+ and Cl^--dependent transporter, specific for imino acids (Kowalczuk et al. 2005). As for Gln, transport of Pro to the blood occurs through 4F2hc/LAT2.

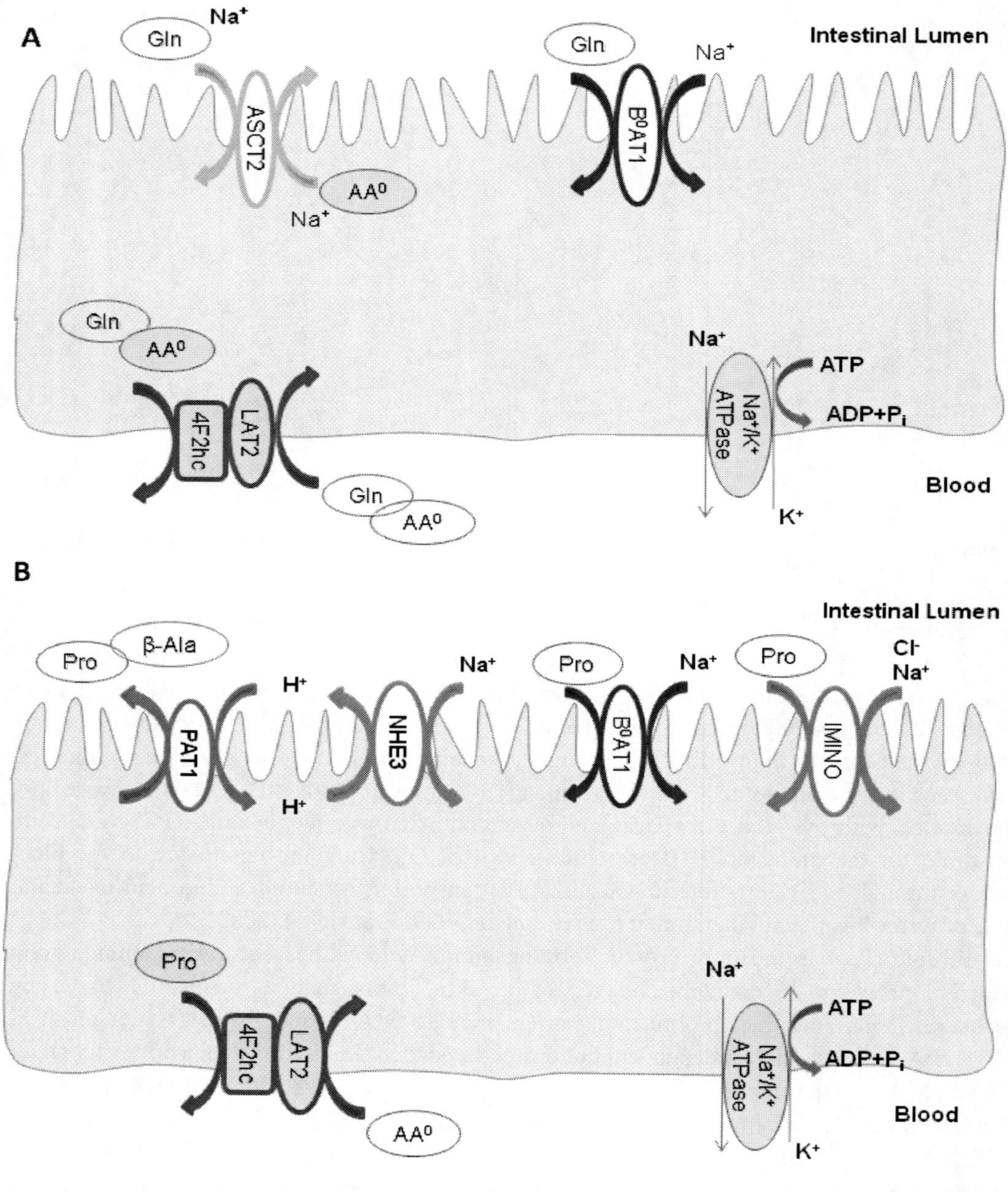

Figure 2. Transporters implicated on intestinal glutamine (Gln; A) and proline (Pro; B) absorption (see text for explanation).

Glutamate (Glu) is one of the most abundant amino acid in the food either in free form or as peptides or proteins (Beyrehuther et al. 2007). Intracellular glutamate increases the antioxidant defense by the generation of glutathione, and participates in the gluconeogenesis in the kidney and in the urea synthesis in the liver (Blachier et al. 2009). Glu intestinal transport takes place by the heterodimeric transporter 4F2hc/xCT, a high affinity Na^+-independent transporter which exchanges Glu and cystine, (Burdo et al. 2006; Broer, 2008), and the high affinity Na^+-dependent transporters for anionic amino acids EAAT1 and EAAT3

(Kanai and Hediger, 1994, Broer, 2008). EAAT1 and EAAT3 belong to the excitatory amino acid transporters family EAATs, which also co-transport H^+ together with Na^+ and Glu. The return of the transporter to its extracellular facing conformational state is facilitated by the intracellular binding of K^+ (Kanai et al. 1994). ASCT2 can also contribute to Glu transport in the intestine because of its acidic microclimate (Christensen, 1984; Munck et al. 1999; Utsunomiya-Tate et al. 1996).

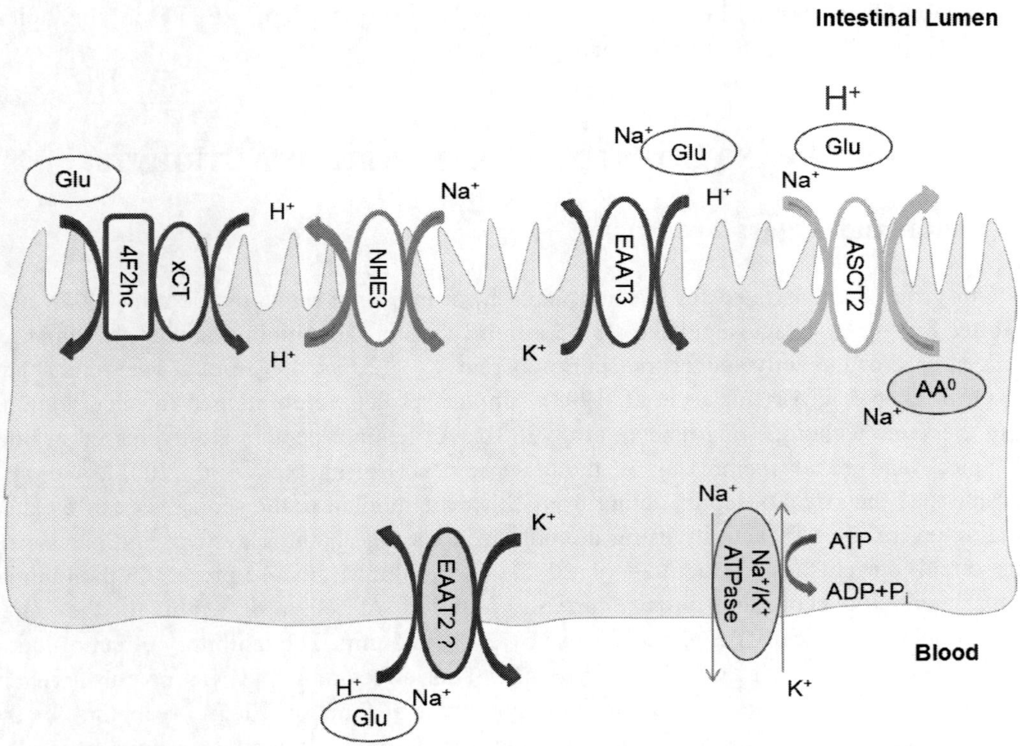

Figure 3. Transporters implicated on intestinal glutamate (Glu) absorption (see text for explanation).

2.3. Regulation of Intestinal Transport of Nutrients

Intestinal absorption can be regulated by several unspecific and specific mechanisms (Ferraris and Carey, 2000; Ferraris, 2001). Unspecific mechanisms include changes in the absorptive surface by increasing the number (hyperplasia) or the size (hypertrophy) of the enterocytes. Diet can also induce changes in the lipid composition of the plasma membrane, altering the lipid environment of the transporters and, in turn, their structure and activity. Another unspecific mechanism is the modification of the Na^+/K^+ ATPase activity, which would change the sodium electrochemical gradient with consequences in the membrane potential and, therefore, in the transporters activity (Ferraris and Diamond, 1997).

Specific regulation of nutrients absorption comprises transcriptional and post-transcriptional mechanisms which, for example, can modify the number of transporters present in the plasma membrane of the enterocytes (Ferraris and Diamond, 1993), through modifications of their synthesis and/or degradation (Tsang et al. 1994). Post-transcriptional regulation of transporters involves activation of protein kinases-dependent pathways which control insertion and recruitment of transporters molecules in the plasma membrane (Wright et al. 1997; Ishikawa et al. 1997; Vayro and Silverman, 1999). In this regard, several hormones such as GLP-2 (Au et al. 2002; Cheeseman et al. 1997), Glucagon-37 (Stümpel et al. 1997), EGF (Chung et al. 1999) and CCK (Hirsh and Cheeseman, 1998) have been found to regulate SGLT1 activity in a short-term manner by regulating its expression in the brush border membrane. Similarly, insulin increases the expression of PEPT1 in the apical membrane of the enterocytes (Thamotharan et al. 1999).

3. Leptin and Intestinal Transport of Nutrients

3.1. Leptin and Sugars Transport

Our group demonstrated for the first time, in rat intestinal rings, that leptin (0.2-78 nM) inhibited by ~40 % galactose uptake after 5 min incubation. That inhibition was accompanied by a decrease of the active sugar transport apparent V_{max} (20 *vs.* 4.8 μmol/g wet weight) and $K_{0,5}$ (15.8 *vs.* 5.3 mM) (Lostao et al. 1998). Similar results were obtained in mice jejunum using the same technique (Barrenetxe et al. 2001). As leptin receptors are expressed in both the apical and basal membrane of the enterocytes (Barrenetxe et al. 2002), we also characterized the effect of leptin, acting from either the luminal or the serosal side of isolated rat jejunum, on SGLT1 activity using the polarized Ussing chamber system, and measuring short-circuit currents (Isc) (Ducroc et al. 2005). Thus, 10 mM glucose present in the luminal compartment induced short-circuit current. Addition of 10 nM leptin to the same compartment dramatically decreased this Isc by 90 % in 5 min. The inhibitory effect of leptin was dose-dependent with an IC50 of 0.13 nM. This effect of leptin was not observed in receptor-deficient *fa/fa* rats, indicating the requirement of functional leptin receptors for the control of SGLT1 activity. In addition, this rapid inhibition was associated with a parallel decrease in the abundance of SGLT1 in the brush-border membrane of the enterocytes as demonstrated by Western-blot. Interestingly, although serosal leptin inhibited glucose Isc after 10 min exposure, this inhibition was blocked by a CCK receptor antagonist, which indicated that the action of leptin from the serosal side of the mucosa was indirect and mediated by the endogenous release of CCK (Ducroc et al. 2005).

A more physiological approach was to study whether luminal leptin could also regulate sugar absorption *in vivo* both at low (basal) and high (post-prandial) sugar concentration. *In vivo* intestinal sugar absorption in rat was measured with the recirculating and single pass perfusion systems and absorption determined by the sugar disappearance from the perfusion medium. Luminal leptin (25 nM) inhibited by 25% sugar absorption at low galactose concentration (1 mM), indicating that the hormone regulated SGLT1 activity (Iñigo et al. 2007). Inhibition was reverted within 15 min when the hormone was eliminated from the perfusion medium. At high glucose concentration (75 mM) leptin also inhibited (~33 %) the phloretin-insensitive component of sugar absorption mediated by SGLT1, but had no effect on the apical passive component of absorption mediated by GLUT2 (Iñigo et al. 2007). This study confirmed our previous findings and supported the view that leptin exerts a regulatory role on intestinal sugar absorption in the post-prandial state by regulating SGLT1.

Similarly to what happens in rodents, in the human model of intestinal epithelial cells Caco-2, where leptin receptors are also expressed (Buyse et al. 2001), apical leptin (0.2 and 8 nM) inhibited by ~30% the uptake of α-methyl-glucoside (α-MG), a specific substrate of SGLT1, after 5 and 30 min treatment. This effect was accompanied by a decrease on SGLT1 protein abundance in the apical membrane of the cells (Fanjul et al. 2012).

Further studies also showed the control by luminal leptin of facilitative glucose transporters of the GLUT family (Sakar et al. 2009; Sakar et al. 2010). In rat intestine, *in vitro* luminal leptin (5 nM) enhanced 100 mM galactose and 30 mM fructose uptake by increasing GLUT2 activity and GLUT5 insertion into the plasma membrane respectively (Sakar et al. 2009). *In vivo* oral fructose administration induced a rapid and potent release of leptin into the gastric juice without any change on leptin plasma levels. Oral administration of leptin, stimulated fructose transport by GLUT5 and fructose-induced increase in blood glucose and mRNA levels of several gluconeogenesis key enzymes (Sakar et al. 2009). These data identified for the first time a positive regulatory control loop between gut leptin and fructose, in which fructose triggers the release of gastric leptin which, in turn, up-regulates GLUT5 and concurrently modulates metabolic functions in the liver.

Table 1. Summary of the main findings on the regulation of sugars transport by leptin. BBM: Brush border membrane; α-MG: α-methyl-D-glucoside; Gal: Galactose; Gluc: Glucose; Fruc: Fructose

Animal/Tissue	Method	Substrate Conc.	Leptin (nM) Exposure time (min)	Effect	Reference
RAT/MOUSE Intestine	Everted jejunal rings	1 mM Gal	Luminal (0.2-78 nM) 5/30 min	↓ SGLT1-mediated sugar uptake	*Lostao et al. 1998* *Barrenetxe et al. 2001*
RAT Intestine	Ussing chambers	10 mM Gluc	Luminal (10 nM) 5 min	↓ SGLT1-mediated sugar Isc ↓ SGLT1 BBM protein expression level	*Ducroc et al. 2005*
RAT Intestine	Ussing chambers	10 mM Gluc	Serosal (10 nM) 10 min	↓ SGLT1-mediated sugar uptake through CCK	*Ducroc et al. 2005*
RAT Intestine	*In vivo*	1 mM Gal 75 mM Gluc	Luminal (25-100 nM) 25 min	↓ SGLT1-mediated sugar absorption (Reversible)	*Iñigo et al. 2007*
RAT Intestine	Jejunal loops	100 mM Gal	Luminal (5 nM) 8 min	↑ GLUT2-mediated sugar uptake	*Sakar et al. 2009*
RAT Intestine	Jejunal loops	30 mM Fruc	Luminal (0.1-10 nM) 8 min	↑ GLUT5- mediated Fructose uptake	*Sakar et al. 2009*
RAT intestine	Western blot	30 mM Fruc	Luminal (1 nM) 8 min	↑ GLUT5 BBM protein expression level	*Sakar et al. 2009*
HUMAN Caco-2 cells	Apical uptake	0.1 mM α-MG	Luminal (0.2- 8 nM) 5/30 min	↓ SGLT1-mediated sugar uptake ↓ SGLT1 BBM protein expression level	*Fanjul et al. 2012*

Since protein kinase C (PKC) and protein kinase A (PKA) are involved in the regulation of SGLT1 (Wright et al. 1997; Ishikawa et al. 1997; Vayro and Silverman, 1999; Ducroc et al. 2005) and it is known that leptin is able to activate these kinases (Sweeney, 2002; Yamagishi et al. 2001; Takekoshi et al. 2001; Maingrette et al. 2003), we investigated whether PKC and PKA could be implicated in the inhibition of sugar absorption by leptin in rat small intestine. Inhibition of 1 mM galactose by 0.2 nM leptin was blocked by chelerythrine, a specific inhibitor of PKC. However H-89, a PKA inhibitor, did not block leptin effect. Biochemical assays showed that the inhibitory effect of leptin was related with a 2-fold increase in PKC and PKA activity. These findings suggested that activation of PKC is more relevant than PKA activation in the inhibition of galactose absorption by leptin (Barrenetxe et al. 2004). In line with these results, in Ussing chambers, the inhibition of glucose-induced Isc by luminal leptin was blunted by an inhibitor of the conventional PKC isoforms (Ducroc et al. 2005). As in rat intestine, H-89 did not block the inhibitory effect of leptin on α-MG uptake in Caco-2 cells, suggesting that PKA is not implicated on the leptin effect in human intestine (Fanjul et al. 2012). Leptin stimulation of fructose uptake in rat was mediated by increase on the phosphorylation/activation of PKCβII and 5′AMP-activated protein kinase (AMPK), that in turn, enhanced GLUT2 and GLUT5 insertion in the brush border membrane of the enterocytes and reduced the insertion of SGLT1 (Sakar et al. 2009).

3.2. Leptin and Amino Acids Transport

In continuation with our studies on leptin effect on intestinal sugars transport, we decided to investigate whether leptin could also regulate amino acids transport using similar approaches. Thus, in rat intestinal everted rings, we demonstrated that leptin (0.2 nM) inhibited by ~ 40-50% the uptake (15 min) of 0.1 mM Gln and Phe (specific substrate of B^0AT1). In Ussing chambers, 10 mM Gln transport followed as Na^+-induced short-circuit current (Isc) was rapidly (2 min) inhibited by luminal leptin in a dose-dependent manner (maximum inhibition at 10 nM; IC_{50}=~ 0.1 nM). Phe-induced Isc was also decreased by leptin. Western blot studies showed that pre-incubation of intestinal loops for 2 min with 1 nM leptin, before 3 min incubation with 10 mM Gln, reduced ASCT2 and B^0AT1 protein expression in the brush border membrane of the enterocytes. Similar results were obtained at the gene expression level after 60 min incubation of the intestine with Gln (Ducroc et al. 2010).

Luminal leptin also regulates amino acids absorption *in vivo*. Using the single pass perfusion system, amino acids absorption was determined by their disappearance from the perfusion medium. Leptin (25 mM) inhibited the absorption of 2 mM Pro, 5 mM β-Ala and 5 mM Gln by ~45% after 5-15 min of leptin perfusion; the effect remained constant until the end of the experiment (80 min) and was rapidly and completely reversed when the hormone was removed from the perfusion medium. Moreover, leptin was able to regulate the absorption of galactose and glutamine in the same animal, indicating leptin direct action on the specific transporters implicated in the absorption of each substrate (Fanjul et al. *unpublished data*).

In Caco-2 cells, apical leptin (0.2 and 8 nM) inhibited by ~40 % Gln and Phe uptake, indicating sensitivity to the hormone of the Na^+-dependent neutral amino acid transporters ASCT2 and B^0AT1. This inhibition was also accompanied by a reduction in amount of the transporters protein at the brush border membrane. Leptin also inhibited 1 mM Pro and β-Ala uptake in Na^+ medium at pH 6, which are the conditions for optimal PAT1 function. Surprisingly, in this case, the abundance of PAT1 in the brush border membrane after leptin treatment was not modified. One explanation would be that leptin could alter the activity of the Na^+/H^+ exchanger NHE3, decreasing the H^+ gradient and thus reducing PAT1activity (Fanjul et al. 2012). Basal leptin (8 nM), in 5 min, also inhibited by ~15-30 % the uptake of 0.1 mM Gln and 1 mM β-Ala. In agreement with the *in vivo* results, apical and basolateral effect of leptin was rapidly and completely reversed when the hormone was removed from the corresponding compartment (Fanjul et al. 2013).

Mordrelle et al. (2000) had reported that in Caco-2 cells the transporters involved on glutamate uptake are the Na^+-dependent transporters EAAT1 and EAAT3. We were able to demonstrate in this cell line that glutamate uptake was both Na^+- and pH-dependent and that this pH dependence could be due to the ASCT2 implication on Glu uptake at acidic pH, as previously mentioned (Utsunomiya-Tate et al. 2006), with the EAAT1/3 transporters being involved in Glu uptake at pH 7. We found that leptin (0.2 nM) inhibited the uptake of Glu at pH 6 (~30%) and pH 7 (15%) in the presence of Na^+, indicating that both EAAT1/3 and ASCT2 were inhibited by the hormone (Fanjul et al. *unpublished data*).

Table 2. Summary of the main findings on the regulation of amino acids transport by leptin. BBM: Brush border membrane

Animal/Tissue	Method	Substrate Conc.	Leptin (nM) Exposure time (min)	Effect	Reference
RAT intestine	Everted jejunal rings	0.5 mM Gln 50 μM Gln	Luminal (0.2nM) 15 min	↓ Gln uptake ↓ ASCT2 and B^0AT1 activity	*Ducroc et al. 2010*
RAT intestine	Everted jejunal rings	0.5 mM Phe	Luminal (0.2 nM) 15 min	↓ Phe uptake	*Ducroc et al. 2010*
RAT intestine	Ussing chambers	10 mM Gln	Luminal (10 nM) 2 min preincubation	↓ ASCT2 and B^0AT1- mediated Gln uptake ↓ ASCT2 and B^0AT1 BBM protein/mRNA expression level	*Ducroc et al. 2010*
RAT intestine	Ussing chambers	10 mM Gln	Serosal (10 nM) 2/10 preincubation	↓ Gln-induced Isc	*Sakar et al. 2009*
RAT intestine	Ussing chambers	10 mM Ala	Luminal (10 nM) 2 min preincubation	↓ Ala-induced Isc	*Ducroc et al. 2010*
RAT intestine	*In vivo*	2 mM Pro 5 mM Gln/ β-Ala	Luminal (25nM) 15 min	↓ Pro /Gln/ β-Ala absorption (Reversible)	*Unpublished data*
HUMAN Caco-2 cells	Apical uptake	0.1 mM Gln	Luminal (0.2/8 nM) 5/30 min	↓ ASCT2 and B^0AT1- mediated Gln uptake ↓ ASCT2 and B^0AT1 BBM protein expression level	*Fanjul et al. 2012*
HUMAN Caco-2 cells	Apical uptake	1 mM Pro pH 6	Luminal (0.2/8 nM) 5/30 min	↓ Pro uptake	*Fanjul et al. 2012*
HUMAN Caco-2 cells	Apical uptake	1 mM β-Ala pH 6	Luminal (0.2/8 nM) 5/30 min	↓ β-Ala uptake No effect PAT1 BBM protein expression level	*Fanjul et al. 2012*
HUMAN Caco-2 cells	Apical uptake	0.1 mM Gln/ 1 mM β-Ala pH 6	Basal (8 nM) 5/30 min	↓ Gln/ β-Ala uptake (Reversible)	*Fanjul et al. 2013*
HUMAN Caco-2 cells	Apical uptake	0.1 mM Gln/ 1 mM β-Ala pH 6	Basal (8 nM) 6 h preincubation	↓ Gln/β-Ala uptake	*Fanjul et al. 2013*
HUMAN Caco-2 cells	Apical uptake	0.1 mM Glu pH 6/ pH 7	Luminal (0.2 nM) 5 min	↓ Glu uptake	*Unpublished data*

3.3. Leptin and Peptides Transport

Contrary to leptin effect on sugars and amino acids transport, the intestinal transport of dipeptides by PEPT-1 is increased by apical leptin. In Caco-2 cells, apical but not basolateral leptin (2 nM) increased uptake of Gly-Sar in 15 min. This effect was associated with an increase on PEPT1 protein expression at the plasma membrane and V_{max}, no change on apparent $K_{0,5}$ and decrease on the intracellular PEPT1 content (Buyse et al. 2001). In the same experimental model, it was also found that leptin transcriptionally enhanced PEPT1 expression and activity via the cAMP-response element-binding protein and Cdx2 transcirption factors (Nduati et al. 2001).

In rat jejunum *in vivo*, intraluminal leptin (100 nM) also induced a rapid 2-fold increase on the intestinal absorption of dipeptides (Buyse et al. 2001).

3.4. Leptin and Fatty Acids and Butyrate Transport

In Caco-2 cells, leptin (200 nM) acting from the basolateral membrane affected lipid handling by decreasing the export of triglycerides to the basolateral medium without affecting monoglyceride, diglyceride and cholesterolester classes. It also decreased the release of *de novo* synthesized apolipoproteins B-100 and B-48, as well as the newly formed chylomicrons and low density lipoproteins (Stan et al. 2001). Interestingly, *in vivo* intravenous injection of leptin attenuated apolipoprotein A-IV transcription elicited by intra-duodenal infusion of lipids (Morton et al. 1998; Doi et al. 2001).

Luminal leptin (10 nM) up-regulated butyrate uptake in Caco-2 cells after 24 h, by increasing its maximal velocity without modification on the apparent $K_{0.5}$. This up-regulation was explained by two mechanisms: 1) the increase of the intracellular pool of the monocarboxylate transporter MCT1, without affecting the expression of CD14, a protein which associates with MCT1 and is required for the butyrate transport activity; 2) the translocation of the CD147/MCT1 to the apical plasma membrane (Buyse et al. 2002).

Table 3. Summary of the main findings on the regulation of peptides and fatty acids transport by leptin. CFX: cephalexin; BBM: Brush border membrane

Animal/Tissue	Method	Substrate Conc.	Leptin (nM) Exposure time (min)	Effect	Reference
RAT Intestine	*In vivo*	1 mM CFX	Luminal (100 nM) 40 min	↑ CFX absorption	*Buyse et al. 2001*
HUMAN Caco-2 cells	Apical uptake	20 µM Gly-Sar (pH 6)	Luminal (2/10 nM)	↑ Gly-Sar uptake ↑ PEPT1 BBM protein expression level	*Buyse et al. 2001*
HUMAN Caco-2 cells	Apical uptake	20 µM Butyrate (pH 6.4)	Apical (10 nM) 1-24 h	↑ Butyrate uptake (12-24h) ↑ translocation of MCT1/CD147 to BBM ↑MCT1 mRNA expression	*Buyse et al. 2002*

4. Leptin Regulation of Nutrients Absorption in Obesity

Leptin major role at the central level is the regulation of appetite and energy expenditure, indicating a clear implication of the hormone in the development of obesity. Since leptin regulates body weight, differences in leptin sensibility or synthesis could lead to differences in body weight.

Obese animals, except the *ob/ob* mice, show higher leptin plasma levels than normal weight animals (Maffei et al. 1995). In this sense, in obese subjects high leptin plasma level is associated with leptin resistance, but little is known about the mechanisms that lead to it. Besides, 10% of the obese population show normal leptin plasma level and, even in some cases, obesity can be due to a diminished leptin production by the adipose tissue (Ioffe et al. 1998).

Our group analyzed the effect of exogenous leptin on intestinal galactose absorption in the genetically obese *ob/ob* (leptin deficient) and *db/db* (leptin-resistant) mice. Although basal galactose uptake was similar in wild-type mice and the two obese groups, contrarily to what happens in wild-type mice, leptin (0.2 and 0.4 nM) increased galactose uptake in *db/db* mice. In the *ob/ob* strain, leptin inhibited galactose uptake only at 0.2 nM (Iñigo et al. 2004). These data indicate that leptin regulation of sugar absorption differ between lean and the genetically obese animals. Since the *db/db* strain is leptin resistant due to the absence of the functional long leptin receptor isoform, the stimulatory effect of leptin on galactose absorption should be mediated by the short receptor isoforms signaling. In contrast, in normal mice, the activation of the long and short receptor isoforms and the resulting cross-talk between their intracellular signaling, in which several kinases are involved, would produce a decrease on galactose uptake (Iñigo et al. 2004). Interestingly, 0.2 nM leptin also increased galactose uptake in *ob/ob* mice. This strain does not secrete leptin suggesting that *ob/ob* mice tissues may have different regulation of leptin receptors expression and, therefore, different sensitivity and response to the hormone (Iñigo et al. 2004). In summary, these data suggest a distinct leptin regulatory mechanism on glucose intestinal absorption in wild-type and obese animals. A study performed in morbid obese subjects showed that they exhibited a different expression pattern of GLUT2 when compared with lean subjects. GLUT2 was present in the apical membrane of the enterocytes in obese individuals even during fasting state, while in lean subjects the presence of GLUT2 in the brush border membrane is usually limited to post-prandial state. This fact is related to the clinical parameters of the obese subjects such as insulin resistance and diabetes (Ait-Omar et al. 2011). In addition, Osswald and colleagues (2005) demonstrated that genetically modified mice lacking RS1, a peptide implicated in the regulation of SGLT1, developed obesity with high levels of the transporter expression associated with increased sugar absorption in the small intestine.

In line with these findings, other authors have shown that intestinal peptides absorption mediated by the H^+-coupled co-transporter PEPT1 was impaired in *ob/ob* mice. While chronic leptin administration increased PEPT1 activity and expression in human and rat intestine, in leptin-deficient *ob/ob* mice the transporter activity and expression were significantly reduced and completely restored after leptin subcutaneous infusion (Hindlet et al. 2007). In addition, in a mice model of diet-induced obesity, it has been shown that 4-week hypercaloric diet resulted in a 46% reduction in PEPT1-specific transport because of a decrease in PEPT1 protein and mRNA levels. These modifications were supported by a parallel reduction in leptin receptor expression, reflecting possible leptin desensitization due to the diet (Hindlet et al. 2009).

Taking together, these findings indicate that the membrane expression of the nutrients transporters and the leptin levels differ between lean and obese subjects. The higher leptin levels found in obese subjects could lead to leptin resistance in the gastrointestinal tract impairing the regulation of nutrients absorption and, therefore, contributing to the onset of obesity.

CONCLUSION

The endocrine and paracrine regulation of the intestinal absorption of nutrients is being subject of intense research, leading to the identification of new actors. In this chapter, we have presented the findings regarding the regulation of intestinal nutrients uptake by leptin.

Leptin, acting from the apical or the basal membrane of the enterocytes, modulates in a short-term manner and in a reversible way *in vivo* and *in vitro* nutrients uptake in rat intestine and human Caco-2 cells. The mechanisms implicated involve direct effect on the transporter membrane expression or indirect processes that lead to modulations of the activity of the implicated transporters.

Interestingly, it has been demonstrated that leptin inhibits Pro and β-Ala uptake through the H^+-dependent, Na^+-independent transporter PAT1, without modifying its expression in the brush border membrane. In this case the mechanism involved seems to be indirect, most probably by alteration of the H^+ gradient through modification of the Na^+/H^+ exchanger activity. In the case of the other H^+-dependent transporters, PEPT1 and CD147/MCT-1, the reduction of the H^+ gradient would be overcompensated by an increase on the amount of the transporters molecules in the apical membrane.

On the view of these data, it seems that the decrease on the expression or activity of the Na^+-dependent transporters (SGLT1, ASCT2, B^oAT1) due to leptin, could be a mechanism for the enterocyte to economize the energy required by the Na^+/K^+-ATPase to maintain the Na^+ gradient during the absorptive period, which demands high energy levels. It is known that leptin delays gastric emptying and transit activity in the jejunum (Martínez et al. 1999; Kiely et al. 2005), therefore, it could be suggested that leptin would slow down the absorption of some nutrients to allow the enterocyte their processing and the energy restoration. As the action of leptin is reversible, this effect would disappear later on and the remaining nutrients in the intestinal lumen would be completely absorbed.

Taken together, the findings presented in this chapter contribute to the vision of leptin as an important hormonal signal for the regulation of intestinal absorption of nutrients, whose impairment may be implicated in the development of different pathologies including obesity.

ACKNOWLEDGMENTS

The works performed by our group here cited were supported by grants PM98-0034 and BFU2007-60420/BFI from the Spanish Government; grants from the "Departamento de Educación y Cultura" of the Navarra Government, PIUNA (University of Navarra) and

"Fundación Marcelino Botín". Our group is a member of Network for Coopertaive Research on membrane transport Proteins (REIT), co-funded by the "Ministerio de Educación y Ciencia" and the European Regional Development Fund (ERDF) (Grant BFU2007-30688-E/BFI).

REFERENCES

Ait-Omar A, Monteiro-Sepulveda M, Poitou C, Le Gall M, Cotillard A, et al. (2011) GLUT2 accumulation in enterocyte apical and intracellular membranes: a study in morbidly obese human subjects and *ob/ob* and high fat-fed mice. *Diabetes* 60: 2598-2607.

Aparicio T, Guilmeau S, Goiot H, Tsocas A, Laigneau JP, et al. (2004) Leptin reduces the development of the initial precancerous lesions induced by azoxymethane in the rat colonic mucosa. *Gastroenterology* 126: 499-510.

Anderson CM, Grenade DS, Boll M, Foltz M, Wake KA, et al. (2004) H^+/amino acid transporter 1 (PAT1) is the imino acid carrier: An intestinal nutrient/drug transporter in human and rat. *Gastroenterol* 127: 1410-1422.

Au A, Gupta A, Schembri P, Cheeseman CI (2002) Rapid insertion of GLUT2 into the rat jejunal brush-border membrane promoted by glucagon-like peptide 2. *The Biochemical Journal* 367: 247-254.

Bado A, Levasseur S, Attoub S, Kermorgant S, Laigneau JP, et al. (1998) The stomach is a source of leptin. *Nature* 394: 790-793.

Banks WA, Kastin AJ, Huang W, Jaspan JB, Maness LM (1996) Leptin enters the brain by a saturable system independent of insulin. *Peptides* 17: 305-311.-1368.

Barone S, Fussell SL, Singh AK, Lucas F, Xu J, et al. (2009) Slc2a5 (Glut5) is essential for the absorption of fructose in the intestine and generation of fructose-induced hypertension. *J Biol Chem* 284: 5056-5066.

Barrenetxe J, Barber A, Lostao MP (2001) Leptin effect on galactose absorption in mice jejunum. *J Physiol Biochem* 57: 345-346.

Barrenetxe J, Villaro AC, Guembe L, Pascual I, Muñoz-Navas M, et al. (2002) Distribution of the long leptin receptor isoform in brush border, basolateral membrane, and cytoplasm of enterocytes. *Gut* 50: 797-802.

Barrenetxe J, Palacios R, Barber A, Lostao MP (2003) Functional expression of the short isoform of the murine leptin receptor Ob-Rc (muB1.219) in *Xenopus laevis* oocytes. *J Physiol Biochem* 59: 119-126.

Barrenetxe J, Sainz N, Barber A, Lostao MP (2004) Involvement of PKC and PKA in the inhibitory effect of leptin on intestinal galactose absorption. *Biochemical and Biophysical Research Communications* 317: 717-721.

Baumann H, Morella KK, White DW, Dembski M, Bailon PS, et al. (1996) The full-length leptin receptor has signaling capabilities of interleukin 6-type cytokine receptors. *Proceedings of the National Academy of Sciences USA* 93: 8374-8378.

Beyreuther K, Biesalski HK, Fernstrom JD, Grimm P, Hammes WP, et al. (2007) Consensus meeting: monosodium glutamate - an update. Eur J Clin Nutr 61:304-313.

Blachier F, Boutry C, Bos C, Tomé D (2009) Metabolism and functions of L-glutamate in the epithelial cells of the small and large intestines. *Am J Clin Nutr* 90(3):814S-821S.

Bjorbaek C, Uotani S, da Silva B, Flier JS (1997) Divergent signaling capacities of the long and short isoforms of the leptin receptor. *J Biol Chem* 272: 32686-32695.

Broer, S. (2008) Amino acid transport across mammalian intestinal and renal epithelia. *Physiol Rev* 88, 249-86.

Burdo J, Dargusch R, Schubert D (2006) Distrinution of the cysteine/glutamate antiporter system Xc- in the rat brain, kidney and duodenum. J Histochem Cytochem 54:549-557.

Buyse M, Berlioz F, Guilmeau S, Tsocas A, Voisin T, et al. (2001) PepT1-mediated epithelial transport of dipeptides and cephalexin is enhanced by luminal leptin in the small intestine. *J Clin Invest* 108: 1483-1494.

Buyse M, Sitaraman SV, Liu X, Bado A, Merlin D (2002) Luminal leptin enhances CD147/MCT-1-mediated uptake of butyrate in the human intestinal cell line Caco2-BBE. *J Biol Chem* 277: 28182-28190.

Cammisotto PG, Renaud C, Gingras D, Delvin E, Levy E, et al. (2005) Endocrine and exocrine secretion of leptin by the gastric mucosa. *J Histochem Cytochem* 53: 851-860.

Cammisotto PG, Gingras D, Renaud C, Levy E, Bendayan M (2006) Secretion of soluble leptin receptors by exocrine and endocrine cells of the gastric mucosa. *Am J Physiol Gastrointest and Liver Physiol* 290: G242-249.

Cammisotto PG, Levy E, Bukowiecki LJ, Bendayan M (2010) Cross-talk between adipose and gastric leptins for the control of food intake and energy metabolism. *Prog Histochem Cytochem* 45: 143-200.

Cammisotto PG, BendayanM (2012) A review on gastric leptin: the exocrine secretion of a gastric hormone. *Anat Cell Biol* 45: 1-16.

Campfield LA, Smith FJ, Mackie G, Tenenbaum R, Sassano ML, et al. (1995) Insulin normalization as an approach to the pharmacological treatment of obesity. *Obesity research* 3 Suppl 4: 591S-603S.

Caprio M, Fabbrini E, Isidori AM, Aversa A, Fabbri A (2001) Leptin in reproduction. *Trends Endocrinol Metab* 12: 65-72.

Ceddia RB, William WN, Jr., Curi R (2001) The response of skeletal muscle to leptin. *Front Biosci* 6: D90-97.

Cheeseman CI (1997) Upregulation of SGLT-1 transport activity in rat jejunum induced by GLP-2 infusion in vivo. *Am J Physiol* 273: R1965-1971.

Cheeseman C (2008) GLUT7: a new intestinal facilitated hexose transporter. *Am J Physiol Endocrinol Metab* 295: E238-241.

Chen H, Charlat O, Tartaglia LA, Woolf EA, Weng X, et al. (1996) Evidence that the diabetes gene encodes the leptin receptor: identification of a mutation in the leptin receptor gene in db/db mice. *Cell* 84: 491-495.

Christensen HN (1984) Organic ion transport *Biochim Biophys Acta* 779 (3):255-69.

Chung BM, Wong JK, Hardin JA, Gall DG (1999) Role of actin in EGF-induced alterations in enterocyte SGLT1 expression. *Am J Physiol* 276: G463-469.

Cinti S, Matteis RD, Picó C, Ceresi E, Obrador A, et al. (2000) Secretory granules of endocrine and chief cells of human stomach mucosa contain leptin. *Int J Obes Relat Metab Disord* 24: 789-793.

Coleman RA, Herrmann TS (1999) Nutritional regulation of leptin in humans. *Diabetologia* 42: 639-646.

Considine RV, Sinha MK, Heiman ML, Kriauciunas A, Stephens TW, et al. (1996) Serum immunoreactive-leptin concentrations in normal-weight and obese humans. *N Engl J Med* 334: 292-295.

Doi T, Liu M, Seeley RJ, Woods SC, Tso P (2001) Effect of leptin on intestinal apolipoprotein AIV in response to lipid feeding. *Am J Physiol Regul Integr Comp Physiol* 281: R753-759.

Ducroc R, Guilmeau S, Akasbi K, Devaud H, Buyse M, et al. (2005) Luminal leptin induces rapid inhibition of active intestinal absorption of glucose mediated by sodium-glucose cotransporter 1. *Diabetes* 54: 348-354.

Ducroc R, Sakar Y, Fanjul C, Barber A, Bado A, et al. (2010) Luminal leptin inhibits L-glutamine transport in rat small intestine: involvement of ASCT2 and B0AT1. *Am J Physiol Gastrointest Liver Physiol* 299: G179-185.

El Homsi M, Ducroc R, Claustre J, Jourdan G, Gertler A, et al. (2007) Leptin modulates the expression of secreted and membrane-associated mucins in colonic epithelial cells by targeting PKC, PI3K, and MAPK pathways. *Am J of Physiol Gastrointest Liver Physiol* 293: G365-373.

Erickson JC, Clegg KE, Palmiter RD (1996) Sensitivity to leptin and susceptibility to seizures of mice lacking neuropeptide Y. *Nature* 381: 415-421.

Fanjul C, Barrenetxe J, Inigo C, Sakar Y, Ducroc R, et al.(2012) Leptin regulates sugar and amino acids transport in the human intestinal cell line Caco-2. *Acta physiologica* (Oxford, England) 205: 82-91.

Fanjul C, Barrenetxe J, & Lostao MP (2013) Basal leptin regulates amino acid uptake in polarized Caco-2 cells. *J Physiol Biochem* (DOI) 10.1007/s13105-013-0239-6.

Fantuzzi G, Faggioni R (2000) Leptin in the regulation of immunity, inflammation, and hematopoiesis. *J Leukoc Biol* 68: 437-446.

Ferraris RP, Diamond JM (1993) Crypt/villus site of substrate-dependent regulation of mouse intestinal glucose transporters. *Proc Natl Acad Sci USA* 90: 5868-5872.

Ferraris RP, Diamond J (1997) Regulation of intestinal sugar transport. *Physiol Rev* 77: 257-302.

Ferraris RP, Carey HV (2000) Intestinal transport during fasting and malnutrition. *Annu Rev Nutr* 20: 195-219.

Ferraris RP (2001)Dietary and developmental regulation of intestinal sugar transport*Biochem J* 360:265-76.

Fleet JC (2000) Leptin and bone: does the brain control bone biology? *Nutr Rev* 58: 209-211.

Fraga S, Pinho MJ, Soares-da-Silva P (2005) Expression of LAT1 and LAT2 amino acid transporters in human and rat intestinal epithelial cells. *Amino Acids* 20: 229-233.

Frank S, Stallmeyer B, Kampfer H, Kolb N, Pfeilschifter J (2000) Leptin enhances wound re-epithelialization and constitutes a direct function of leptin in skin repair. *J Clin Invest* 106: 501-509.

Frühbeck G (2006) Intracellular signalling pathways activated by leptin. *Biochem J* 393: 7-20.

Goïot H, Laigneau JP, Devaud H, Sobhani I, Bado A (2005) Similarities and differences in the transcriptional regulation of the leptin gene promoter in gastric and adipose cells. *FEBS Lett* 579: 1911-1916.

Golden PL, Maccagnan TJ, Pardridge WM (1997) Human blood-brain barrier leptin receptor. Binding and endocytosis in isolated human brain microvessels. *J Clin Investn* 99: 14-18.

Gonzalez RR, Caballero-Campo P, Jasper M, Mercader A, Devoto L, et al.(2000) Leptin and leptin receptor are expressed in the human endometrium and endometrial leptin secretion is regulated by the human blastocyst. *J Clin Endocrinol Metab* 85: 4883-4888.

Guilmeau S, Buyse M, Tsocas A, Laigneau JP, Bado A (2003) Duodenal leptin stimulates cholecystokinin secretion: evidence of a positive leptin-cholecystokinin feedback loop. *Diabetes* 52: 1664-1672.

Guilmeau S, Buyse M, Bado A (2004) Gastric leptin: a new manager of gastrointestinal function. *Current opinion in pharmacology* 4: 561-566.

Hindlet P, Bado A, Farinotti R, Buyse M (2007) Long-term effect of leptin on H^+-coupled peptide co-transporter 1 activity and expression in vivo: evidence in leptin-deficient mice. *J Pharmacol Exp Ther.* 323(1):192-201.

Hindlet P, Bado A, Kamenicky P, Deloménie C, Bourasset F et al. (2009) Reduced intestinal absorption of dipeptides via PepT1 in mice with diet-induced obesity is associated with leptin receptor down-regulation. *J Biol Chem.* 13; 284(11):6801-8.

Hirsh AJ, Cheeseman CI (1998) Cholecystokinin decreases intestinal hexose absorption by a parallel reduction in SGLT1 abundance in the brush-border membrane. *The Journal of Biological Chemistry* 273: 14545-14549.

Hynes GR, Jones PJ (2001) Leptin and its role in lipid metabolism. *Curr Opin Lipidol* 12: 321-327.

Iñigo C, Barber A, Lostao MP (2004) Leptin effect on intestinal galactose absorption in *ob/ob* and *db/db* mice. *J Physiol Biochem* 60: 93-97.

Iñigo C, Barber A, Lostao MP (2006) Na^+ and pH dependence of proline and β-alanine absorption in rat small intestine. *Acta Physiol* (Oxford, England) 186: 271-278.

Iñigo C, Patel N, Kellett GL, Barber A, Lostao MP (2007) Luminal leptin inhibits intestinal sugar absorption in vivo. *Acta Physiol* (Oxford, England) 190: 303-310.

Ioffe E, Moon B, Connolly E, Friedman JM (1998) Abnormal regulation of the leptin gene in the pathogenesis of obesity. *Proc Natl Acad Sci USA* 95: 11852-11857.

Ishikawa Y, Eguchi T, Ishida H (1997) Mechanism of beta-adrenergic agonist-induced transmural transport of glucose in rat small intestine. Regulation of phosphorylation of SGLT1 controls the function. *Biochim Biophys Acta* 1357: 306-318.

Kanai Y, Stelzner M, Nussberger S, Khawaja S, Hebert SC et al. (1994) The neuronal and epithelial human high affinity glutamate transporter. Insights into structure and mechanisms of transport. *J Biol Chem* 269: 20599-20606.

Kanai Y, Hediger MA (2004) The glutamate/neutral amino acid transporter family SLC1: molecular, physiological and pharmacological aspects. *Pflugers Arch-Eur J Physiol* 447:469-479.

Kellett GL, Helliwell PA (2000) The diffusive component of intestinal glucose absorption is mediated by the glucose-induced recruitment of GLUT2 to the brush-border membrane. *The Biochem Journal* 350 Pt 1: 155-162.

Kellett GL, Brot-Laroche E (2005) Apical GLUT2: a major pathway of intestinal sugar absorption. *Diabetes* 54: 3056-3062.

Kellett GL, Brot-Laroche E, Mace OJ, Leturque A (2008) Sugar absorption in the intestine: the role of GLUT2. *Annual Review of Nutrition* 28: 35-54.

[1] Kennedy A, Gettys TW, Watson P, Wallace P, Ganaway E, et al. (1997) The metabolic significance of leptin in humans: gender-based differences in relationship to adiposity, insulin sensitivity, and energy expenditure. *J Clin Endocrinol Metab* 82: 1293-1300.

Kiely JM, Noh JH, Graewin SJ, Pitt HA, Swartz-Basile DA (2005) Altered intestinal motility in leptin-deficient obese mice.*J Surg Res*. 124(1):98-103.

Kowalczuk S, Bröer A, Munzinger M, Tietze N, Klingel K, Bröer S (2005) Molecular cloning of the mouse IMINO system: an Na^+- and Cl^--dependent proline transporter. *Biochem J* 386: 417-422.

Lee GH, Proenca R, Montez JM, Carroll KM, Darvishzadeh JG, et al. (1996) Abnormal splicing of the leptin receptor in diabetic mice. *Nature* 379: 632-635.

Lostao MP, Urdaneta E, Martinez-Ansó E, Barber A, Martinez JA (1998) Presence of leptin receptors in rat small intestine and leptin effect on sugar absorption. *FEBS letters* 423: 302-306.

Maffei M, Halaas J, Ravussin E, Pratley RE, Lee GH, et al. (1995) Leptin levels in human and rodent: measurement of plasma leptin and ob RNA in obese and weight-reduced subjects. *Nat Med* 1: 1155-1161.

Maingrette F, Renier G (2003) Leptin increases lipoprotein lipase secretion by macrophages: involvement of oxidative stress and protein kinase C. *Diabetes* 52: 2121-2128.

Martínez V, Barrachina MD, Wang L, Taché Y (1999) Intracerebroventricular leptin inhibits gastric emptying of a solid nutrient meal in rats. *Neuroreport* 10(15):3217-21.

Martinez-Ansó E, Lostao MP, Martinez JA (1999) Immunohistochemical localization of leptin in rat kidney. *Kidney Int* 55: 1129-1130.

Masuzaki H, Ogawa Y, Sagawa N, Hosoda K, Matsumoto T, et al.(1997) Nonadipose tissue production of leptin: leptin as a novel placenta-derived hormone in humans. *Nat Med* 3: 1029-1033.

Matarese G (2000) Leptin and the immune system: how nutritional status influences the immune response. *Eur Cytokine Netw* 11: 7-14.

Meister B (2000) Control of food intake via leptin receptors in the hypothalamus. Vitamins and Hormones 59: 265-304.

Mordrelle A, Jullian E, Costa C, Cormet-Bocaya E, Benamouzigm R et al. (2000) EAAT1 is involved in transport of L-glutamate during differentiation of the Caco-2 cell line. *Am J Physiol Gastrointest Liver Physiol* 279:366-373.

Morton NM, Emilsson V, Liu YL, Cawthorne MA (1998) Leptin action in intestinal cells. *J Biol Chem* 273: 26194-26201.

Munck BG, Munck LK (1999) Effects of pH changes on systems ASC and B in rabbit ileum. *Am J Physiol* 276:G173- 84.

Nduati V, Yan Y, Dalmasso G, Driss A, Sitaraman S, Merlin D (2007). Leptin transcriptionally enhances peptide *J Biol Chem* 282(2):1359-73.

Osswald C, Baumgarten K, Stumpel F, Gorboulev V, Akimjanova M, et al. (2005) Mice without the regulator gene Rsc1A1 exhibit increased Na+-D-glucose cotransport in small intestine and develop obesity. *Molecular and Cellular Biology* 25: 78-87.

Park HY, Kwon HM, Lim HJ, Hong BK, Lee JY, et al. (2001) Potential role of leptin in angiogenesis: leptin induces endothelial cell proliferation and expression of matrix metalloproteinases *in vivo* and *in vitro*. *Exp Mol Med* 33: 95-102.

Pelleymounter MA, Cullen MJ, Baker MB, Hecht R, Winters D, et al. (1995) Effects of the obese gene product on body weight regulation in *ob/ob* mice. *Science* (New York, NY) 269: 540-543.

Ryan NK, Woodhouse CM, Van der Hoek KH, Gilchrist RB, Armstrong DT, et al. (2002) Expression of leptin and its receptor in the murine ovary: possible role in the regulation of oocyte maturation. *Biol Reprod* 66: 1548-1554.

Sakar Y, Nazaret C, Letteron P, Ait-Omar A, Avenati M, et al. (2009) Positive regulatory control loop between gut leptin and intestinal GLUT2/GLUT5 transporters links to hepatic metabolic functions in rodents. *PloS one* 4: e7935.

Sakar Y, Nazaret C, Bado A, Ducroc R (2010) Leptin and insulin control the activity and expression of intestinal hexose transporter GLUT7. *Gene & Nutrition*, 5(1), S71 European Intestinal Transport Group, 23th meeting, Salerno, Italy.

Schwartz MW, Seeley RJ, Woods SC, Weigle DS, Campfield LA, et al. (1997) Leptin increases hypothalamic pro-opiomelanocortin mRNA expression in the rostral arcuate nucleus. *Diabetes* 46: 2119-2123.

Segawa H, Fukusawa Y, Miyamoto K, Takeda E, Endou H, Kanai Y (1999) identification and functional characterization of a Na+-indeoendent neutral amino acid transporter with broad substrate selectivity. *J Biol Chem* 274: 19745-19751.

Shimon I, Yan X, Magoffin DA, Friedman TC, Melmed S (1998) Intact leptin receptor is selectively expressed in human fetal pituitary and pituitary adenomas and signals human fetal pituitary growth hormone secretion. *J Clin Endocrinol Metab* 83: 4059-4064.

Sobhani I, Bado A, Vissuzaine C, Buyse M, Kermorgant S, et al. (2000) Leptin secretion and leptin receptor in the human stomach. *Gut* 47: 178-183.

Sobhani I, Buyse M, Goiot H, Weber N, Laigneau JP, et al. (2002) Vagal stimulation rapidly increases leptin secretion in human stomach. *Gastroenterology* 122: 259-263.

Stan S, Levy E, Bendayan M, Zoltowska M, Lambert M, et al. (2001) Effect of human recombinant leptin on lipid handling by fully differentiated Caco-2 cells. *FEBS Lett* 508: 80-84.

Stümpel F, Scholtka B, Jungermann K (1997) A new role for enteric glucagon-37: acute stimulation of glucose absorption in rat small intestine. FEBS Lett 410: 515-519.

Sweeney G (2002) Leptin signalling. *Cell Signal* 14: 655-663.

Takekoshi K, Ishii K, Nanmoku T, Shibuya S, Kawakami Y, et al. (2001) Leptin stimulates catecholamine synthesis in a PKC-dependent manner in cultured porcine adrenal medullary chromaffin cells. *Endocrinology* 142: 4861-4871.

Tartaglia LA, Dembski M, Weng X, Deng N, Culpepper J, et al. (1995) Identification and expression cloning of a leptin receptor, OB-R. *Cell* 83: 1263-1271.

Tartaglia LA (1997) The leptin receptor. *The Journal of Biological Chemistry* 272: 6093-6096.

Thamotharan M, Bawani SZ, Zhou X, Adibi SA (1999) Hormonal regulation of oligopeptide transporter Pept-1 in a human intestinal cell line. *Am J Physiol.* 276: C821-6.

Thwaites DT, Kennedy DJ, Raldua D, Anderson CM, Mendoza ME, et al. (2002) H/dipeptide absorption across the human intestinal epithelium is controlled indirectly via a functional Na^+/H^+ exchanger. *Gastroenterology* 122 (5):1322-33.

Thwaites DT, Anderson CM (2007a) H+-coupled nutrient *Exp Physiol* 92(4):603-19.

Thwaites DT, Anderson CM (2007b) Deciphering the mechanisms of intestinal imino (and amino *Biochem Biophys Acta* 1768 (2):179-97

Tsang R, Ao Z, Cheeseman C (1994) Influence of vascular and luminal hexoses on rat intestinal basolateral glucose transport. *Canadian Journal of Physiology and Pharmacology* 72: 317-326.

Tu H, Pan W, Feucht L, Kastin AJ (2007) Convergent trafficking pattern of leptin after endocytosis mediated by ObRa-ObRd. *J Cell Physiol* 212: 215-222.

Utsunomiya-Tate N, Endou H, Kanai Y (1996) Cloning and functional characterization of a system ASC-like Na^+-dependent neutral amino acid transporter. *J Biol Chem* 271: 14883-14890.

Vayro S, Silverman M (1999) PKC regulates turnover rate of rabbit intestinal Na+-glucose transporter expressed in COS-7 cells. *Am J Physiol* 276: C1053-1060.

Wang J, Liu R, Hawkins M, Barzilai N, Rossetti L (1998) A nutrient-sensing pathway regulates leptin gene expression in muscle and fat. *Nature* 393: 684-688.

Wright EM, Hirsch JR, Loo DD, Zampighi GA (1997) Regulation of Na+/glucose cotransporters. *J Exp Biol* 200: 287-293.

Wright EM, Hirayama BA & Loo DF (2007) Active sugar transport in health and disease. *J Int Med* 261, 32-43.

Wright EM, Loo DD, Hirayama BA (2011) Biology of human sodium glucose transporters. *Physiol Rev* 91: 733-794.

Yamagishi SI, Edelstein D, Du XL, Kaneda Y, Guzman M, et al.(2001) Leptin induces mitochondrial superoxide production and monocyte chemoattractant protein-1 expression in aortic endothelial cells by increasing fatty acid oxidation via protein kinase A. *J Biol Chem* 276: 25096-25100.

Yamashita T, Murakami T, Otani S, Kuwajima M, Shima K (1998) Leptin receptor signal transduction: OBRa and OBRb of fa type. *Biochem Biophys Res Commun* 246: 752-759.

Yang G, Ge H, Boucher A, Yu X, Li C (2004) Modulation of direct leptin signaling by soluble leptin receptor. *Mol Endocrinol* 18: 1354-1362.

Yarandi SS, Hebbar G, Sauer CG, Cole CR, Ziegler TR (2011) Diverse roles of leptin in the gastrointestinal tract: modulation of motility, absorption, growth, and inflammation. *Nutrition* 27(3): 269-75.

Zhang Y, Proenca R, Maffei M, Barone M, Leopold L, et al.(1994) Positional cloning of the mouse obese gene and its human homologue. *Nature* 372: 425-432.

In: Leptin: Biosynthesis, Functions and Clinical Significance ISBN: 978-1-62948-801-1
Editor: Edward L. Blum

Chapter 7

IMPLICATIONS OF LEPTIN IN MALE REPRODUCTIVE FUNCTION

Luc J. Martin*
Biology Department, Université de Moncton, Moncton, New-Brunswick, Canada

ABSTRACT

Obesity is associated with reduced quality of life, increased subfertility, and increased morbidity for diseases as a result of reduced testosterone production in aging males. Leptin is a metabolic hormone produced by white adipose tissue whose production is directly correlated with the level of obesity. It is well documented that leptin has influences on the physiology of reproduction. Indeed, leptin interacts with its receptor at every levels of the hypothalamus-pituitary-gonads (HPG) axis in males. However, most obese individuals develop a functional leptin resistance, rendering them insensitive to increased endogenous leptin concentrations. Such alterations in leptin signaling can lead to abnormal functioning of the endocrine and reproductive systems. In males, an inability of leptin action may contribute to hypogonadism and male infertility. Indeed, leptin resistance or leptin insufficiency impairs the hypothalamic function and normal physiology of the testis. In this chapter, we will do an update on the mechanisms of action of leptin at each components of the HPG axis. Furthermore, the effects of leptin on testosterone production and spermatogenesis in relation to male reproduction will be discussed.

* Corresponding author: Dr. Luc J. Martin, Biology Department, Université de Moncton, 18, avenue Antonine Maillet, Moncton, New-Brunswick, CANADA E1A 3E9, Tel: 506-858-4937, Fax: 506-858-4541, E-mail: Luc.Martin@umoncton.ca.

INTRODUCTION

Incidence of Obesity

Obesity, defined by a body mass index (BMI) of more than 30 kg/m^2, is a major health problem having variable incidences worldwide, depending on social, cultural and economic factors. According to a study from the World Health Organization in 2008, more than 35 % of adults aged 20 and over were overweight (BMI over 25 kg/m^2) and 11 % were obese (BMI over 30 kg/m^2). In the U.S., the obesity level in adult men reaches more than 35 % [1]. Negative impact of obesity on health is linked to body fat accumulation in the central abdominal region, suggesting that waist circumference should be a more appropriate indicator of obesity than BMI.

Health Impact of Obesity

Individuals suffering from obesity have increased susceptibility for several diseases, including type 2 diabetes, cardiovascular diseases, respiratory disorders, immune malfunction, endocrine disorders, certain hormone-dependent cancers (such as endometrial, breast and prostate) and decreased fertility [2]. In recent years, male sperm counts has been estimated to decline by nearly 1.5% per year in the North American population and this tendency may be attributed to increased obesity incidence [3]. Indeed, obesity might contribute to male subfertility, particularly in young men (20-30 years old) where total sperm counts are inversely correlated to BMI [4]. Although obese men have reduced sperm concentration, sperm morphology and motility appear unaffected [5], suggesting that the condition of obesity has no major effect on sperm quality. Reduced testosterone levels in obese men may be associated to delayed onset and maintenance of sperm production, resulting in a subfertility condition.

In men, abdominal obesity is correlated with lower testosterone levels and a greater decrease in testosterone production with aging [6,7]. Indeed, free testosterone decreases by 1.2%, and albumin-bound testosterone by 1.0% per year in aging men [8]. In addition, obesity is also linked to a reduction in levels of sex hormone-binding globulin (SHBG) [9,10]. Such decline in SHBG synthesis and secretion by the liver may be associated to hyperinsulinemia, secondary to obesity-related insulin resistance [11,12]. Decreased SHBG binding capacity may be a consequence of low serum testosterone concentrations [13] as a result of a direct action of leptin and other adipose-derived hormones on testicular function [14–16]. To exacerbate this condition, low testosterone concentrations may contribute to the accumulation of abdominal fat [17–19] by reducing lipolysis in the abdominal region [20], thus creating a cycle exacerbating the condition of obesity in men.

In addition to a good maintenance of reproductive function, appropriate levels of testosterone in men are also important to avoid the onset of conditions related to aging, generally known as andropause. Indeed, lower testosterone levels are associated to the development of cardiovascular diseases and shorter life expectancy in men [21]. The inhibitory effect of obesity on female reproduction has been well covered [22,23]. The current chapter will highlight recent findings on molecular mechanisms initiated by leptin at each components of the HPG axis. Furthermore, the effects of leptin on testosterone production and spermatogenesis in relation to male reproduction will be covered.

LEPTIN

The adipose-derived hormone leptin, encoded by the *Ob* gene, is known to regulate feeding behavior and energy metabolism, as well as to have a significant impact on reproduction and fertility in mammals. Different animal models were used to establish the significance of leptin in the regulation of the hypothalamic-pituitary-gonadal (HPG) axis (reviewed in [24]). In addition, human families with congenital leptin deficiency have been reported with symptoms such as childhood obesity, hyperphagia, hypogonadotropic hypogonadism and delayed onset of puberty [25–27]. Interestingly, human leptin receptor mutations usually results in less severe phenotypes than those with leptin deficiency [28]. In genetically obese *Ob/Ob*$^{(-/-)}$ male mice, leptin treatment not only reduces food consumption and body weight gain, but also restores reproductive function [29,30]. In humans, normal sex hormones production and fertility require adequate leptin secretion. Increased leptin circulating levels, leading to hormonal resistance in obese individuals, may contribute to the development of androgen deficiency in obese men [16].

Recently, it has been demonstrated that inhibition of the action of ghrelin in *Ob/Ob*$^{(-/-)}$ mice improved male infertility [31], suggesting that the reproductive phenotype of leptin deficiency is in part associated to ghrelin. The hormone ghrelin is expressed primarily in the stomach and hypothalamus and has the ability to stimulate food intake and release of growth hormone [32]. In addition, ghrelin has also been localized in fetal and adult-type Leydig cells of the rat testis [33], thus suggesting a paracrine action of this hormone at the testicular level. In human testis, ghrelin production by Leydig cells is inversely correlated to serum testosterone concentrations [34]. In the *Ob/Ob*$^{(-/-)}$ testis, ghrelin signaling is up-regulated, contributing to reduced androgen synthesis and increased germ cell apoptosis [31].

In human testis, leptin can be found in seminiferous tubules and spermatozoa [35]. However, the source of leptin involved in the regulation of male reproductive function may come from the testis itself and/or other body regions, since this hormone is able to pass through the blood-testis barrier [36]. The leptin receptor has been characterized on different cell types of the testis, including Leydig, Sertoli and testicular germ cells in rodents [14,37], and cells from the seminiferous tubules in humans [35,38]. Together, these results support a possible role of leptin in the modulation of testicular functions [39,40].

Leptin Receptors (Ob-R)

Six isoforms are obtained from alternative splicing of the *Ob-R* gene transcript and are classified as long (Ob-Rb), short (Ob-Ra, Ob-Rc, Ob-Rd and Ob-Rf) and secreted (Ob-Re) receptor types. With the longest intracellular domain, Ob-Rb is the only functional isoform of the hypothalamus able to activate cell signaling in this tissue [41]. The shortest isoform, Ob-Re, lacks the trans-membrane and intracellular domains and is a soluble leptin receptor isoform that might interact with circulating leptin to regulate its bioavailability [42]. While

Ob-Rb is mainly expressed in the hypothalamus, Ob-Ra is rather found in peripheral tissues of most species investigated [43]. Moreover, leptin activates signal transducer and activator of transcription 3 (STAT3) in the hypothalamus, whereas such regulation is not consistent in other cell types. Thus, Ob-Ra may activate STAT transcription factors other than STAT3 in peripheral tissues and may involve the mitogen-activated protein kinase (MAPK) signaling pathway.

Expression profiles for leptin and Ob-R in the testis appear to be species-specific (Table 1). In the rat testis, Ob-R is detected only on Leydig cells [14]. However, others have shown that *Ob-R* mRNA is transcribed in adult rats Sertoli cells using *in situ* hybridization [44]. Thus, the lack of protein detection inside seminiferous tubules suggests that the antibody used against Ob-R in immunohistochemistry might not be sensitive enough for proper detection on Sertoli cells. In contrast to rat testis, Ob-R protein is detected only in seminiferous tubules and is located on germ cells in neonatal and adult mouse testis [37]. In fertile men, Ob-R protein is restricted to Leydig cells, whereas leptin is produced by spermatocytes [35]. Ob-R expression in Leydig cells is inversely correlated to circulating testosterone levels. In addition, increases in testicular leptin and Ob-R expression levels is correlated with abnormalities in sperm production [35]. In pigs, the expressions of leptin and of its receptor are limited to the interstitial compartment of the immature testis, whereas both proteins are detected in Leydig cells and seminiferous tubules of mature gonads [45]. This suggests a potential role of leptin in endocrine and/or autocrine/paracrine regulation of porcine male reproduction. In addition to its role in pig testis, leptin might also be involved in sperm capacitation by interacting with its receptor on the acrosome [46]. A similar regulatory mechanism could be attributed to leptin in human as leptin and its receptor have also been identified in human spermatozoa [47].

Since Ob-R has been characterized in different cell types of the testis, its leptin dependent activation might involve cell-specific signal transduction pathways. However, testicular action of leptin might also involve specific isoforms, such as Ob-Ra. Nonetheless, the expression pattern of this isoform is not sufficiently documented to show its involvement in leptin regulation of testicular function. Interestingly, perinatal malnutrition seems to have a stimulatory effect on the expression of leptin receptors isoforms in the testis of adult rats [57]. Indeed, maternal nutritional restrictions affect sexual maturation, testosterone and LH serum levels, as well as testicular function and fertility in male rats [58].

Ob-Rb isoform has three conserved tyrosine residues (Y985, Y1077 and Y1138 according to mouse receptor sequence) important for cytoplasmic signal transduction. The critical role of Y1138 is underscored by the severe phenotype of obesity observed in male and female knock-in mice harboring a Y1138S mutation in Ob-Rb [59]. Phosphorylation of Y985 of Ob-Rb contributes to the recruitment of the suppressor of cytokine signaling (SOCS)-3 protein, a potent inhibitor of leptin signaling [60].

Cell signaling involved following activation of Ob-R

More research is needed to better define leptin receptor signaling in peripheral tissues and the involvement of members of the STAT family of transcription factors. In male rodents, activation of Ob-Rb by leptin modulates a cascade of intracellular signal transduction pathways, including the Janus kinase 2 (JAK2)/STAT3 [61], PI3K [62], 5'-AMP-activated protein kinase (AMPK) [63,64] and MAPK pathways such as extracellular signal-related kinases 1 and 2 (ERK1/2), c-Jun amino-terminal kinases (JNK), and p38 [65,66].

Table 1. Expression profiles of leptin and its functional receptor (Ob-Rb) in male gonads according to species

Cell types	Species	Experimental evidences*	References
Leptin			
Seminiferous tubules (spermatocytes) (adults)	Human, Rat	IH	[35,48]
Leydig cells (2-3 and 18-24 months old, adults)	Pig, Rat	IH	[45,48]
Elongated spermatids and epididymis (18-24 months old)	Pig	IH	[45]
Spermatozoa	Human, Pig	RT-PCR, WB, IF	[47,49]
Spermatocytes (PND20, adult)	Mouse	IH	[50]
Leptin receptor (Ob-R)			
Fetal Leydig cells (E19.5)	Rat	IH	[14]
Prepubertal and adult Leydig cells (PND 21, 35, 60 and 90)	Rat	IH, RT-PCR	[14,48,51,52]
Adult Leydig and Sertoli cells (PND 75)	Rat	ISH	[44]
Type A spermatogonia (PND5 and 20)	Mouse	IH	[37]
Leydig cells (PND5 and 20, adult)	Mouse	IH	[37,53]
Adult Leydig cells	Human	IH	[35]
Leydig cells and epididymis (2-3 and 18-24 months old)	Pig	IH	[45]
Spermatozoa	Boar	IF, RT-PCR	[46]
Spermatozoa and epididymis	Pig	RT-PCR, WB, IF	[49]
Spermatozoa	Bovine	RT-PCR	[54,55]
Spermatozoa	Human	IF, WB	[56]

*IH, immunohistochemistry; IF, immunofluorescence; ISH, *in situ* hybridization; WB, western blot; RT-PCR, reverse transcriptase PCR.

For the JAK2/STAT3 pathway, leptin-induced grouping of Ob-Rb activates JAK2 [67] (see Figure 1). Activated JAK2 phosphorylates Ob-Rb on Y985, Y1077 and Y1138 of the intracellular domain [68]. Phosphorylated Y1138 recruits STAT3 to the Ob-Rb-JAK2 complex [69–71], where JAK2 phosphorylates it at Y705 (of the murine STAT3 sequence). The subsequent dimerization and nuclear translocation of STAT3 result in the alteration of target cell transcription and function [72]. Interestingly, genetically modified male mice with Ob-Rb neurons having STAT3 disruption on a mixed genetic background exhibit severe obesity and normal fertility [73]. Although the genetic background of mice models might influence STAT3 inactivation phenotypes, these results indicate that leptin's effects on male reproduction involve signaling pathways other than STAT3 and/or that leptin-dependent regulation of reproduction at the CNS level might involve a mechanism independent of Ob-Rb.

Following Ob-Rb activation, leptin signaling is subject to negative feedback regulation, especially with obesity and resulting hyperleptinemia [74]. Expression of a major inhibitor of leptin signaling, SOCS3, is induced by the JAK2/STAT3 pathway. Once activated, SOCS3 inhibits the phosphorylation and activation of JAK2 and Ob-Rb tyrosine residue Y985 [75], contributing to leptin resistance. Indeed, leptin administration to SOCS3 male and female knockout mice results in increased STAT3 expression and greater weight loss [76,77]. Another negative regulator of STAT3-dependent gene regulation is the SH2-containing phosphatase-2 (SHP-2), which is also activated by leptin [78]. The phosphorylated Y985 site of Ob-Rb is involved in the recruitment and association of SHP-2 [78,79].

In addition to its repressive effects, SHP-2 might also act as a positive regulator of leptin signaling through activation of the MAPK pathway. Indeed, interaction between SHP-2 and phosphorylated Y985 may be followed by recruitment of the adapter protein growth receptor bound 2 (Grb-2) and activation of the Ras/Raf pathway [80,81]. This secondary pathway for leptin involves the recruitment of JAK2 and the phosphatase activity of SHP-2. The MAPK pathway is involved in leptin-induced cFos activation in male rat subcutaneous preadipocytes [82], in placental BeWo cells [83] and mouse neurotensin-expressing hypothalamic neurons [84]. Interestingly, cFos has been shown to repress steroidogenic gene expression in adrenal [85] and Leydig cells [86], raising a possibility that leptin represses testosterone production in the testis through cFos activation. In addition, SOCS3 may also function as an adapter protein to other signaling pathways involved in the inhibition of testosterone production from Leydig cells.

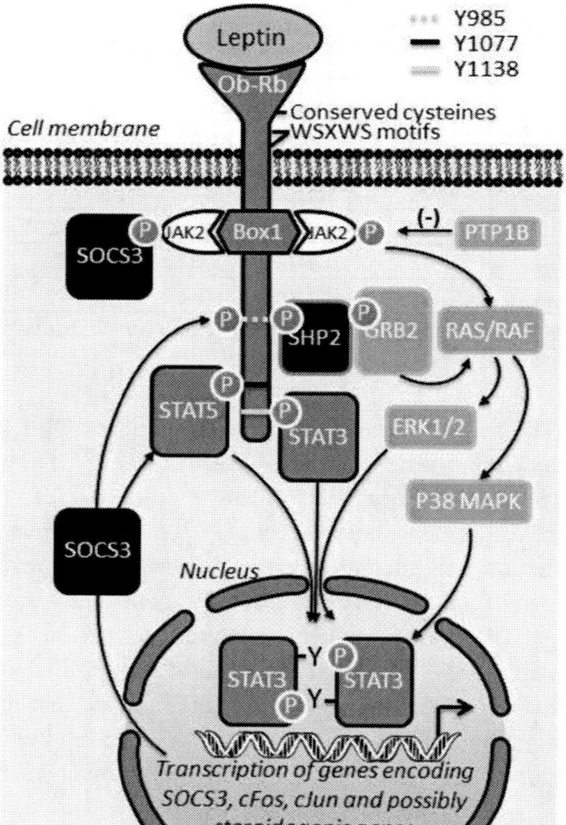

Figure 1. Leptin-dependent activation of its receptor Ob-Rb resulting in modulation of various signal transduction pathways and transcriptional regulation of target genes, which may be involved in the regulation of testicular steroidogenesis. See text for a detailed description.

Although disruption of Ob-Rb/STAT3 signaling contributes to obesity in mice, fertility in these mice models seems normal, suggesting the involvement of additional leptin-dependent regulators. Indeed, inactivation of the cyclic AMP responsive element-binding protein-1 (Creb1)-regulated transcription coactivator-1 (Crtc1) in male and female *Crtc1*$^{(-/-)}$ mice results in hyperphagia, obesity and infertility [87]. This Creb1-Crtc1 pathway might contribute to the action of leptin on energy balance and fertility at the hypothalamic level.

Activated Ob-Rb, resulting in phosphorylation of its Y1077, might also lead to recruitment and activation of STAT5. Indeed, leptin stimulation of STAT5 phosphorylation and nuclear translocation has been reported in the hypothalamus [88,89]. In addition, leptin also activated STAT1 and AP-1 family members in mouse adipose tissue [90]. Since STAT1/3/5 and AP-1 members are being expressed in testicular Leydig cells [91,92], these transcription factors might be involved in leptin dependent regulation of testosterone production in males.

Factors contributing to leptin resistance

With obesity, most individuals become insensitive to circulating leptin and develop a functional leptin resistance. Several mechanisms may be implicated in leptin resistance: Saturation of leptin transport across the blood-brain barrier, inhibition of leptin receptor activation and/or signal transduction and increased leptin receptor degradation [80,93].

Leptin's transport through the blood-brain barrier involves the short isoform of leptin receptor (Ob-Ra), found in the choroid plexus [94]. This transport saturates at a leptin concentration of 5-10 ng/ml [95]. However, several factors may influence the transport of leptin across the blood-brain barrier. Indeed, increased circulating triglycerides levels during obesity have an inhibitory effect on the accumulation of leptin in the cerebrospinal fluid [96]. Moreover, leptin transport across the blood-brain barrier might be influenced by hormonal changes, as shown with increased prolactin levels during pregnancy [97].

Leptin receptor signal transduction is downregulated by two mediators, SOCS3 and PTP1B, leading to leptin resistance. Indeed, SOCS3 inhibits JAK2/STAT3 [75] and AMPK [98] activations in response to leptin interaction with its receptor. In mouse NPY neurons, overexposure to leptin results in reduced AMPK signaling and NPY secretion [99]. Others have shown that activation of hypothalamic cAMP-regulated guanine nucleotide exchange factor for the small G protein Rap1 (cAMP-Epac) pathway, independent of PKA activation, is sufficient to induce leptin resistance [100]. In addition, direct inhibition of the receptor via other mechanisms, including receptor targeting to the proteasome, might also be involved in leptin resistance.

PTP1B, also involved in leptin resistance, decreases JAK2 phosphorylation, resulting in lower phosphorylation of STAT3 [101]. Moreover, PTP1B is also involved in a specific form of leptin resistance caused by stress signals disrupting the endoplasmic reticulum function, leading to accumulation of unfolded proteins [102]. The implications of PTP1B in regulation of male reproduction remain to be investigated.

In the testis, the blood-testis barrier may not contribute to local leptin resistance [103]. As opposed to the blood-brain barrier, leptin transport through the blood-testis barrier appears to be nonsaturable [36]. Thus, this would mean that when plasma leptin concentrations increase, Sertoli, germinal and Leydig cells would be exposed to increasing concentrations of leptin.

Regulation of Hypothalamus and Pituitary Functions by Leptin

In addition to its effects on eating behavior and energy regulation, leptin also affects reproduction, immunity, and inflammation through actions on the hypothalamus and pituitary. The HPG axis plays a major role in the regulation of testicular function. Hypothalamic neurons release gonadotropin-releasing hormone (GnRH), which stimulates the secretion of pituitary gonadotropins, luteinizing hormone (LH) and follicle-stimulating hormone (FSH) (Figure 2). These hormones regulate testicular steroidogenesis and spermatogenesis, respectively. In morbidly obese men, central leptin insufficiency triggers the development of hypogonadotropic hypogonadism by decreasing circulating gonadotropins [104–106] and subsequently inducing the apoptosis of testicular cells [107]. In *Ob/Ob*$^{(-/-)}$ mice, gonadotropins and sex-steroid hormones are low, consistent with the developing condition of hypogonadotropic hypogonadism and a role for leptin in the regulation of the HPG axis [39].

In the hypothalamus and pituitary, leptin modulates the secretions of GnRH, FSH, LH, ACTH, cortisol, and GH [39,108]. In the absence of leptin resistance, leptin stimulates GnRH secretion by the hypothalamus and gonadotropins LH and FSH secretions by the pituitary [109,110] (Figure 2). Leptin's action on the modulation of GnRH secretion is indirect, since leptin receptors are not present on GnRH secreting neurons [111–113].

Leptin might regulate reproductive function by influencing the activity of neurons linked to hypothalamic GnRH secreting neurons [114], such as agouti-related peptide/neuropeptide Y (AgRP/NPY) and proopiomelanocortin/cocaine- and amphetamine-regulated transcript (POMC/CART) neurons (Figure 3). Leptin inhibits neuropeptide Y (NPY) release, which is involved in the downregulation of gonadotropin secretion [115]. In addition, melanocortin (MC) signaling also plays a major role in this indirect action of leptin on the hypothalamus [116]. However, the actions of leptin on POMC/CART neurons producing melanocortin are not critical for reproductive function, as shown using conditional *Ob-R* knockouts specific to POMC neurons [117]. In the arcuate nucleus, Ob-R co-localizes with POMC, AgRP/NPY and kisspeptins (Kiss1) neurons [118–120]. Therefore, leptin may also act indirectly to regulate gonadotropin secretion in the hypothalamus by modulating kisspeptins secretion in the arcuate nucleus [121]. Indeed, leptin-deficient *Ob/Ob*$^{(-/-)}$ male mice also exhibit reduced expression of the *Kiss1* gene in the arcuate nucleus, which is partially restored by leptin treatment [120]. However, total hypothalamic expression of Kiss1 (which includes the preoptic area and the arcuate nucleus) was not affected in *Ob/Ob*$^{(-/-)}$ mice, except when combined with food-restriction [122].

Using the *SF-1* gene promoter to control Cre expression in ventromedial nucleus of the hypothalamus (VMH), a physiological role of the VMH in leptin's effect on energy homeostasis has been demonstrated [123,124]. However, cell-specific deletion of *Ob-R* in VMH neurons did not affect reproduction, suggesting that leptin signaling in the VMH is not required for leptin's effects on reproduction in mice. Interestingly, bilateral lesions of the ventral premammillary nucleus (PMV) in *Ob/Ob*$^{(-/-)}$ mice reduced the actions of leptin treatments on sexual maturation [125]. Therefore, the PMV is a critical site for the permissive action of leptin to initiate puberty.

In addition to its stimulatory effect on the hypothalamus, leptin also has direct actions on the anterior pituitary [110]. Ob-R is expressed in nearly 90% of the gonadotropes in the pars tuberalis and 30% of the gonadotropes in the pars distalis [126]. Interestingly, leptin is also produced by gonadotropes and somatotropes in response to GnRH, NPY and growth-hormone-releasing hormone (GHRH) [127–129], suggesting autocrine and/or paracrine actions of leptin in the pituitary. In male pituitary, leptin is mainly produced by somatotropes [128]. Leptin may directly stimulate LH and FSH secretions from the pituitary, possibly through nitric oxide synthase activation in gonadotrope cells [130]. In pituitary of pro-estrus rats, use of a competitive inhibitor of NO synthase (NOS), N^G-monomethyl-L-arginine (NMMA), completely suppressed leptin dependent secretion of LH [131]. However, the signaling mechanisms involved in leptin's action in the pituitary and the implications in male reproduction remain to be determined.

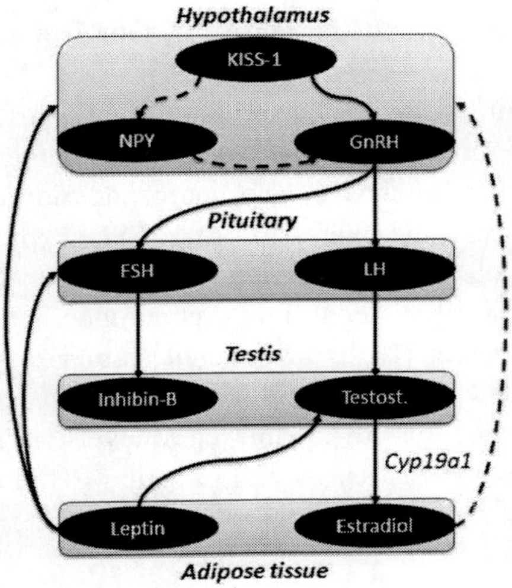

Figure 2. Influences of normal leptin levels on the male hypothalamus-pituitary-gonadal axis. Stimulatory and inhibitory actions are denoted with solid and dashed lines, respectively.

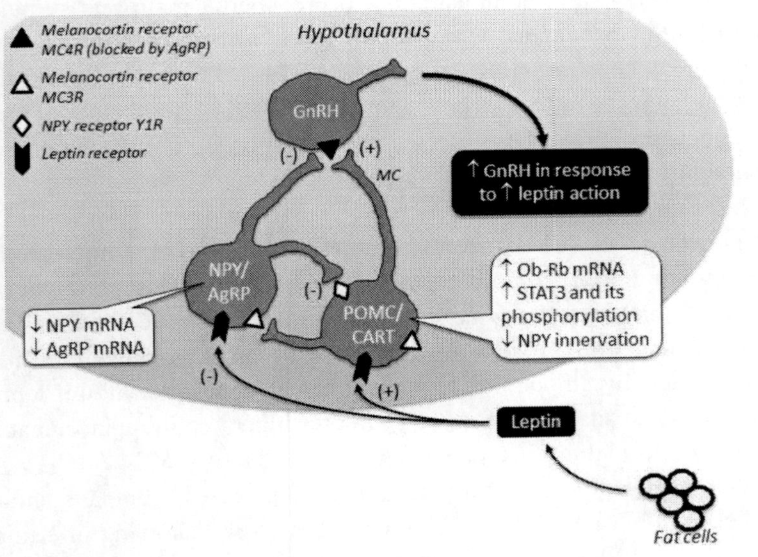

Figure 3. Regulation of GnRH secretion by leptin at the hypothalamic level. Under normal conditions, leptin is produced by the adipocytes and influences several groups of neurons from the hypothalamus, leading to an increase in GnRH production. See text for description.

Leptin regulates a population of neurons located mainly in the arcuate nucleus, expressing either orexigenic (NPY and AgRP) or anorexigenic (POMC and CART) peptides [132]. Leptin alters the state of hypogonadism in lean animals by increasing the expression of *POMC* gene, transport and acylation of melanocortins in the brain [133]. Food restriction leads to a modulation of the expression of *NPY* gene during the phase of low leptin production [134] and the action of leptin on LH secretion also depends on the availability of glucose [135]. Indeed, the increase in hypothalamic *NPY* gene expression by caloric restriction may result from the coordinated action of several factors, including the decrease in serum levels of leptin and insulin [136]. Others have shown that increased levels of NPY can stimulate feeding behavior and inhibit the release of GnRH during certain periods of food supply [114,137].

Kisspeptin and NPY neurons are considered good candidates for linking perturbations in the energy balance with alterations in proper functioning of the reproductive axis. NPY, a potent orexigenic neuropeptide involved in the neuroendocrine control of the reproductive axis, may metabolically regulate the expression of KISS-1 expression in the hypothalamus [122,138]. In addition, the role of KISS-1/kisspeptin/GPR54 system as protector of GnRH neurons and involved in the metabolic control of the reproductive axis has been demonstrated [139,140]. The short-term fasting (72 h) in pubertal animals causes a decrease in KISS-1 mRNA expression, associated with reduced LH in both males and females rats [139]. However, others have suggested that low serum leptin levels are not entirely responsible for the inhibitions of the arcuate nucleus Kiss-1 and of serum LH levels during negative energy balance [141].

Leptin as an initiator of puberty

Leptin is known to be an important modulator of the onset of puberty [142–144]. Indeed, early onset of reproductive function has been observed following leptin treatment of normal female mice [108,145]. Leptin administration to prepubertal male rats stimulated pulsatile GnRH secretion [146]. In humans, leptin serum levels in boys peaked just before puberty, reaching an average concentration of 3.6 ng/ml [147,148]. Prepubertal peak of serum leptin levels precedes the increase in free serum testosterone [149]. After the initial prepubertal rise, serum leptin concentration in boys decreases in response to the suppressive action of testosterone on leptin production, whereas higher serum leptin levels during the late stages of puberty in girls may be associated to the increase in estrogen levels [148,150,151]. According to age and body mass index (BMI), serum leptin concentrations in women are higher than in men [152], suggesting that sex differences in leptin concentrations may result from differences in sex hormones, such as estradiol and testosterone [153–155]. Indeed, sex steroids do modulate leptin production and secretion in an opposite manner: estrogens stimulate leptin release by adipocytes *in vitro*, whereas androgens inhibit leptin production and secretion from white adipose tissue [156]. Interestingly, leptin replacement has also been linked to recovery of normal testosterone levels in starved men [157].

The implication of leptin in puberty is further supported by humans and mice lacking leptin or Ob-R (*Ob/Ob*$^{(-/-)}$ and *Obr/Obr*$^{(-/-)}$ mice, respectively) showing infertility and failure to begin puberty [125]. Overall, low leptin concentrations serves as a nutrient sensor to provide a hormonal signal to the brain that the environmental conditions may not be favorable for reproduction due to limited food availability [158], leading to a decrease in testosterone production in the male. According to this, restoring normal leptin levels in animal and human models results in normalization of the HPG axis, reversal of infertility and recovery of delayed puberty [29,30,159,160]. In obese adolescents, hyperleptinemia (10-45 ng/ml) is inversely correlated with insulin-like factor 3 (INSL3) serum levels, suggesting that testicular Leydig cells' are functionally impaired during puberty in boys suffering from obesity [161]. Interestingly, stimulation of prepubertal Leydig cells with leptin has been shown to decrease cell division through increased cyclin D1 expression [51], supporting steroidogenic genes expression. Altogether, leptin is a permissive factor to the onset of puberty, and, although some minimal threshold level of leptin is required for pubertal development, leptin is not sufficient to initiate puberty.

Regulation of Steroidogenesis by Leptin

In males, increased serum leptin levels associated with obesity (usually more than two times the normal leptin concentrations at prepubertal stage) has deleterious effects on androgen production and spermatogenesis [16]. Indeed, increased leptin concentrations to 20 ng/ml results in decreased serum concentrations of testosterone through a Ob-R mediated inhibition of Leydig cells' function [16,52]. Leydig cells are the main cells synthesizing androgens in the male gonads. Regulated by pituitary LH, testosterone is synthesized from cholesterol under the action of a cascade of steroidogenic enzymes. In older men, testicular testosterone production and its serum concentrations decline gradually, possibly involving altered Leydig cells function. This decrease results in changes in the proportion of body fat, decreased energy and muscle strength, as well as subfertility [162]. A condition precipitating such age related symptoms might be the increase in obesity and the resulting changes in hormones production by adipocytes, leading to repression of steroidogenesis in Leydig cells.

Regulation of normal male reproduction by the hormone leptin may include actions at every levels of the hypothalamus-pituitary-testicular axis. Indeed, high levels of leptin also appears to have inhibitory effects on testicular steroidogenesis, which may explain the link between hyperleptinaemia and decreased testosterone levels in obese men [40]. It has been shown that leptin inhibits hCG-induced testosterone production in prepubertal and adult male rats' testes [163]. In adult rat testis, mRNA expressions of several steroidogenic genes, such as steroidogenic factor-1 (*Nr5a1*), steroidogenic acute regulatory protein (*StAR*) and cytochrome P450 cholesterol side-chain cleavage enzyme (*Cyp11a1*), are decreased in response to leptin, leading to reduced testosterone production [44,164]. Moreover, hCG-stimulated cytochrome P450 17α-hydroxylase/17,20 lyase/17,20 desmolase (*Cyp17a1*) steroidogenic enzyme expression is also inhibited by leptin in rat Leydig cells [52]. Leptin actions in rodent models are consistent with those observed in humans where obese men have elevated leptin serum concentrations inversely correlated with androgen levels [165]. However, the signal transduction pathways implicated after Ob-R activation in the testis remain to be characterized. In other types of cells, leptin signaling usually activates the JAK/STAT signaling pathway [80,166].

In Leydig cells, potential interplay between the JAK/STAT pathway and the adenylate cyclase-cAMP-PKA pathway, stimulated by leptin and LH, respectively, might regulate testosterone production. In granulosa cells, STAT3 activation modulates the expressions of steroidogenic genes including *Nr5a1*, *StAR* and *Cyp11a1* [167]. In the human granulosa cells, leptin inhibition of steroidogenesis involves downregulation of cAMP signaling through the

MAPK pathway, leading to decreased StAR protein expression and reduced progesterone production [168]. The involvement of such signaling pathways in the regulation of Leydig cells steroidogenesis by leptin remains to be elucidated.

Recently, it has been suggested that hypoxia might induce leptin expression and modulate steroidogenic gene expression, thus leading to increased testosterone (by up-regulating *cyp11a* and *hsd3b*) and decreased estradiol (by down-regulating *cyp19a*) productions in zebrafish [169]. This transcriptional regulation of leptin in response to hypoxia might be mediated by the hypoxia-inducible factor 1 (HIF-1), a transcription factor that plays a central role in regulation of oxygen homeostasis [170]. Interestingly, hypoxia and HIF-1 can increase the expression of leptin in trophoblast-derived BeWo cells [171]. Such leptin dependent regulation of testicular steroidogenesis in response to hypoxia needs further investigation.

In the presence of increased leptin levels, leptin's repressive action on steroidogenic gene expression will reduce LH-mediated testosterone production. Leptin's inhibitory action on steroidogenesis in Leydig cells constitutes another regulatory mechanism of reproductive functions. Leptin is not only released in the bloodstream, but also secreted in seminiferous tubules as well as from germ cells, while its receptor is expressed on Leydig cells (see Table 1). Being able to cross the blood-testis barrier [36], leptin might have paracrine actions in the testis leading to regulation of testosterone production by influences on testicular Leydig cells. Indeed, leptin receptors are expressed in rodents [14,37,52,53] and human [35] Leydig cells (see Table 1), thus supporting the presence of a leptin regulatory mechanism for the modulation of Leydig cell functions in these species. According to Ob-R expression profiles during development, Leydig cells exhibit different levels of sensitivity to leptin, such that embryonic and adult but not prepubertal rat Leydig cells show leptin inhibitory actions on hCG-induced testosterone production [14,172].

Another element reducing testosterone levels in obese men is the increased aromatization of testosterone to estradiol in peripheral fat tissues [17], leading to modulations of the HPG axis [173,174] (see Figure 2). Furthermore, such conversion might contribute to decreased plasma testosterone concentrations [175,176]. Low testosterone levels may increase the activity of the hypothalamic–pituitary–adrenal axis and trigger the development of visceral obesity [18] by reducing abdominal fat lipolysis [177]. Low testosterone levels may also contribute to the development of insulin resistance and type 2 diabetes [178,179]. In addition, men with various levels of glucose tolerance show a consistent reduction in total and free testosterone levels following standard glucose load ingestion [180], implementing a feedback loop aggravating the condition. In men, low testosterone serum concentrations are associated with increased risk of developing metabolic syndrome with aging [181].

In infertile men with disorders such as obstructive azoospermia, Sertoli cell-only syndrome and varicocele, Ob-R expression in Leydig cells is inversely correlated with the serum testosterone levels [35]. Thus, over-expression of Ob-R in Leydig cells appears to inhibit testosterone production in such conditions. Therefore, leptin does not only have stimulatory effects on pituitary secretions of LH and FSH [110,128,130,131,182], but also on Leydig cells to regulate steroidogenesis. However, the molecular mechanism(s) and signaling pathway(s) implicated in leptin's influence on gene expression in Leydig cells needs further investigation.

Interestingly, increased serum testosterone concentrations may lead to reduced leptin levels in the bloodstream. Indeed, this may be attributed to the suppressive effect of testosterone and of its biologically active metabolite dihydrotestosterone (DHT) on leptin production [19,183].

Regulation of Spermatogenesis by Leptin

In men and rodents, obesity results in altered spermatic function with reduced sperm concentration, motility and viability [184–186]. Lower sperm quality causes a reduction in fertility potential [184], supporting that obesity may result in subfertility in males. The production and secretion of leptin in bovine, pig and human spermatozoa [54] suggests a paracrine/autocrine action of this hormone in sperm physiology. Moreover, prostate gland and seminal vesicles may be other sources of leptin in seminal plasma, as shown using immunohistochemical localization [187].

Interestingly, leptin deficiency in mice results in impaired spermatogenesis and infertility, likely due to insufficient gonadotropin support of spermatogenesis and increased germ cell death by apoptosis [188,189]. Indeed, testicular sections from $Ob/Ob^{(-/-)}$ male mice display reduced seminiferous tubule area, fewer pachytene spermatocytes, and fewer tubules with elongated spermatids and mature spermatozoa [188]. Leptin-deficient $Ob/Ob^{(-/-)}$ mice also show upregulated expression of nine testicular pro-apoptotic genes [188]. Impaired spermatogenesis, as observed in leptin deficient mice, might explain, in part, the reduced quality of sperm resulting from obesity and leptin resistance. The leptin-receptor-deficient Zucker rat is known for complete sterility of females [190] and reduced reproductive capacity of males in an age-dependent manner [191,192]. This experimental model has been shown to present alterations in spermatogenesis, as observed in histological sections of the testis, leading to increased sperm DNA fragmentation and subfertility of obese Zucker rats [193]. Interestingly, others have shown that leptin can affect sperm quality by inducing the production of reactive oxygen species in adult rats [194].

It has been suggested that leptin may have different effects on proliferation and differentiation of germ cells at different stages. Indeed, leptin acts on spermatogonia through phosphorylation of STAT3 to prevent cell differentiation and allowing the population of spermatogonial germ cells to renew itself. For spermatocytes, leptin rather stimulates the cells to develop into spermatids [37].

Inhibin-B, a peptide hormone produced by Sertoli cells of the seminiferous tubules, is found in lower plasma concentrations in obese young adult men compared to normal-weight men [24]. Therefore, Sertoli cells proliferation and function may be inhibited during obesity, contributing to male reproductive dysfunction. Moreover, there is a negative correlation between serum levels of leptin and inhibin B [36,195], suggesting that leptin may regulate Sertoli cells function.

Leptin has been detected in human seminal plasma [38,56,196] and its levels are inversely related to sperm concentration and sperm motility [48]. Moreover, leptin has also been detected on human ejaculated spermatozoa [47]. No major effects of leptin on motility and capacitation/acrosome reaction has been observed in human ejaculated mature spermatozoa [197]. Interestingly, combination of insulin and leptin improved human sperm motility, acrosome reaction and nitric oxide production [198], contributing to enhanced fertilization capacity of human spermatozoa through hormonal cross-talk. Interestingly, leptin concentration in seminal plasma is positively correlated with sperm concentration and motility but not with BMI [199]. However, the mechanisms of how leptin influences sperm function remain to be determined with more experiments.

Conclusion

Subfertility is a major health issue affecting more than 10% of the population in developed countries [200]. Moreover, an increasing proportion of women and men of reproductive age are overweight or obese [201]. Obese men have an increased risk of subfertility due to various factors (physical, genetic, environmental, nutritional, hormonal) resulting in endocrine disruption and abnormal semen parameters [202]. The common effect of this endocrine disturbance is the disregulation of the HPG axis. Several explanations may be obtained from animal models, showing that reduced leptin signaling in the hypothalamus leads to reduced GnRH secretion. Increased leptin resistance associated with obesity, resulting in modulation of LH and FSH secretions, may explain the correlations between BMI, altered semen parameters and subfertility. More research linking obesity to male infertility should be undertaken, especially with the increasing prevalence of this condition worldwide [202].

Lastly, a better understanding of the regulatory mechanisms of adipose derived hormones on gonadal steroidogenesis is required to ascertain the consequences of obesity on men's health. In men, the decrease of testosterone production during aging is enhanced with obesity. A decrease in testosterone production is associated with the development of certain conditions related to aging, including neurodegenerative and cardiovascular diseases, and shorter life expectancy. However, normal weight loss through changes in lifestyle results in increased total androgen concentrations and improved semen parameters in obese men [203–206].

Acknowledgments

Current work was funded by the New Brunswick Health Research Foundation (NBHRF), Canada.

Disclosure

The author declares that there is no conflict of interest that would prejudice his impartiality.

References

[1] Flegal, KM; Carroll, MD; Kit, BK; Ogden, CL. Prevalence of obesity and trends in the distribution of body mass index among US adults, 1999-2010. *JAMA*, 2012, 307, 491–7.

[2] Pi-Sunyer, FX. The obesity epidemic: pathophysiology and consequences of obesity. Obes Res 2002, 10 Suppl 2, 97S–104S.

[3] Swan, SH; Elkin, EP; Fenster, L. The question of declining sperm density revisited: an analysis of 101 studies published 1934-1996. *Environ Health Perspect*, 2000, 108, 961–6.

[4] Paasch, U; Grunewald, S; Kratzsch, J; Glander, H-J. Obesity and age affect male fertility potential. *Fertil Steril*, 2010, 94, 2898–901.

[5] Mah, PM; Wittert, GA. Obesity and testicular function. *Mol Cell Endocrinol*, 2010, 316, 180–6.

[6] Derby, CA; Zilber, S; Brambilla, D; Morales, KH; McKinlay, JB. Body mass index, waist circumference and waist to hip ratio and change in sex steroid hormones: the Massachusetts Male Ageing Study. *Clin Endocrinol*, (Oxf) 2006, 65, 125–31.

[7] Tan, RS; Pu, SJ. Impact of obesity on hypogonadism in the andropause. *Int J Androl*, 2002, 25, 195–201.

[8] Gray, A; Feldman, HA; McKinlay, JB; Longcope, C. Age, disease, and changing sex hormone levels in middle-aged men: results of the Massachusetts Male Aging Study. *J Clin Endocrinol Metab*, 1991, 73, 1016–25.

[9] Haffner, SM; Valdez, RA; Stern, MP; Katz, MS. Obesity, body fat distribution and sex hormones in men. *Int J Obes Relat Metab Disord*, 1993, 17, 643–9.

[10] Vermeulen, A. Ageing, hormones, body composition, metabolic effects. *World J Urol*, 2002, 20, 23–7.

[11] Plymate, SR; Matej, LA; Jones, RE; Friedl, KE. Inhibition of sex hormone-binding globulin production in the human hepatoma (Hep G2) cell line by insulin and prolactin. *J Clin Endocrinol Metab*, 1988, 67, 460–4.

[12] Hautanen, A. Synthesis and regulation of sex hormone-binding globulin in obesity. *Int J Obes Relat Metab Disord*, 2000, 24 Suppl 2, S64–70.

[13] Giagulli, VA; Kaufman, JM; Vermeulen, A. Pathogenesis of the decreased androgen levels in obese men. *J Clin Endocrinol Metab*, 1994, 79, 997–1000.

[14] Caprio, M; Fabbrini, E; Ricci, G; Basciani, S; Gnessi, L; Arizzi, M, et al. Ontogenesis of leptin receptor in rat Leydig cells. *Biol Reprod*, 2003, 68, 1199–207.

[15] Caminos, JE; Nogueiras, R; Gaytán, F; Pineda, R; González, CR; Barreiro, ML, et al. Novel expression and direct effects of adiponectin in the rat testis. *Endocrinology*, 2008, 149, 3390–402.

[16] Isidori, AM; Caprio, M; Strollo, F; Moretti, C; Frajese, G; Isidori, A, et al. Leptin and androgens in male obesity: evidence for leptin contribution to reduced androgen levels. *J Clin Endocrinol Metab*, 1999, 84, 3673–80.

[17] Cohen, PG. Aromatase, adiposity, aging and disease. The hypogonadal-metabolic-atherogenic-disease and aging connection. *Med Hypotheses*, 2001, 56, 702–8.

[18] Mårin, P; Arver, S. Androgens and abdominal obesity. *Baillières Clin Endocrinol Metab*, 1998, 12, 441–51.

[19] De Maddalena, C; Vodo, S; Petroni, A; Aloisi, AM. Impact of testosterone on body fat composition. *J Cell Physiol*, 2012, 227, 3744–8.

[20] Xu, X; De, Pergola, G; Björntorp, P. The effects of androgens on the regulation of lipolysis in adipose precursor cells. *Endocrinology*, 1990, 126, 1229–34.

[21] Bray, GA. Medical consequences of obesity. *J Clin Endocrinol Metab*, 2004, 89, 2583–9.

[22] Mitchell, M; Armstrong, DT; Robker, RL; Norman, RJ. Adipokines: implications for female fertility and obesity. *Reprod*, 2005, 130, 583–97.

[23] Metwally, M; Ledger, WL; Li, TC. Reproductive *Endocrinology*, and clinical aspects of obesity in women. *Ann N Y Acad Sci*, 2008, 1127, 140–6.

[24] Teerds, KJ, de Rooij, DG; Keijer, J. Functional relationship between obesity and male reproduction: from humans to animal models. *Hum Reprod Update*, 2011, 17, 667–83.

[25] Strobel, A; Issad, T; Camoin, L; Ozata, M; Strosberg, AD. A leptin missense mutation associated with hypogonadism and morbid obesity. *Nat Genet*, 1998, 18, 213–5.

[26] Ozata, M; Ozdemir, IC; Licinio, J. Human leptin deficiency caused by a missense mutation: multiple endocrine defects, decreased sympathetic tone, and immune system dysfunction indicate new targets for leptin action, greater central than peripheral resistance to the effects of leptin, and spontaneous correction of leptin-mediated defects. *J Clin Endocrinol Metab*, 1999, 84, 3686–95.

[27] Clément, K; Vaisse, C; Lahlou, N; Cabrol, S; Pelloux, V; Cassuto, D, et al. A mutation in the human leptin receptor gene causes obesity and pituitary dysfunction. *Nature*, 1998, 392, 398–401.

[28] Farooqi, IS; Wangensteen, T; Collins, S; Kimber, W; Matarese, G; Keogh, JM, et al. Clinical and molecular genetic spectrum of congenital deficiency of the leptin receptor. *N Engl J Med*, 2007, 356, 237–47.

[29] Mounzih, K; Lu, R; Chehab, FF. Leptin treatment rescues the sterility of genetically obese ob/ob males. *Endocrinology*, 1997, 138, 1190–3.

[30] Chehab, FF; Lim, ME; Lu, R. Correction of the sterility defect in homozygous obese female mice by treatment with the human recombinant leptin. *Nat Genet*, 1996, 12, 318–20.

[31] Zhu, C-C; Zhang, H; Zhang, J-S; Li, Z; Zhao, J; Li, W; et al. Inhibition of ghrelin signaling improves the reproductive phenotype of male ob/ob mouse. *Fertil Steril*, 2013, 99, 918–26.

[32] Kirchner, H; Heppner, KM; Tschöp, MH. The role of ghrelin in the control of energy balance. *Handb Exp Pharmacol*, 2012, 161–84.

[33] Tena-Sempere, M; Barreiro, ML; González, LC; Gaytán, F; Zhang, F-P; Caminos, JE, et al. Novel expression and functional role of ghrelin in rat testis. *Endocrinology*, 2002, 143, 717–25.

[34] Ishikawa, T; Fujioka, H; Ishimura, T; Takenaka, A; Fujisawa, M. Ghrelin expression in human testis and serum testosterone level. *J Androl*, 2007, 28, 320–4.

[35] Ishikawa, T; Fujioka, H; Ishimura, T; Takenaka, A; Fujisawa, M. Expression of leptin and leptin receptor in the testis of fertile and infertile patients. *Andrologia*, 2007, 39, 22–7.

[36] Banks, WA; McLay, RN; Kastin, AJ; Sarmiento, U; Scully, S. Passage of leptin across the blood-testis barrier. *Am J Physiol*, 1999, 276, E1099–1104.

[37] El-Hefnawy, T; Ioffe, S; Dym, M. Expression of the leptin receptor during germ cell development in the mouse testis. *Endocrinology*, 2000, 141, 2624–30.

[38] Glander, H-J; Lammert, A; Paasch, U; Glasow, A; Kratzsch, J. Leptin exists in tubuli seminiferi and in seminal plasma. *Andrologia*, 2002, 34, 227–33.

[39] Cunningham, MJ; Clifton, DK; Steiner, RA. Leptin's actions on the reproductive axis: perspectives and mechanisms. *Biol Reprod*, 1999, 60, 216–22.

[40] Tena-Sempere, M; Barreiro, ML. Leptin in male reproduction: the testis paradigm. *Mol Cell Endocrinol*, 2002, 188, 9–13.

[41] Tartaglia, LA. The leptin receptor. *J Biol Chem*, 1997, 272, 6093–6.

[42] Lammert, A; Kiess, W; Bottner, A; Glasow, A; Kratzsch, J. Soluble leptin receptor represents the main leptin binding activity in human blood. *Biochem Biophys Res Commun*, 2001, 283, 982–8.

[43] Margetic, S; Gazzola, C; Pegg, GG; Hill, RA. Leptin: a review of its peripheral actions and interactions. *Int J Obes Relat Metab Disord*, 2002, 26, 1407–33.

[44] Tena-Sempere, M; Manna, PR; Zhang, FP; Pinilla, L; González, LC; Diéguez, C, et al. Molecular mechanisms of leptin action in adult rat testis: potential targets for leptin-induced inhibition of steroidogenesis and pattern of leptin receptor messenger ribonucleic acid expression. *J Endocrinol*, 2001, 170, 413–23.

[45] Rago, V; Aquila, S; Guido, C; Carpino, A. Leptin and its receptor are expressed in the testis and in the epididymis of young and adult pigs. *Anat Rec Hoboken NJ*, 2007 2009, 292, 736–45.

[46] De, Ambrogi, M; Spinaci, M; Galeati, G; Tamanini, C. Leptin receptor in boar spermatozoa. *Int J Androl*, 2007, 30, 458–61.

[47] Aquila, S; Gentile, M; Middea, E; Catalano, S; Morelli, C; Pezzi, V, et al. Leptin secretion by human ejaculated spermatozoa. *J Clin Endocrinol Metab*, 2005, 90, 4753–61.

[48] Chen, B; Guo, J-H; Lu, Y-N; Ying, X-L; Hu, K; Xiang, Z-Q, et al. Leptin and varicocele-related spermatogenesis dysfunction: animal experiment and clinical study. *Int J Androl*, 2009, 32, 532–41.

[49] Aquila, S; Rago, V; Guido, C; Casaburi, I; Zupo, S; Carpino, A. Leptin and leptin receptor in pig spermatozoa: evidence of their involvement in sperm capacitation and survival. *Reprod*, 2008, 136, 23–32.

[50] Herrid, M; O'Shea, T; McFarlane, JR. Ontogeny of leptin and its receptor expression in mouse testis during the postnatal period. *Mol Reprod Dev*, 2008, 75, 874–80.

[51] Fombonne, J; Charrier, C; Goddard, I; Moyse, E; Krantic, S. Leptin-mediated decrease of cyclin A2 and increase of cyclin D1 expression: relevance for the control of prepubertal rat Leydig cell division and differentiation. *Endocrinology*, 2007, 148, 2126–37.

[52] Caprio, M; Isidori, AM; Carta, AR; Moretti, C; Dufau, ML; Fabbri, A. Expression of functional leptin receptors in rodent Leydig cells. *Endocrinology*, 1999, 140, 4939–47.

[53] De Matteis, R; Dashtipour, K; Ognibene, A; Cinti, S. Localization of leptin receptor splice variants in mouse peripheral tissues by immunohistochemistry. *Proc Nutr Soc*, 1998, 57, 441–8.

[54] Abavisani, A; Baghbanzadeh, A; Shayan, P; Dehghani, H. Leptin mRNA in bovine spermatozoa. *Res Vet Sci*, 2011, 90, 439–42.

[55] Nikbakht, G; Mehr, MRA; Baghbanzadeh, A; Tajik, P; Tamanini, C; Emam, M. Leptin receptor mRNA in bull ejaculated spermatozoa. *Reprod Domest Anim*, 2010, 45, 237–42.

[56] Jope, T; Lammert, A; Kratzsch, J; Paasch, U; Glander, H-J. Leptin and leptin receptor in human seminal plasma and in human spermatozoa. *Int J Androl*, 2003, 26, 335–41.

[57] Gombar, FM; Ramos, CF. Perinatal malnutrition programs gene expression of leptin receptors isoforms in testis and prostate of adult rats. *Regul Pept*, 2013, 184, 115–20.

[58] Zambrano, E; Rodríguez-González, GL; Guzmán, C; García-Becerra, R; Boeck, L; Díaz, L, et al. A maternal low protein diet during pregnancy and lactation in the rat impairs male reproductive development. *J Physiol*, 2005, 563, 275–84.
[59] Bates, SH; Stearns, WH; Dundon, TA; Schubert, M; Tso, AWK; Wang, Y; et al. STAT3 signalling is required for leptin regulation of energy balance but not reproduction. *Nature*, 2003, 421, 856–9.
[60] Bjorbak, C; Lavery, HJ; Bates, SH; Olson, RK; Davis, SM; Flier, JS, et al. SOCS3 mediates feedback inhibition of the leptin receptor via Tyr985. *J Biol Chem*, 2000, 275, 40649–57.
[61] Gao, Q; Horvath, TL. Cross-talk between estrogen and leptin signaling in the hypothalamus. *Am J Physiol Endocrinol Metab*, 2008, 294, E817–826.
[62] Kim, YB; Uotani, S; Pierroz, DD; Flier, JS; Kahn, BB. In vivo administration of leptin activates signal transduction directly in insulin-sensitive tissues: overlapping but distinct pathways from insulin. *Endocrinology*, 2000, 141, 2328–39.
[63] Minokoshi, Y; Kim, Y-B; Peroni, OD; Fryer, LGD; Müller, C; Carling, D, et al. Leptin stimulates fatty-acid oxidation by activating AMP-activated protein kinase. *Nature*, 2002, 415, 339–43.
[64] Lim, CT; Kola, B; Korbonits, M. AMPK as a mediator of hormonal signalling. *J Mol Endocrinol*, 2010, 44, 87–97.
[65] Séverin, S; Ghevaert, C; Mazharian, A. The mitogen-activated protein kinase signaling pathways: role in megakaryocyte differentiation. *J Thromb Haemost*, 2010, 8, 17–26.
[66] Sharma, V; Mustafa, S; Patel, N; Wambolt, R; Allard, MF; McNeill, JH. Stimulation of cardiac fatty acid oxidation by leptin is mediated by a nitric oxide-p38 MAPK-dependent mechanism. *Eur J Pharmacol*, 2009, 617, 113–7.
[67] Kloek, C; Haq, AK; Dunn, SL; Lavery, HJ; Banks, AS; Myers, MG Jr. Regulation of Jak kinases by intracellular leptin receptor sequences. *J Biol Chem*, 2002, 277, 41547–55.
[68] Villanueva, EC; Myers, MG Jr. Leptin receptor signaling and the regulation of mammalian physiology. *Int J Obes*, 2005 2008, 32 Suppl 7, S8–12.
[69] Banks, AS; Davis, SM; Bates, SH; Myers, MG Jr. Activation of downstream signals by the long form of the leptin receptor. *J Biol Chem*, 2000, 275, 14563–72.
[70] Baumann, H; Morella, KK; White, DW; Dembski, M; Bailon, PS; Kim, H, et al. The full-length leptin receptor has signaling capabilities of interleukin 6-type cytokine receptors. *Proc Natl Acad Sci U S A*, 1996, 93, 8374–8.
[71] White, DW; Kuropatwinski, KK; Devos, R; Baumann, H; Tartaglia, LA. Leptin receptor (OB-R) signaling. Cytoplasmic domain mutational analysis and evidence for receptor homo-oligomerization. *J Biol Chem*, 1997, 272, 4065–71.
[72] Schindler, C; Darnell, JE Jr. Transcriptional responses to polypeptide ligands: the JAK-STAT pathway. *Annu Rev Biochem*, 1995, 64, 621–51.
[73] Piper, ML; Unger, EK; Myers, MG, Jr; Xu, AW. Specific physiological roles for signal transducer and activator of transcription 3 in leptin receptor-expressing neurons. *Mol Endocrinol*, 2008, 22, 751–9.
[74] Oswal, A; Yeo, G. Leptin and the control of body weight: a review of its diverse central targets, signaling mechanisms, and role in the pathogenesis of obesity. *Obes*, 2010, 18, 221–9.

[75] Myers, MG; Cowley, MA; Münzberg, H. Mechanisms of leptin action and leptin resistance. *Annu Rev Physiol*, 2008, 70, 537–56.
[76] Howard, JK; Cave, BJ; Oksanen, LJ; Tzameli, I; Bjørbaek, C; Flier, JS. Enhanced leptin sensitivity and attenuation of diet-induced obesity in mice with haploinsufficiency of Socs3. *Nat Med*, 2004, 10, 734–8.
[77] Mori, H; Hanada, R; Hanada, T; Aki, D; Mashima, R; Nishinakamura, H, et al. Socs3 deficiency in the brain elevates leptin sensitivity and confers resistance to diet-induced obesity. *Nat Med*, 2004, 10, 739–43.
[78] Carpenter, LR; Farruggella, TJ; Symes, A; Karow, ML; Yancopoulos, GD; Stahl, N. Enhancing leptin response by preventing SH2-containing phosphatase 2 interaction with Ob receptor. *Proc Natl Acad Sci U S A*, 1998, 95, 6061–6.
[79] Li, C; Friedman, JM. Leptin receptor activation of SH2 domain containing protein tyrosine phosphatase 2 modulates Ob receptor signal transduction. *Proc Natl Acad Sci U S A*, 1999, 96, 9677–82.
[80] Zabeau, L; Lavens, D; Peelman, F; Eyckerman, S; Vandekerckhove, J; Tavernier, J. The ins and outs of leptin receptor activation. *FEBS Lett*, 2003, 546, 45–50.
[81] Bjørbaek, C; Buchholz, RM; Davis, SM; Bates, SH; Pierroz, DD; Gu, H, et al. Divergent roles of SHP-2 in ERK activation by leptin receptors. *J Biol Chem*, 2001, 276, 4747–55.
[82] Machinal-Quélin, F; Dieudonné, MN; Leneveu, MC; Pecquery, R; Giudicelli, Y. Proadipogenic effect of leptin on rat preadipocytes in vitro: activation of MAPK and STAT3 signaling pathways. *Am J Physiol Cell Physiol*, 2002, 282, C853–863.
[83] Caüzac, M; Czuba, D; Girard, J; Hauguel-de, Mouzon, S. Transduction of leptin growth signals in placental cells is independent of JAK-STAT activation. *Placenta*, 2003, 24, 378–84.
[84] Cui, H; Cai, F; Belsham, DD. Leptin signaling in neurotensin neurons involves STAT, MAP kinases ERK1/2, and p38 through c-Fos and ATF1. *FASEB J*, 2006, 20, 2654–6.
[85] Shea-Eaton, W; Sandhoff, TW; Lopez, D; Hales, DB; McLean, MP. Transcriptional repression of the rat steroidogenic acute regulatory (StAR) protein gene by the AP-1 family member c-Fos. *Mol Cell Endocrinol*, 2002, 188, 161–70.
[86] Manna, PR; Stocco, DM. Crosstalk of CREB and Fos/Jun on a single cis-element: transcriptional repression of the steroidogenic acute regulatory protein gene. *J Mol Endocrinol*, 2007, 39, 261–77.
[87] Altarejos, JY; Goebel, N; Conkright, MD; Inoue, H; Xie, J; Arias, CM, et al. The Creb1 coactivator Crtc1 is required for energy balance and fertility. *Nat Med*, 2008, 14, 1112–7.
[88] Gong, Y; Ishida-Takahashi, R; Villanueva, EC; Fingar, DC; Münzberg, H; Myers, MG Jr. The long form of the leptin receptor regulates STAT5 and ribosomal protein S6 via alternate mechanisms. *J Biol Chem*, 2007, 282, 31019–27.
[89] Mütze, J; Roth, J; Gerstberger, R; Hübschle, T. Nuclear translocation of the transcription factor STAT5 in the rat brain after systemic leptin administration. *Neurosci Lett*, 2007, 417, 286–91.
[90] Bendinelli, P; Maroni, P; Pecori, Giraldi, F; Piccoletti, R. Leptin activates Stat3, Stat1 and AP-1 in mouse adipose tissue. *Mol Cell Endocrinol*, 2000, 168, 11–20.

[91] Jean, S; Landry, D; Daigle, M; Martin, LJ. Influence of the adipose derived hormone resistin on STAT factors, steroidogenesis and proliferation of Leydig cells. *Asian Pac J Reprod*, 2012, 1, 1–6.

[92] Martin, LJ; Tremblay, JJ. The nuclear receptors NUR77 and SF1 play additive roles with c-JUN through distinct elements on the mouse Star promoter. *J Mol Endocrinol*, 2009, 42, 119–29.

[93] El-Haschimi, K; Pierroz, DD; Hileman, SM; Bjørbaek, C; Flier, JS. Two defects contribute to hypothalamic leptin resistance in mice with diet-induced obesity. *J Clin Invest*, 2000, 105, 1827–32.

[94] Hileman, SM; Pierroz, DD; Masuzaki, H; Bjørbaek, C; El-Haschimi, K; Banks, WA; et al. Characterizaton of short isoforms of the leptin receptor in rat cerebral microvessels and of brain uptake of leptin in mouse models of obesity. *Endocrinology*, 2002, 143, 775–83.

[95] Banks, WA. Role of the blood-brain barrier in the evolution of feeding and cognition. *Ann N Y Acad Sci*, 2012, 1264, 13–9.

[96] Banks, WA; Coon, AB; Robinson, SM; Moinuddin, A; Shultz, JM; Nakaoke, R; et al. Triglycerides induce leptin resistance at the blood-brain barrier. *Diabetes*, 2004, 53, 1253–60.

[97] Trujillo, ML; Spuch, C; Carro, E; Señarís, R. Hyperphagia and central mechanisms for leptin resistance during pregnancy. *Endocrinology*, 2011, 152, 1355–65.

[98] Steinberg, GR; McAinch, AJ; Chen, MB; O'Brien, PE; Dixon, JB; Cameron-Smith, D; et al. The suppressor of cytokine signaling 3 inhibits leptin activation of AMP-kinase in cultured skeletal muscle of obese humans. *J Clin Endocrinol Metab*, 2006, 91, 3592–7.

[99] Dhillon, SS; McFadden, SA; Chalmers, JA; Centeno, M-L; Kim, GL; Belsham, DD. Cellular leptin resistance impairs the leptin-mediated suppression of neuropeptide Y secretion in hypothalamic neurons. *Endocrinology*, 2011, 152, 4138–47.

[100] Fukuda, M; Williams, KW; Gautron, L; Elmquist, JK. Induction of leptin resistance by activation of cAMP-Epac signaling. *Cell Metab*, 2011, 13, 331–9.

[101] Lund, IK; Hansen, JA; Andersen, HS; Møller, NPH; Billestrup, N. Mechanism of protein tyrosine phosphatase 1B-mediated inhibition of leptin signalling. *J Mol Endocrinol*, 2005, 34, 339–51.

[102] Hosoi, T; Sasaki, M; Miyahara, T; Hashimoto, C; Matsuo, S; Yoshii, M, et al. Endoplasmic reticulum stress induces leptin resistance. *Mol Pharmacol*, 2008, 74, 1610–9.

[103] Von Sobbe, H-U; Koebnick, C; Jenne, L; Kiesewetter, F. Leptin concentrations in semen are correlated with serum leptin and elevated in hypergonadotrophic hypogonadism. *Andrologia*, 2003, 35, 233–7.

[104] Banks, WA; Kastin, AJ; Huang, W; Jaspan, JB; Maness, LM. Leptin enters the brain by a saturable system independent of insulin. *Peptides*, 1996, 17, 305–11.

[105] Banks, WA. The blood-brain barrier as a cause of obesity. *Curr Pharm Des*, 2008, 14, 1606–14.

[106] Caro, JF; Kolaczynski, JW; Nyce, MR; Ohannesian, JP; Opentanova, I; Goldman, WH, et al. Decreased cerebrospinal-fluid/serum leptin ratio in obesity: a possible mechanism for leptin resistance. *Lancet*, 1996, 348, 159–61.

[107] Tapanainen, JS; Tilly, JL; Vihko, KK; Hsueh, AJ. Hormonal control of apoptotic cell death in the testis: gonadotropins and androgens as testicular cell survival factors. *Mol Endocrinol*, 1993, 7, 643–50.

[108] Chehab, FF; Mounzih, K; Lu, R; Lim, ME. Early onset of reproductive function in normal female mice treated with leptin. *Science*, 1997, 275, 88–90.

[109] Nagatani, S; Guthikonda, P; Thompson, RC; Tsukamura, H; Maeda, KI; Foster, DL. Evidence for GnRH regulation by leptin: leptin administration prevents reduced pulsatile LH secretion during fasting. *NeuroEndocrinology*, 1998, 67, 370–6.

[110] Yu, WH; Kimura, M; Walczewska, A; Karanth, S; McCann, SM. Role of leptin in hypothalamic-pituitary function. *Proc Natl Acad Sci U S A*, 1997, 94, 1023–8.

[111] Håkansson ML, Brown H, Ghilardi N, Skoda RC, Meister B. Leptin receptor immunoreactivity in chemically defined target neurons of the hypothalamus. *J Neurosci*, 1998, 18, 559–72.

[112] Louis, GW; Greenwald-Yarnell, M; Phillips, R; Coolen, LM; Lehman, MN; Myers, MG Jr. Molecular mapping of the neural pathways linking leptin to the neuroendocrine reproductive axis. *Endocrinology*, 2011, 152, 2302–10.

[113] Quennell, JH; Mulligan, AC; Tups, A; Liu, X; Phipps, SJ; Kemp, CJ, et al. Leptin indirectly regulates gonadotropin-releasing hormone neuronal function. *Endocrinology*, 2009, 150, 2805–12.

[114] Hill, JW; Elmquist, JK; Elias, CF. Hypothalamic pathways linking energy balance and reproduction. *Am J Physiol Endocrinol Metab*, 2008, 294, E827–832.

[115] Sainsbury, A; Schwarzer, C; Couzens, M; Herzog, H. Y2 receptor deletion attenuates the type 2 diabetic syndrome of ob/ob mice. *Diabetes*, 2002, 51, 3420–7.

[116] Israel, DD; Sheffer-Babila, S; de, Luca, C; Jo, Y-H; Liu, SM; Xia, Q; et al. Effects of leptin and melanocortin signaling interactions on pubertal development and reproduction. *Endocrinology*, 2012, 153, 2408–19.

[117] Shi, H; Sorrell, JE; Clegg, DJ; Woods, SC; Seeley, RJ. The roles of leptin receptors on POMC neurons in the regulation of sex-specific energy homeostasis. *Physiol Behav*, 2010, 100, 165–72.

[118] Baskin, DG; Breininger, JF; Schwartz, MW. Leptin receptor mRNA identifies a subpopulation of neuropeptide Y neurons activated by fasting in rat hypothalamus. *Diabetes*, 1999, 48, 828–33.

[119] Cheung, CC; Clifton, DK; Steiner, RA. Proopiomelanocortin neurons are direct targets for leptin in the hypothalamus. *Endocrinology*, 1997, 138, 4489–92.

[120] Smith, JT; Acohido, BV; Clifton, DK; Steiner, RA. KiSS-1 neurones are direct targets for leptin in the ob/ob mouse. *J Neuroendocrinol*, 2006, 18, 298–303.

[121] Gottsch, ML; Cunningham, MJ; Smith, JT; Popa, SM; Acohido, BV; Crowley, WF, et al. A role for kisspeptins in the regulation of gonadotropin secretion in the mouse. *Endocrinology*, 2004, 145, 4073–7.

[122] Luque, RM; Kineman, RD; Tena-Sempere, M. Regulation of hypothalamic expression of KiSS-1 and GPR54 genes by metabolic factors: analyses using mouse models and a cell line. *Endocrinology*, 2007, 148, 4601–11.

[123] Bingham, NC; Anderson, KK; Reuter, AL; Stallings, NR; Parker, KL. Selective loss of leptin receptors in the ventromedial hypothalamic nucleus results in increased adiposity and a metabolic syndrome. *Endocrinology*, 2008, 149, 2138–48.
[124] Dhillon, H; Zigman, JM; Ye, C; Lee, CE; McGovern, RA; Tang, V, et al. Leptin directly activates SF1 neurons in the VMH, and this action by leptin is required for normal body-weight homeostasis. *Neuron*, 2006, 49, 191–203.
[125] Donato, J, Jr; Cravo, RM; Frazão, R; Gautron, L; Scott, MM; Lachey, J; et al. Leptin's effect on puberty in mice is relayed by the ventral premammillary nucleus and does not require signaling in Kiss1 neurons. *J Clin Invest*, 2011, 121, 355–68.
[126] Iqbal, J; Pompolo, S; Considine, RV; Clarke, IJ. Localization of leptin receptor-like immunoreactivity in the corticotropes, somatotropes, and gonadotropes in the ovine anterior pituitary. *Endocrinology*, 2000, 141, 1515–20.
[127] Akhter, N; Johnson, BW; Crane, C; Iruthayanathan, M; Zhou, Y-H; Kudo, A, et al. Anterior pituitary leptin expression changes in different reproductive states: in vitro stimulation by gonadotropin-releasing hormone. *J Histochem Cytochem*, 2007, 55, 151–66.
[128] Akhter, N; Crane, C; Childs, GV. Pituitary leptin-A paracrine regulator of gonadotropes: A review. *Open Neuroendocrology J*, 2011, 4, 25–42.
[129] McDuffie, IA; Akhter, N; Childs, GV. Regulation of leptin mRNA and protein expression in pituitary somatotropes. *J Histochem Cytochem*, 2004, 52, 263–73.
[130] Yu, WH; Walczewska, A; Karanth, S; McCann, SM. Nitric oxide mediates leptin-induced luteinizing hormone-releasing hormone (LHRH) and LHRH and leptin-induced LH release from the pituitary gland. *Endocrinology*, 1997, 138, 5055–8.
[131] De, Biasi, SN; Apfelbaum, LI; Apfelbaum, ME. In vitro effect of leptin on LH release by anterior pituitary glands from female rats at the time of spontaneous and steroid-induced LH surge. *Eur J Endocrinol*, 2001, 145, 659–65.
[132] Zigman, JM; Elmquist, JK. Minireview: From anorexia to obesity--the yin and yang of body weight control. *Endocrinology*, 2003, 144, 3749–56.
[133] Backholer, K; Smith, JT; Rao, A; Pereira, A; Iqbal, J; Ogawa, S, et al. Kisspeptin cells in the ewe brain respond to leptin and communicate with neuropeptide Y and proopiomelanocortin cells. *Endocrinology*, 2010, 151, 2233–43.
[134] Archer, ZA; Findlay, PA; McMillen, SR; Rhind, SM; Adam, CL. Effects of nutritional status and gonadal steroids on expression of appetite-regulatory genes in the hypothalamic arcuate nucleus of sheep. *J Endocrinol*, 2004, 182, 409–19.
[135] Nagatani, S; Thompson, RC; Foster, DL. Prevention of glucoprivic stimulation of corticosterone secretion by leptin does not restore high frequency luteinizing hormone pulses in rats. *J Neuroendocrinol*, 2001, 13, 371–7.
[136] Sucajtys-Szulc, E; Goyke, E; Korczynska, J; Stelmanska, E; Rutkowski, B; Swierczynski, J. Chronic food restriction differentially affects NPY mRNA level in neurons of the hypothalamus and in neurons that innervate liver. *Neurosci Lett*, 2008, 433, 174–7.
[137] Bojkowska, K; Hamczyk, MM; Tsai, H-W; Riggan, A; Rissman, EF. Neuropeptide Y influences acute food intake and energy status affects NPY immunoreactivity in the female musk shrew (Suncus murinus). *Horm Behav*, 2008, 53, 342–50.

[138] Castellano, JM; Roa, J; Luque, RM; Dieguez, C; Aguilar, E; Pinilla, L; et al. KiSS-1/kisspeptins and the metabolic control of reproduction: physiologic roles and putative physiopathological implications. *Peptides*, 2009, 30, 139–45.
[139] Fernandez-Fernandez, R; Martini, AC; Navarro, VM; Castellano, JM; Dieguez, C; Aguilar, E, et al. Novel signals for the integration of energy balance and reproduction. *Mol Cell Endocrinol*, 2006, 254-255, 127–32.
[140] Smith, JT; Rao, A; Pereira, A; Caraty, A; Millar, RP; Clarke, IJ. Kisspeptin is present in ovine hypophysial portal blood but does not increase during the preovulatory luteinizing hormone surge: evidence that gonadotropes are not direct targets of kisspeptin in vivo. *Endocrinology*, 2008, 149, 1951–9.
[141] True, C; Kirigiti, MA; Kievit, P; Grove, KL; Smith, MS. Leptin is not the critical signal for kisspeptin or luteinising hormone restoration during exit from negative energy balance. *J Neuroendocrinol*, 2011, 23, 1099–112.
[142] Farooqi, IS. Leptin and the onset of puberty: insights from rodent and human genetics. Semin *Reprod*, Med 2002, 20, 139–44.
[143] Urbanski, HF. Leptin and puberty. *Trends Endocrinol Metab*, 2001, 12, 428–9.
[144] Vogel, G. Leptin: a trigger for puberty? *Science*, 1996, 274, 1466–7.
[145] Ahima, RS; Dushay, J; Flier, SN; Prabakaran, D; Flier, JS. Leptin accelerates the onset of puberty in normal female mice. *J Clin Invest*, 1997, 99, 391–5.
[146] Parent, AS; Lebrethon, MC; Gérard, A; Vandersmissen, E; Bourguignon, JP. Leptin effects on pulsatile gonadotropin releasing hormone secretion from the adult rat hypothalamus and interaction with cocaine and amphetamine regulated transcript peptide and neuropeptide Y. *Regul Pept*, 2000, 92, 17–24.
[147] Brandão, CMA; Lombardi, MT; Nishida, SK; Hauache, OM; Vieira, JGH. Serum leptin concentration during puberty in healthy nonobese adolescents. *Braz J Med Biol Res*, 2003, 36, 1293–6.
[148] Mantzoros, CS; Flier, JS; Rogol, AD. A longitudinal assessment of hormonal and physical alterations during normal puberty in boys. V. Rising leptin levels may signal the onset of puberty. *J Clin Endocrinol Metab*, 1997, 82, 1066–70.
[149] Roemmich, JN; Huerta, MG; Sundaresan, SM; Rogol, AD. Alterations in body composition and fat distribution in growth hormone-deficient prepubertal children during growth hormone therapy. *Metabolism*, 2001, 50, 537–47.
[150] Budak, E; Fernández, Sánchez, M; Bellver, J; Cerveró, A; Simón, C; Pellicer, A. Interactions of the hormones leptin, ghrelin, adiponectin, resistin, and PYY3-36 with the reproductive system. *Fertil Steril*, 2006, 85, 1563–81.
[151] Horlick, MB; Rosenbaum, M; Nicolson, M; Levine, LS; Fedun, B; Wang, J, et al. Effect of puberty on the relationship between circulating leptin and body composition. *J Clin Endocrinol Metab*, 2000, 85, 2509–18.
[152] Mantzoros, CS; Moschos, SJ. Leptin: in search of role(s) in human physiology and pathophysiology. *Clin Endocrinol*, (Oxf) 1998, 49, 551–67.
[153] Lin, KC. Increase of leptin levels following exogenous administration of estrogen in women with normal menstruation. *Kaohsiung J Med Sci*, 2000, 16, 13–9.
[154] Chan, JL; Blüher, S; Yiannakouris, N; Suchard, MA; Kratzsch, J; Mantzoros, CS. Regulation of circulating soluble leptin receptor levels by gender, adiposity, sex steroids, and leptin: observational and interventional studies in humans. *Diabetes*, 2002, 51, 2105–12.

[155] Shimizu, H; Shimomura, Y; Nakanishi, Y; Futawatari, T; Ohtani, K; Sato, N, et al. Estrogen increases in vivo leptin production in rats and human subjects. *J Endocrinol*, 1997, 154, 285–92.

[156] Wauters, M; Considine, RV; Van, Gaal, LF. Human leptin: from an adipocyte hormone to an endocrine mediator. *Eur J Endocrinol Eur*, 2000, 143, 293–311.

[157] Chan, JL; Heist, K; DePaoli, AM; Veldhuis, JD; Mantzoros, CS. The role of falling leptin levels in the neuroendocrine and metabolic adaptation to short-term starvation in healthy men. *J Clin Invest*, 2003, 111, 1409–21.

[158] Burney, BO; Garcia, JM. Hypogonadism in male cancer patients. *J Cachexia Sarcopenia Muscle*, 2012, 3, 149–55.

[159] Ahima, RS; Prabakaran, D; Mantzoros, C; Qu, D; Lowell, B; Maratos-Flier, E, et al. Role of leptin in the neuroendocrine response to fasting. *Nature*, 1996, 382, 250–2.

[160] Farooqi, IS; Jebb, SA; Langmack, G; Lawrence, E; Cheetham, CH; Prentice, AM, et al. Effects of recombinant leptin therapy in a child with congenital leptin deficiency. *N Engl J Med*, 1999, 341, 879–84.

[161] Taneli, F; Ersoy, B; Ozhan, B; Calkan, M; Yılmaz, O; Dinç, G, et al. The effect of obesity on testicular function by insulin-like factor 3, inhibin B, and leptin concentrations in obese adolescents according to pubertal stages. *Clin Biochem*, 2010, 43, 1236–40.

[162] Matsumoto, AM. Andropause: clinical implications of the decline in serum testosterone levels with aging in men. *J Gerontol A Biol Sci Med Sci*, 2002, 57, M76–99.

[163] Tena-Sempere, M; Pinilla, L; González, LC; Diéguez, C; Casanueva, FF; Aguilar, E. Leptin inhibits testosterone secretion from adult rat testis in vitro. *J Endocrinol*, 1999, 161, 211–8.

[164] Tena-Sempere, M; Pinilla, L; Zhang, FP; González, LC; Huhtaniemi, I; Casanueva, FF, et al. Developmental and hormonal regulation of leptin receptor (Ob-R) messenger ribonucleic acid expression in rat testis. *Biol Reprod*, 2001, 64, 634–43.

[165] Tchernof, A; Després, JP; Bélanger, A; Dupont, A; Prud'homme, D; Moorjani, S, et al. Reduced testosterone and adrenal C19 steroid levels in obese men. *Metabolism*, 1995, 44, 513–9.

[166] Bjørbaek, C; Uotani, S; da, Silva, B; Flier, JS. Divergent signaling capacities of the long and short isoforms of the leptin receptor. *J Biol Chem*, 1997, 272, 32686–95.

[167] Ruiz-Cortés, ZT; Martel-Kennes, Y; Gévry, NY; Downey, BR; Palin, M-F; Murphy, BD. Biphasic effects of leptin in porcine granulosa cells. *Biol Reprod*, 2003, 68, 789–96.

[168] Lin, Q; Poon, SL; Chen, J; Cheng, L; HoYuen, B; Leung, PCK. Leptin interferes with 3',5'-cyclic adenosine monophosphate (cAMP) signaling to inhibit steroidogenesis in human granulosa cells. *Reprod Biol Endocrinol*, 2009, 7, 115.

[169] Yu, RMK; Chu, DLH; Tan, T; Li, VWT; Chan, AKY; Giesy, JP, et al. Leptin-mediated modulation of steroidogenic gene expression in hypoxic zebrafish embryos: implications for the disruption of sex steroids. *Environ Sci Technol*, 2012, 46, 9112–9.

[170] Semenza, GL; Jiang, BH; Leung, SW; Passantino, R; Concordet, JP; Maire, P, et al. Hypoxia response elements in the aldolase A, enolase 1, and lactate dehydrogenase A gene promoters contain essential binding sites for hypoxia-inducible factor 1. *J Biol Chem*, 1996, 271, 32529–37.

[171] Grosfeld, A; Andre, J; Hauguel-De, Mouzon, S; Berra, E; Pouyssegur, J; Guerre-Millo, M. Hypoxia-inducible factor 1 transactivates the human leptin gene promoter. *J Biol Chem*, 2002, 277, 42953–7.

[172] Giovambattista, A; Suescun, MO; Nessralla, CCDL; França, LR; Spinedi, E; Calandra, RS. Modulatory effects of leptin on leydig cell function of normal and hyperleptinemic rats. *NeuroEndocrinology*, 2003, 78, 270–9.

[173] Vermeulen, A. Decreased androgen levels and obesity in men. *Ann Med*, 1996, 28, 13–5.

[174] Vermeulen, A; Kaufman, JM. Ageing of the hypothalamo-pituitary-testicular axis in men. *Horm Res*, 1995, 43, 25–8.

[175] Corbould, AM; Judd, SJ; Rodgers, RJ. Expression of types 1, 2, and 3 17 beta-hydroxysteroid dehydrogenase in subcutaneous abdominal and intra-abdominal adipose tissue of women. *J Clin Endocrinol Metab*, 1998, 83, 187–94.

[176] Schneider, G; Kirschner, MA; Berkowitz, R; Ertel, NH. Increased estrogen production in obese men. *J Clin Endocrinol Metab*, 1979, 48, 633–8.

[177] Mårin, P. Testosterone and regional fat distribution. *Obes Res*, 1995, 3 Suppl 4, 609S–612S.

[178] Lazarus, R; Sparrow, D; Weiss, S. Temporal relations between obesity and insulin: longitudinal data from the Normative Aging Study. *Am J Epidemiol*, 1998, 147, 173–9.

[179] Goodman-Gruen, D; Barrett-Connor, E. Sex differences in the association of endogenous sex hormone levels and glucose tolerance status in older men and women. *Diabetes Care*, 2000, 23, 912–8.

[180] Caronia, LM; Dwyer, AA; Hayden, D; Amati, F; Pitteloud, N; Hayes, FJ. Abrupt decrease in serum testosterone levels after an oral glucose load in men: implications for screening for hypogonadism. *Clin Endocrinol (Oxf)*, 2013, 78, 291–6.

[181] Kupelian, V; Page, ST; Araujo, AB; Travison, TG; Bremner, WJ; McKinlay, JB. Low sex hormone-binding globulin, total testosterone, and symptomatic androgen deficiency are associated with development of the metabolic syndrome in nonobese men. *J Clin Endocrinol Metab*, 2006, 91, 843–50.

[182] Avelino-Cruz, JE; Flores, A; Cebada, J; Mellon, PL; Felix, R; Monjaraz, E. Leptin increases L-type Ca2+ channel expression and GnRH-stimulated LH release in LbetaT2 gonadotropes. *Mol Cell Endocrinol*, 2009, 298, 57–65.

[183] Luukkaa, V; Pesonen, U; Huhtaniemi, I; Lehtonen, A; Tilvis, R; Tuomilehto, J, et al. Inverse correlation between serum testosterone and leptin in men. *J Clin Endocrinol Metab*, 1998, 83, 3243–6.

[184] Fernandez, CDB; Bellentani, FF; Fernandes, GSA; Perobelli, JE; Favareto, APA, Nascimento AF, et al. Diet-induced obesity in rats leads to a decrease in sperm motility. *Reprod Biol Endocrinol*, 2011, 9, 32.

[185] Hammoud, AO; Wilde, N; Gibson, M; Parks, A; Carrell, DT; Meikle, AW. Male obesity and alteration in sperm parameters. *Fertil Steril*, 2008, 90, 2222–5.

[186] Vigueras-Villaseñor, RM; Rojas-Castañeda, JC; Chávez-Saldaña, M; Gutiérrez-Pérez, O; García-Cruz, ME; Cuevas-Alpuche, O, et al. Alterations in the spermatic function generated by obesity in rats. Acta Histochem 2011, 113, 214–20.

[187] Sayed-Ahmed, A; Abd-Elmaksoud, A; Elnasharty, M; El-Magd, MA. In situ hybridization and immunohistochemical localization of leptin hormone and leptin

receptor in the seminal vesicle and prostate gland of adult rat. *Acta Histochem*, 2012, 114, 185–91.

[188] Bhat, GK; Sea, TL; Olatinwo, MO; Simorangkir, D; Ford, GD; Ford, BD, et al. Influence of a leptin deficiency on testicular morphology, germ cell apoptosis, and expression levels of apoptosis-related genes in the mouse. *J Androl*, 2006, 27, 302–10.

[189] Lee, J; Richburg, JH; Younkin, SC; Boekelheide, K. The Fas system is a key regulator of germ cell apoptosis in the testis. *Endocrinology*, 1997, 138, 2081–8.

[190] Chelich, AM; Edmonds, ES. Copulatory behavior and reproductive capacity of the genetically obese female Zucker rat. *Physiol Behav*, 1981, 27, 331–5.

[191] Edmonds, ES; Dallie, SK; Withyachumnarnkul, B. Reproductive system of the obese male zucker rat. Reproductive capacity, artificial insemination and plasma testosterone levels. *Biol Reprod*, 1982, 27, 891–7.

[192] Piser, JA; Edmonds, ES; Hoftiezer, V. Sperm Motility and Histomorphometry of the Testis of the Genetically Obese Zucker Rat. *J Androl*, 1981, 2, 200–4.

[193] Vendramini, V; Cedenho, AP; Miraglia, SM; Spaine, DM. Reproductive Function of the Male Obese Zucker Rats: Alteration in Sperm Production and Sperm DNA Damage. Reprod Sci 2013 ahead of print.

[194] Abbasihormozi, S; Shahverdi, A; Kouhkan, A; Cheraghi, J; Akhlaghi, AA; Kheimeh, A. Relationship of leptin administration with production of reactive oxygen species, sperm DNA fragmentation, sperm parameters and hormone profile in the adult rat. *Arch Gynecol Obstet*, 2013, 287, 1241–9.

[195] Zorn, B; Osredkar, J; Meden-Vrtovec, H; Majdic, G. Leptin levels in infertile male patients are correlated with inhibin B, testosterone and SHBG but not with sperm characteristics. *Int J Androl*, 2007, 30, 439–44.

[196] Camiña, JP; Lage, M; Menendez, C; Graña, M; García-Devesa, J; Dieguez, C, et al. Evidence of free leptin in human seminal plasma. *Endocrine*, 2002, 17, 169–74.

[197] Li, HWR; Chiu, PCN; Cheung, MPL; Yeung, WSB; O, WS. Effect of leptin on motility, capacitation and acrosome reaction of human spermatozoa. *Int J Androl*, 2009, 32, 687–94.

[198] Lampiao, F; du, Plessis, SS. Insulin and leptin enhance human sperm motility, acrosome reaction and nitric oxide production. Asian *J Androl*, 2008, 10, 799–807.

[199] Thomas, S; Kratzsch, D; Schaab, M; Scholz, M; Grunewald, S; Thiery, J, et al. Seminal plasma adipokine levels are correlated with functional characteristics of spermatozoa. *Fertil Steril*, 2013, 99, 1256–1263.e3.

[200] Taylor, A. ABC of subfertility: extent of the problem. *BMJ*, 2003, 327, 434–6.

[201] Pasquali, R; Patton, L; Gambineri, A. Obesity and infertility. *Curr Opin Endocrinol Diabetes Obes*, 2007, 14, 482–7.

[202] Cabler, S; Agarwal, A; Flint, M; du, Plessis, SS. Obesity: modern man's fertility nemesis. *Asian J Androl*, 2010, 12, 480–9.

[203] Kasturi, SS; Tannir, J; Brannigan, RE. The metabolic syndrome and male infertility. *J Androl*, 2008, 29, 251–9.

[204] Chavarro, JE; Toth, TL; Wright, DL; Meeker, JD; Hauser, R. Body mass index in relation to semen quality, sperm DNA integrity, and serum reproductive hormone levels among men attending an infertility clinic. *Fertil Steril*, 2010, 93, 2222–31.

[205] Kaukua, J; Pekkarinen, T; Sane, T; Mustajoki, P. Sex hormones and sexual function in obese men losing weight. *Obes Res*, 2003, 11, 689–94.

[206] Niskanen, L; Laaksonen, DE; Punnonen, K; Mustajoki, P; Kaukua, J; Rissanen, A. Changes in sex hormone-binding globulin and testosterone during weight loss and weight maintenance in abdominally obese men with the metabolic syndrome. *Diabetes Obes Metab*, 2004, 6, 208–15.

In: Leptin: Biosynthesis, Functions and Clinical Significance ISBN: 978-1-62948-801-1
Editor: Edward L. Blum

Chapter 8

Role of Leptin in Early Life Increases the Metabolic Vulnerability in Adults: Physiological, Pathological and Potential Therapeutic Implications[†]

***L. Manuel Apolinar*[1,*] *and E. de la Chesnaye Caraveo*[2]**
[1]Endocrine Research Unit, Centro Médico Nacional,
Instituto Mexicano del Seguro Social (IMSS), Mexico City, Mexico
[2]Cardiovascular and Metabolic Diseases Research Unit, Centro Médico Nacional,
Instituto Mexicano del Seguro Social (IMSS), Mexico City, Mexico

Abstract

Leptin, the protein product of the *obese (ob* or *Lep)* gene, is a hormone synthesized by adipocytes that signals available energy reserves to the brain, thereby influencing development, growth, metabolism and reproduction. In mammals, leptin acts as an adiposity signal: circulating leptin fluctuates in proportion to fat mass, exerting its action on the hypothalamus to suppress food intake. In this manner, central leptin signaling plays a pivotal role in the regulation of ~~the~~ metabolic activity. More importantly, leptin levels during the perinatal period are essential for the development of metabolic systems involved in energy homeostasis. Moreover, maternal nutrition and the hormonal environment during pregnancy and lactation may also modulate the offspring's response to postnatal modifications in leptin levels.

There are several reports showing that hyperleptinemia positively correlates with atherogenic processes including promotion of platelet aggregation and thrombosis, as well as with hypertension, production of inflammatory cytokines and metabolic syndrome. Thereby endothelial dysfunction takes place and underlies metabolic and vascular alterations that contribute to the development of both cardiovascular disease and type 2 diabetes. In fact, it has been demonstrated that an increase of leptin serum levels in

---

† This research was supported by FIS/IMSS.
* Corresponding author: PhD Leticia Manuel Apolinar. Email: letymanu@yahoo.com.mx.

humans, are also associated with a higher risk of myocardial infarction and stroke independent of obesity and obesity-related cardiovascular risk factors.

The present study highlights the importance of leptin levels during the perinatal period in the development of metabolic systems that control energy homeostasis and how modifications of these levels may induce long-lasting and potentially irreversible effects on metabolism, which in turn may contribute to the development of different cardio-metabolic diseases.

Keywords: Leptin, fetal programming, obesity, diabetes

INTRODUCTION

The discovery of leptin has led to a new era in nutrition biology. Leptin was discovered in mice in 1994 by Jeffrey M. Friedman. The word Leptin is derived from the Greek ~~word~~ leptos, which means ‘thin’. The serum concentrations of leptin are predominantly defined by body fat mass [1]. Leptin was the first adipocytokine identified, its primary structure is composed of 167 amino acids, and it is mainly expressed in adipose tissue. Leptin regulates energy homeostasis and interferes with several neuroendocrine and immune functions [2]. A higher amount of leptin is secreted by subcutaneous adipocytes than by the visceral adipocytes. Its presence has also been detected in many other tissues, including the placenta, mammary glands, breast milk, testes, ovaries, endometrium, stomach, hypothalamus, and pituitary gland. Leptin exerts pleiotropic effects by binding and activating specific leptin receptors (obR) in the hypothalamus and other organs. It has direct and indirect effects in different metabolically active tissues and also regulates several neuroendocrine axes [3, 4]. Early research focused on leptin and its receptors in the hypothalamus region led to the belief that leptin is an important regulatory hormone for signaling body fat status.

On the other hand, various studies have shown the promotion of inflammation by elevating levels of leptin. It is conceivable that the control of leptin circulating levels might prevent metabolic diseases. However, many questions need to be address~~ed~~ before leptin can be used as a therapeutic target in metabolic and inflammatory complications.

CHARACTERISTICS AND FUNCTIONS OF LEPTIN

Leptin was the first adipokine to be characterized. This hormone was discovered by Jeffrey M. Friedman in mice with several abnormalities derived from a point mutation in the *ob* gene, including diabetes, hyperphagia, infertility, high bone mass, as well as a less efficient immune system and impaired thermogenesis [1, 5, 6]; The altered phenotype in *ob/ob* mice, was completely rescued when the recombinant hormone was administered. Moreover, similar results were reported for obese individuals with a homozygous mutation in the leptin gene, who received leptin therapy [7], demonstrating a direct participation of leptin and its receptor in body weight regulation and energy homeostasis [8, 9]. Upon the cloning of leptin and the identification of its receptors (OB-R), a remarkable progress has been made in the understanding of the molecular mechanisms that act in concert to maintain the fine balance between appetite and satiety signaling in the brain.

Leptin is comprised of 167 aminoacids and is primarily synthesized in the subcutaneous white adipose tissue [10], but it has also been identified in many other tissues, like placenta, mammary glands, breast, gonads, endometrium, stomach, as welll as the hypothalamus and the pituitary gland [11]. Leptin is secreted to the circulatory system, where its concentration is directly proportional to body fat, in a range from 5 to 10 ng/ml in healthy subjects and from 40 to 100 ng/ml in obese individuals [12]. This 16 kDa peptide hormone presents six different isoforms that exert different biological actions through leptin receptors (ObRa through ObRf, being ObRb the predominant) in many organs. In fact different studies have implicated leptin in cellular proliferation, apoptosis inhibition and angiogenesis stimulation [13, 14]. Nonetheless, its fundamental role in metabolic homeostasis and regulation of energy expenditure is the most extensively studied. It is now well established that leptin´s pleiotropic effects occur through leptin specific receptors located in the arcuate, dorso-medial and ventro-medial areas of the hypothalamus [12]. In particular, the arcuate nucleous of the hypothalamus (ARC), which is the primary target organ of leptin, has an important role in sensing long-term energy stores, thereby regulating food intake. Leptin acts by modulating the activity of two main neuronal populations, expressing either the proopiomelanocortin (POMC) or Y (NPY) neuropeptides [15]. Both POMC and NYP neurons express the active form of the leptin receptor (ObRb), which after binding to its ligand, activates in both neuronal types, the JAK/STAT, AMPK and PI3kinase/AKT signal transduction pathways [16], both of which can be inhibited by the suppressor of cytokine signaling (SOCS), leading to leptin resistance and obesity [17]. The inhibition of the STAT3 and PI3kinase/AKT signal transduction pathways, upregulates the vascular endothelial growth factor, thereby enhancing angiogenesis in adipocytes [12]. In mice, disruption of the JAK/STAT pathway results in an increment of food intake and adipose tissue [18].

In order to promote the activation of different anorexigenic pathways, leptin favors POMC neuron activity upon the respective for NYP cells. In fact, leptin signaling in the ARC leads to the transcriptional repression of the NYP gene, whereas the transcriptional activity of POMC is increased [16]. The latter is supported by studies demonstrating that both, gene ablation of POMC neurons as well as optogenetic activation of AgRP/NYP neurons cause hyperphagia [19, 20]. Interestingly, pharmacological activation of POMC neurons has demonstrated a gradual effect upon food intake and body weight regulation. This subtler role of POMC cells in food intake repression is in contrast with the immediate effect of hyperphagia generated after NYP neurons activation [20].

In addition, studies conducted on leptin deficient ob/ob mice, have shown that leptin is able to modulate the synaptic pattern of the ARC neurons, that is, ob/ob mice exhibit an increase in NYP excitatory synapses and conversely a decrease in excitatory synapses on the POMC neurons. Leptin replacement in these mice normalized these synaptic alterations, which demonstrated that the adult hypothalamus presents neuronal plasticity [21]. In this context, studies on experience induced neuronal plasticity have revealed an important participation of neurotrophins, in particular the brain derived neurotrophic factor (BDNF) which mediates leptin´s control over neuronal plasticity and food intake. The latter is supported by the fact that BDNF deficient mice are obese [22]. BDNF is synthesized and transported anterogradely, through the activation of the melanocortin-4 receptor on the ventro-medial hypothalamic nucleus (VMH), due to the action of POMC neuron projections from the ARC to the VMH [23]. When synaptically released, BDNF facilitates the consolidation of neuronal circuits, by establishing long-term potentiation [24]. Moreover, increasing evidence suggests leptin regulates other neuronal circuits apart from the hypothalamic and metabolism related [15]. Of note, it has been demonstrated that calorie restriction in itself induces neural plasticity in adult rats [25], whereas leptin supplementation exerts a positive effect on pediatric neural plasticity and cognitive performance [26].

LEPTIN IN PROGRAMMING FETAL AND METABOLISM

The term "programming" has been used to describe the process by which stimuli or nutritional manipulation exerted during critical or decisive stages of development that may cause short-, medium- or long-term changes either in the structure or function of the organism, with a possible compromise of health. Fetal programming was first studied during the 1970s and, during that time, the notion that not only genetics influenced the life and health of an individual was already taken into consideration [27, 28]. Fetal programming implies that during critical periods of prenatal growth, some changes in hormonal and nutritional environment of the embryo can alter fetal genome expression in tissues with physiological and metabolic functions in adulthood. Thus, metabolic changes *in utero* induce long-term physiological and structural patterns that can "program" health in adulthood, a theory popularly known as "Barker hypothesis". Evidence suggests that pathologies like vascular disease (eg, hypertension), metabolic syndrome and type 2 diabetes mellitus, may be "programmed" during the early stages of fetal development and manifest in later stages, when interacting with lifestyle and other conventionally acquired environmental risk factors. Barker et al. in 1993 proposed that low birth weight (LBW) infants were at an increased risk for developing obesity, hypertension and type 2 diabetes [29]. Various studies in populations and animal models have revealed critical periods when offspring are most vulnerable to environmental influences, including maternal nutritional imbalance [30, 31, 32]. In rats, malnutrition during select periods of pregnancy causes newborns to have LBW [33]. Thus, fetal programming is considered to be a potential mechanism that contributes to the development of metabolism of alterations.

Hales et al. evaluated glucose tolerance in 64-year-old individuals and the results showed a strong association between LBW and metabolic diseases. Neonates with birth weight <2500 g had 7.5 times predisposition to develop diabetes or glucose intolerance compared with neonates who weighed >4000 g. That report was considered the origin of the "thrifty" genotype-phenotype saver theory [34]. There is also evidence that early postnatal growth acceleration, which would normally be considered desirable, may exacerbate metabolic dysfunction in later life [35] because excessive calorie intake and subsequent obesity increases the risk of developing chronic disease and decrease life expectancy.

Likewise, the degree of nutrient enhancement during the newborn period may modulate appetite programming with regulating hormones and neurotransmitters, body composition, and diminished propensity to adult obesity in newborns with undernutrition. In rodent models, calorie restriction with adequate nutrient intake decreases the risk of developing chronic disease and extends maximum life span. Prevalence of obesity has increased markedly over the last several decades worldwide. However, there is a well-recognized epidemic of adult obesity in United States. Current data indicate that >20% of adults are clinically obese (body mass index ≥ 30 kg/m^2 (BMI)), and an additional 30% are overweight (body mass index ≥25 kg/m^2), 15% of children and adolescents are obese [31]. Thus, maternal malnutrition has defined time windows with long term effects on weight gain and metabolism in infants. In addition, lactation is a critical period for the programming of adult life; suggesting that overfeeding immediately after fetal growth retardation induces "catch-up growth".

Alongside the diverse beliefs and conceptions regarding the a etiology of type 2 diabetes and metabolic syndrome, there was a strong polarization of views in the 1980s and 1990s concerning the roles of muscle insulin resistance, defective pancreatic insulin secretion and elevated hepatic glucose production in the pathophysiology of type 2 diabetes. This debate has now been settled by a uniform agreement that glucose intolerance, ranging from the prediabetic states of impaired fasting glucose and impaired glucose tolerance to overt type 2 diabetes, constitutes heterogeneous dysmetabolic states involving multiple organ dysfunction including liver, muscle, pancreas, adipose tissue, gut, kidney and brain [36]. It is of interest that the concept of fetal programming, with its ideas of organ plasticity, may represent the most plausible hypothesis of a common ground for the underlying etiology and molecular mechanisms of type 2 diabetes. Thus, the multiple organ dysfunctions in type 2 diabetes, time and age associated changes, and differences in magnitude between type 2 diabetic patients within and among societies, require a comprehensive conceptual framework such as developmental programming.

During recent years, numerous studies have added to a body of evidence showing that the effect of leptin in early life is quite distinct from that in the adult. Recent studies suggest that hyperphagia is a consequence of fetal programming. Hyperphagia also contributes to obesity in the adult offspring of undernourished mothers [37]. The hypothalamus is considered to be the main integrator and processor of peripheral metabolic information. Also, leptin is a hormone expressed in a variety of tissues, mainly in adipocytes, and it is a key hormone in the regulation of food intake and energy expenditure in the hypothalamus via the long form of the leptin receptor (ObRb). Leptin has a profound effect on the proliferation, maintenance, and differentiation of neuronal and glial cells and is required for the formation of neuronal circuitry involved in functions ranging from cognition and memory to energy homeostasis [38].

In rodent the fetal malnutrition has effect on birth weight and neonatal body weight. Thus, offspring with undernutrition at birth but with *ad libitum* feeding showed catch-up growth at 2 weeks of age. Dietary fat and fructose, which do not increase insulin secretion, lead to reduced leptin production, suggesting a mechanism for high-fat/high-sugar diets to increase energy intake and weight gain [39].

Thus, early postnatal catch-up growth occurring after fetal malnutrition favors the programming of obesity in adult life. An increase in the hypothalamic ObRb receptor expression was observed in the offspring with undernutrition at birth, which may be due to developmental adaptation to ensure fetal survival induced by fetal undernutrition. Moreover, an increase in body weight was present in postnatal life at 2 weeks of age and 3 months of age, with a continued accelerated weight gain after weaning. Because ObRb expression increased in parallel, it may be hypothesized that leptin plays a key role in the etiology of hyperphagia and obesity as a consequence of altered fetal development. [40].

In the adult brain, leptin regulates energy homeostasis primarily via the hypothalamic circuit that affects food intake and energy expenditure [2]. Evidence from rodent models has demonstrated that during early postnatal life, leptin is relatively ineffective in modulating these pathways, despite the high circulating levels and the presence of leptin receptors within the central nervous system (CNS) [41]. Some studies show serum leptin levels are significantly increased during rat gestation [42-44]. This increase is due to a hyperproduction of leptin by the placenta and adipose tissue as pregnancy progresses and to an increase in the plasma leptin-binding activity [45, 46]. This paradoxical increase in leptin concentration during gestation suggests that a physiological state of leptin resistance may exist at the hypothalamic level that may explain the hyperphagia observed in pregnant rats [47]. Moreover, although the cellular and molecular mechanisms that determine hyperphagia and leptin resistance during pregnancy are not completely understood, evidence exists for a reduction in the hypothalamic expression of receptor ObRb [48], a suppression of hypothalamic leptin-induced STAT3 signaling in midgestation [49], and an increase in orexigenic neuropeptides in the hypothalamus of late pregnant rats [50]. Also, it seems likely that these adaptive mechanisms will be driven by the hormonal changes characteristic of pregnancy, including increased levels of progesterone, prolactin, or placental lactogen, and a loss of the cyclic elevations of serum estradiol. In fact, it has been demonstrated that the chronic activation of the prolactin receptor due to the production of placental lactogens in mid- and late pregnancy is one of the factors involved in leptin resistance during gestation [47].

Other studies associate fetal state nutritional with impact of development, Vickers et al. indicated that severe fetal undernutrition-programmed hyperleptinemia leads to leptin resistance, hyperphagia, and obesity in adult life. Many of the effects of leptin on food intake and body fat storage have been attributed to its actions on hypothalamic neurons that coordinate behavioral and metabolic controls of energy balance [51]. All of these changes were amplified by postnatal hypercaloric nutrition. Also, several studies on rodents suggest that a defective programming of these hypothalamic circuits may begin *in utero* and continue in early postnatal life throughout the suckling period, leading to a disturbed organization and, consequently, long-lasting dysfunction in adulthood [52].

In the rodent, hypothalamic energy balance circuits are still forming during the early postnatal period, and in the leptin-deficient *ob/ob* mouse, there is reduced axonal projection from the ARC to the downstream paraventricular nucleus in the neonate, which can be rescued by leptin administration exclusively during this perinatal period [53]. There is a restricted period of functional leptin receptor expression in the ventricular region of the hypothalamus during the early postnatal period. This receptor may provide a substrate basis for the neurotrophic actions of leptin during this early period of life that are important in the establishment of hypothalamic energy balance circuitry. The initially low expression levels and the lack of regulation of neuropeptide mRNA by leptin in the ARC until the end of the second postnatal week also suggest that ARC cells are relatively insensitive to endogenous leptin during this time. This may reflect postnatal changes in neuronal distribution and also suggests a functional uncoupling of leptin receptor to neuropeptide mRNA regulation, until neurons are appropriately positioned in their respective nuclei [41].

In the fetus, leptin levels follow the evolution of adipose tissue development, with low levels being found during the first half of gestation and dramatically increasing during the latter part of the third trimester [54]. Shortly after birth, circulating leptin levels decline. The conversion of preadipocytes into mature adipocytes is accompanied by an increase in leptin gene expression [55], and abundance of leptin in fetal adipose tissue is related to fetal body weight [56]. Indeed, children born small for gestational age have lower cord blood leptin levels than those born normal for gestational age [57]. Leptin levels in cord blood have been suggested to predict adiposity in later years [58], suggesting that *in utero* leptin levels also have long-term influences on metabolism in humans.

Leptin also exhibits significant effects on lipid metabolism, platelet aggregation, hematopoiesis, smooth muscle cell proliferation, pancreatic cell function, and thermogenesis as well as on the response to bacterial lipopolysaccharide. Other emerging data suggest that leptin may accelerate vascular disease in an "over-flow" situation, i.e. in association with increased body weight when leptin levels are elevated [53].

Leptin concentrations are higher in females than in males, and an age dependence was shown in children and adolescents. Reference intervals referring to measures of body fat should therefore be stratified according to gender and pubertal development. Similar to other hormones, leptin secretion shows circadian rhythm and oscillatory pattern. The nocturnal increase of leptin secretion is entrained by mealtime, probably as a result of the cumulative hyperinsulinemia that occurs during the entire day.

Moreover, in experimental models, leptin has been shown to have angiogenic activity, to increase oxidative stress in endothelial cells as well as to promote vascular cell calcification and smooth muscle cell proliferation and migration [59]. Increased circulating leptin levels have also been correlated with aging and higher inflammatory markers independent of body fat mass [60].

Role of Leptin Resistance in the Development of Obesity

It is now well established that white adipose tissue functions as an active endocrine organ to modulate physiological metabolic processes. As adipose tissue contains various cell types such as adipocytes, immune cells, endothelial cells, and fibroblasts, it produces and releases diverse secretory proteins called adipocytokines into the systemic circulation. The adipocytokines interact with metabolic, endocrine and immune functions and may contribute to the development of obesity. Clinical studies also link the accumulation of intraabdominal visceral fat and central adiposity to coronary heart disease, metabolic syndrome, and risk of type 2 diabetes [61].

Although adipokines have multiple metabolic functions, we will mainly discuss the inflammatory functions of adipokines that play important roles in mediating obesity induced insulin resistance. In this regard, adipokines are classified as pro- and anti-inflammatory adipokines according to their effects on inflammatory responses in adipose tissues.

The association of obesity with chronic low grade inflammation and insulin resistance is well established [62]. The facts that obesity is the most powerful risk factor for type 2 diabetes and that increased concentrations/expression of inflammatory mediators in the obese predicts the occurrence of future diabetes are also well established. In addition, type 2 diabetes is also known to be associated with chronic inflammation. Recent data also demonstrate that inflammatory mediators may interfere with insulin signal transduction. These facts reinforce the importance of inflammation in the pathogenesis of insulin resistance and type 2 diabetes [63, 64].

Thus, obesity is frequently associated with adipocytokines and includes high plasma leptin concentrations and leptin resistance and metabolic syndrome and has been shown as an independent risk factor for coronary heart disease. The pro-inflammatory adipokines (leptin) are increased whereas the anti-inflammatory adipokines associated with insulin resistance are decreased in obese rodents and humans. The most important variable that determines circulating leptin concentrations is body fat mass [65]. Leptin circulates in the plasma as a free adipokine or bound to leptin-binding proteins, mainly its soluble receptor. In lean individuals, the great majority of leptin circulates in the bound form whereas it circulates in the free form in obese individuals. The structure of leptin is similar to pro-inflammatory helical cytokines including IL-2, IL-6, and granulocyte-colony stimulating factor (G-CSF), and leptin indeed induces inflammatory responses through the long isoform of the Ob-Rb and its proximal Janus kinase 2 (JAK2) and signal transducer and activator of transcription 3 (STAT3) signaling pathway [66].

Obviously, under conditions of regular eating cycles, leptin reflects the proportion of adipose tissue [67], showing an exponential relationship. This constitutive synthesis of leptin is modulated by several nonhormonal and hormonal variables. Stimulators in both rodents and humans are overfeeding, insulin, and glucocorticoids [68]. Suppression has been shown for fasting, cAMP, and β3-adrenoreceptor agonists. However, leptin levels in circulation are increased in obese rodents and humans suggesting that obese subjects display leptin resistance. Also, leptin was initially considered for treatment of obesity. Obese individuals, however, often have increased leptin concentrations, and leptin administration shows only very limited effects. Recent data have indicated that this is likely the result of desensitization for the leptin signal, a phenomenon now often referred to as “leptin resistance”. This may occur on at least two distinct levels: saturable transport of leptin across the blood–brain barrier and abnormalities in the extent of leptin receptor activation and/or signal transduction. In addition to its role via the CNS, leptin also has direct effects on a series of peripheral tissues, implying a much more complex leptin axis than was originally hypothesized [64, 69].

Thus, hyperleptinemia is an essential feature of human obesity. The BMI is the best predictor of circulating leptin concentrations. Although the *ob* gene is differentially expressed in different fat compartments, apart from total body fat, upper or lower body adiposity and visceral fat do not influence basal leptin concentrations. Similarly, age, basal glucose concentrations, and ethnicity do not influence circulating leptin concentrations. Only in insulin-sensitive individuals do basal concentrations of insulin and leptin correlate positively even after factoring in body fat. Diabetes does not influence leptin secretion in both lean and obese individuals. In the eating disorders anorexia nervosa and bulimia, leptin concentrations are not up-regulated but simply reflect BMI and, probably, body fat [70]. Despite a strong correlation between body fat and leptin concentrations, there is great heterogeneity in leptin concentrations at any given index of body fat. Approximately 5% of obese populations can be regarded as “relatively” leptin deficient and could benefit from leptin therapy.

Leptin in Diabetes and Obesity

Classically in mammals, there are two functional and developmental defined types of adipose tissue, white and brown. White adipose tissue is located throughout the body. Subcutaneous and visceral adipose tissues are major adipocyte depots, with additional adipose depots distributed at various organs such as heart, lung, and kidney. Subcutaneous and visceral adipose tissues have differences in gene expression, hypertrophy, and hyperplasia in obesity and differentially contribute to obesity-induced insulin resistance. Subcutaneous adipose tissue has high capacity for adipocytes differentiation and cell size expansion to store large amounts of triacylglycerol. This storage capacity serves to reduce visceral adipose tissue mass and lipid deposition in liver and muscle. The inability to convert excess carbohydrate to lipid for storage in subcutaneous adipose tissue (decreased gene expression such as SREBP-1 and ChREBP) is associated with diabetes in obese humans. In contrast, visceral adipose tissue is positively associated with risk of insulin resistance and shows higher monocytes infiltration and IL-6 production than subcutaneous adipose tissue to induce inflammation in obese subjects [71].

Because the relationship between obesity and insulin resistance is a dynamic one and weight gain leads to increased resistance and weight loss to a reduction in insulin resistance, it is possible that macronutrient intake may be crucial and central to these relationships. This concept led us to investigate whether macronutrient intake leads to an increase in inflammation and caloric restriction leads to a reduction in inflammation. Thus, dietary factors may also potentially influence adipokine levels and insulin sensitivity. There is a growing body of literature showing that higher consumption of foods with high glycemic index/glycemic load values is associated with lower adiponectin levels in both healthy and diabetic individuals and higher leptin levels. Glycemic foods are known to induce both hyperglycemia and hyperinsulinemia [69]. Conversely, high intake of fiber may attenuate the glycemic effect of a full meal, and cereal fiber intake is positively associated with adiponectin. Previous studies have shown that ethnic populations at higher risk for metabolic syndrome–related conditions largely consume a diet consisting of foods with a high glycemic index [72]. It is not known whether a higher consumption of glycemic foods influences adipokine levels and insulin resistance in these populations.

Another interesting way to determine the effects of leptin resistance during aging is to study the leptin receptor deficient *db/db* mice longitudinally. In this model, young animals (5–6 weeks) are normoglycemic because their peripheral insulin resistance is overcome by an increase in insulin secretion. This hyperinsulinemia usually occurs for 2 to 3 months and is then followed by a rapid increase in glycemia, reflecting a defect in β-cells secretion. Aging in *db/db* mice is also characterized by an important increase in plasma lipids, higher mean arterial pressure, and lower hepatic insulin-binding capacity. Associated with the already well described important weight gain of *db/db* mice, these metabolic factors contribute to the alteration of cardiac metabolism in favor of fatty acid oxidation and the progressive development of a cardiomyopathy [73].

Recombinant leptin administration has been shown to promote atherosclerosis in mice and endogenous leptin levels have been associated with arterial stiffness, insulin resistance, inflammation, and metabolic syndrome-associated cardiometabolic risk factors in children. Similarly, low levels of adiponectin are mechanistically linked to increased clearance rate of HDL-C (i.e., reduced numbers of this lipoprotein) and are associated with increased progression of coronary artery calcification in adults and increased carotid intima media thickness in children. Together, these data suggest that leptin and adiponectin may play prominent roles in the early disease processes of type 2 diabetes mellitus and cardiovascular disease and abnormal levels of these adipokines in childhood may reflect increased risk for developing these chronic diseases. Abnormal levels of leptin and adiponectin may signal increased risk for type 2 diabetes mellitus and cardiovascular disease.

Leptin and Inflammation

It is well established that in patients with obesity or obesity-related metabolic and cardiovascular diseases, serum concentrations of different adipokines such as tumor necrosis factor α, C-reactive protein, interleukin-1, -6, -8, plasminogen activator inhibitor, retinol binding protein, resistin, adiponectin, leptin and others, are either elevated or reduced and directly linked with chronic inflammation [74]. The adipokine leptin is considered a proinflammatory protein that induces T helper 1 cells responses, natural killer cell (NK) cytotoxicity and increased secretion of other inflammatory cytokines like, C-reactive protein, interleukin-6 (IL-6), tumor necrosis factor alpha (TNFα) and serum amyloid A [12]. Moreover, leptin receptor is also up-regulated in response to these inflammatory signals [75]. Leptin induces inflammatory responses, through the long isoform of the leptin receptor b, which in turn activates the Janus kinase 2, a signal transducer and activator of the STAT3 signaling pathway [76]. In order to promote synthesis of IL-6, IL-12 and TNFα, this adipokine also activates monocytes, macrophages, and stimulates the production of the chemokine CCL-2 and the vascular endothelial growth factor in hepatic stellate cells [77, 78]. It has been demonstrated that peripheral treatment with leptin, significantly increase granulocyte numbers as well as NK cells and monocytes. Furthermore, leptin treatment promoted NK cell differentiation and maturation in the bone marrow of leptin receptor deficient db/db mice [79]. Leptin treatment also increases the differentiation and proliferation of CD4+ and T cells [80]. Moreover, the fact that db/db mice suffer thymus atrophy and that ob/ob mice are immunodeficient, supports the statement that leptin plays an important role in both the immune system and energy homeostasis [76]. The latter also explains why in cases of reduced food intake or acute starvation, both circulating levels of leptin and the immune system condition are diminished. This last one is reverted with the administration of exogenous leptin [81].

Leptin in Hypertension and Cardiovascular Disease

Cardiovascular disease represents the first leading cause of death worldwide. According to the World Heart Federation, the risk factors associated to it include: hypertension, smoking, poor lifestyle condition, being overweight, family history of cardiovascular events, and metabolic alterations [81]. All of these are related to systemic inflammation which is characterized by hyperplasia and hypertrophy of adipose cells, leading to an altered pattern of adipokines synthesis and secretion, which in turn gives way to different cardiovascular anomalies, including vascular contractility and atherosclerosis; underlied by an altered expression of different pro-angiogenic and pro-atherogenic factors [82]. In these context, studies performed in the general population, have associated hyperleptinaemia with atherosclerosis, hypertension and metabolic syndrome. Both leptin and its receptors have been identified in the cardiovascular system [83]. It has been demonstrated that leptin regulates in cardiomyocytes, cardiac contractility, metabolism, cell size, as well as the production of extracellular matrix substances [84-86]. Within the vascular system, this hormone exerts its action via PI3-Akt and MAPK pathways, which are involved in the reperfusion injury salvation kinase pathway (RISC pathway), protecting the myocardium against ischemia reperfusion injury generated by either mechanical or chemical insults. Nonetheless, leptin also appears to participate in the pro-atherogenic pathway by stimulating the hypertrophy and proliferation of the vascular smooth muscle cells, as well as promoting the synthesis of metalloproteinase 2 and the proliferation of profibrinotic cytokines [87]. Leptin is also involved in the development of atherosclerosis by recruiting leukocytes and macrophages to the endothelial wall, through the induction of both superoxide production and monocyte chemoattractant protein-1 in endothelial cells [81]. This last statement is supported by the fact that ob/ob mice are resistant to atherosclerosis [87]. In humans, increased serum leptin concentrations are associated with an increased risk of myocardial infarction and stroke independent of obesity [81].

On the other hand, leptin presents a positive correlation with blood pressure which would suggest, this adipokine promotes the development of hypertension; interestingly, it has been demonstrated that leptin phosphorylates eNOS, which in turn releases nitric oxide, thereby relaxing the smooth muscle cells of the vascular system [88]. The latter is somewhat contradictory, because even-though hyperleptinaemia induces vasodilation, hypertension often coexist; both acute and chronic effects of leptin on the vasculature, could be the cause of hypertension in hyperleptinaemic patients [81].

Considering the above, Leptin exerts a dual role in cardiovascular diseases, that is, it reduces infarct size by protecting against ischemia/reperfusion injury as well as decreasing damage in cardiomyocytes generated by hypoxia, but at the vascular level, its actions are detrimental, since leptin promotes hypertension, atherosclerosis, vascular inflammation and hypertrophy, as well as endothelial dysfunction.

Conclusion

In summary, enhanced sensitivity to environmental stimuli during critical periods of development implies that insults or adverse conditions experienced in early life may have long-term effects on health subsequently. Different studies have shown that changes in the nutritional or hormonal environment during the first weeks of life can affect the development of central energy balance circuits. It is important to associate the role of leptin in the mechanisms controlling energy homeostasis which, to date, have only focused on brain receptors and neuroendocrine pathways that regulate feeding behavior and sympathetic nervous system activity. Therefore, knowing that stressful stimuli generated by increased leptin levels during pre- and postnatal periods promote a stronger susceptibility to obesity in later life, leptin may be considered as a therapeutic target in some clinical situations, such as proinflammatory states or metabolic diseases.

Acknowledgments

We wish to acknowledge support of the Instituto Mexicano del Seguro Social (FIS/IMSS) and National Council for Technology and Research (CONACYT).

Disclosure Statement

The authors have nothing to declare.

References

[1] Friedman J. M., Halaas J. L. (1998) Leptin and the regulation of body weight in mammals. *Nature* 395, 763-770.

[2] Ahima R. S., Prabakaran D., Mantzoros C., Qu. D., Lowell B., Maratos-Flier E., Flier J. S. (1996) Role of leptin in the neuroendocrine response to fasting. *Nature* 382, 250–252.

[3] Konturek P. C., Konturek J. W., Czesnikiewicz-Guzik M., Brzozowski T., Sito E., Konturek S. J. (2005) Neuro-hormonal control of food intake: basic mechanisms and clinical implications. *J. Physiol. Pharmacol.* 56, 5–25.

[4] Hegyi K., Fulop K., Kovacs K., Toth S., Falus A. (2004) Leptin-induced signal transduction pathways. *Cell Biol. Int.* 28, 159–169.

[5] Lindström P. (2007). The physiology of obese-hyperglycemic mice [ob/ob mice]. *Scientific World J.* 7, 666-685.

[6] Yadav V. K., Oury E., Suda N. et al. (2009). A serotonin-dependent mechanism explains the leptin regulation of bone mass, appetite, and energy expenditure. *Cell* 138, 976-989.

[7] Sadaf Farooqi I., O'Rahilly S. (2009). Leptin: a pivotal regulator of human energy homeostasis. *Am. J. Clin. Nutrit.* 89, 980S-984S.

[8] Pelleymounter M. A., Cullen M. J., Baker M. B. et al. (1995). Effects of the obese gene product on body weight regulation in ob/ob mice. *Science* 269, 540-543.

[9] Salvador J., Gomez-Ambrosi J., Fühbeck G. (2001). Perspectives in the therapeutic use of leptin. *Expert Opinion Pharmacother.* 2, 1615-1622.

[10] Zhang Y., Proenca R., Maffei M., Barone M., Leopold L., Friedman J. M. (1994). Positional cloning of the mouse obese gene and its human homologue. *Nature* 372, 425-432.

[11] Van Harmelen V., Reynisdottir S., Eriksson P., Thorne A., Hoffstedt J., Lonnqvist F., Arner P. (1998). Leptin secretion from subcutaneous and visceral adipose tissue in women. *Diabetes* 47, 913-917.

[12] Al-Suhaimi E.A., Shehzad A. (2013). Leptin, resistin and visfatin: the missing link between endocrine metabolic disorders and immunity. *Eur. J. Med. Res.* 18, 12.

[13] Tsuchiya T., Shimizu H., Horie T., Mori M. (1999). Expression of leptin receptor in lung: leptin as a growth factor. *Eur. J. Pharmacol.* 365, 273-279.

[14] Artwohl M., Roden M., Hoizenbein T., Freudenthaler A., Waldaldhausl W., Baurngartner Parzer. S. M. (2002). Modulation by leptin of proliferation and apoptosis in vascular endothelial cells. *Int. J. Obes. Metab. Disord.* 26, 577-580.

[15] Mainardi M., Pizzorusso T., Maffei M. (2013). Environment, leptin sensitivity, and hypothalamic plasticity. *Neural Plasticity* ID 438072, 8 pages.

[16] Plum 1., Belgardt B.E., Brüning J.C. (2006). Central insulin action in energy and glucose homeostasis. *J. Clin. Invest.* 116, 1761-1766.

[17] Sahu A. (2011). Intracellular leptin-signaling pathways in hypothalamic neurons: the emerging role of phosphatidyl inositol-3 kinase-phosphodiesterase-3B- cAMP pathway. *Neuroendocrinol.* 93, 201-210.

[18] Munzberg H., Huo L., Nillni E. A., Hollenberg A. N., Bjorbaek C. (2003). Role of Signal transducer and activator of transcription 3 in regulation of hypothalamic pro-opiomelanocortin gene expression by leptin. *Endocrinol.* 144, 2121-2131.

[19] Yaswen L., Diehl N., Brennan M.B., Hochgeschwender U. (1999). Obesity in the mouse model of pro-opiomelanocortin deficiency responds to peripheral melanocortin. *Nature Med.* 5, 1066-1070.

[20] Aponte Y., Atasoy D., Sternson S. M. (2011). AGRP neurons are sufficient to orchestate feeding behavior rapidly and without training. *Nature Neuroscie.* 14, 351-355.

[21] Pinto S., Roseberry A.G., Liu H., et al. (2004) Rapid rewiring of arcuate nucleus feeding circuits by leptin. *Science* 34, 110-115.

[22] Gray J., Yeo G. S. H., Cox J. J., et al. (2006) Hyperphagia, severe obesity, impaired cognitive function, and hyperactivity associated with functional loss of one copy of the brain-derived neurotrophic factor (BDNF) gene. *Diabetes* 55, 3366-3371.

[23] Altar C. A., Distefano P. S. (1998). Neurotrophin trafficking by anterograde transport. *Trends Neurosci.* 21, 433-437.

[24] Barco A., Patterson S., Alarcon J. M., et al. (2005) Gene expression profiling of facilitated L-LTP in VP16-CREB mice reveals that BDNF is critical for the maintenance of LTP and its synaptic captur. *Neuron* 48, 441-448.

[25] Spolidoro M., Baroncelli L., Putignano E., Maya-Vetencourt J. F., Viegi A., Maffei I. (2011). Food restriction enhances visual cortex plasticity in adulthood. *Nature Communications* 2, 320.

[26] Paz-Filho G. J., Babikian T., Asarnow R., et al. (2008) Leptin replacement improves cognitive development. *PLoS One* 3: ID e3098.

[27] Barker D. J. (1992). The fetal origins of diseases of old age. *Eur. J. Clin. Nutr.* 46, S3-S9.

[28] Lucas A. (1994). Role of nutritional programming in determining adult morbidity. *Arch. Dis. Child.* 71, 288-290.

[29] Barker D. J. P., Hales C. N., Fall C. H.D., Osmond C., Phipps K., Clark P. M. S. (1993). Type 2 (non-insulin-dependent) diabetes mellitus, hypertension and hyperlipidaemia (syndrome X): relation to reduced fetal growth. *Diabetologia* 36, 62–67.

[30] Fontaine K. R., Redden D. T., Wang C., Westfall A. O., Allison D. B. (2003). Years of life lost due to obesity. *JAMA* 289, 187-193.

[31] Fontana L., Klein S. (2007). Aging, Adiposity, and Calorie Restriction. *JAMA* 297, 986-994.

[32] Poston L. (2010). Developmental programming and diabetes. The human experience and insight from animal models. *Best Pract. Res. Clin. Endocrinol. Metab.* 24, 541-552.

[33] Desai M., Gayle D., Babu J., Ross G. M. (2005). Programmed obesity in intrauterine growth-restricted newborns: modulation by newborn nutrition. *Am. J. Physiol. Regul. Integr. Comp. Physiol.* 288, R91-R96.

[34] Hales C. N., Barker D. J. (2001). The thrifty phenotype hypothesis. *Br. Med. Bull.* 60, 5-20.

[35] Eleftheriades M., Creatsas G., Nicolaides K. (2006). Fetal growth restriction and postnatal development. *Ann. N. Y. Acad. Sci.* 1092, 319-30.
[36] DeFronzo R. (2009). Banting lecture. From the triumvirate to the ominous octet: a new paradigm for the treatment of type 2 diabetes mellitus. *Diabetes* 58, 773-795.
[37] Gluckman P. D., Cutfield W., Hofman P., et al. (2005). The fetal, neonatal, and infant environments-the long-term consequences for disease risk. *Early Hum. Dev.* 81, 51-59.
[38] Udagawa J., Hatta T., Hashimoto R., Otani H. (2007). Roles of leptin in prenatal and perinatal brain development. *Congen. Anom.* 47, 77-83.
[39] Havel P. J. (2004). Update on adipocyte hormones: regulation of energy balance and carbohydrate/ lipid metabolism. *Diabetes* 53(Suppl 1), S143-51.
[40] Manuel-Apolinar L., Zarate A., Rocha L., Hernández-Valencia M. (2010). Fetal malnutrition affects hypothalamic leptin receptor expression after birth in mice. *Arch. Med. Res.* 41, 240-245.
[41] Cottrell E. C., Cripps R. L., Duncan J. S., Barrett P., Mercer J. G., Herwig A., Ozanne S. E. (2009). Development al changes in hypothalamic leptin receptor: relationship with the postnatal leptin surge and energy balance neuropeptides in the postnatal rat. *Am. J. Physiol. Regul. Integr. Comp. Physiol.* 296, R631-9.
[42] Chien E. K., Hara M., Rouard M., Yano H., Phillippe M., Polonsky K. S., Bell G. I. (1997). Increase in serum leptin and uterine leptin receptor messenger RNA levels during pregnancy in rats. *Biochem. Biophys. Res. Commun.* 237, 476-480.
[43] Kawai M., Yamaguchi M., Murakami T., Shima K., Murata Y., Kishi K. (1997) The placenta is not the main source of leptin production in pregnant rat: gestational profile of leptin in plasma and adipose tissues. *Biochem. Biophys. Res. Commun.* 240, 798-802.
[44] Gavrilova O., Barr V., Marcus-Samuels B., Reitman M. (1997) Hyperleptinemia of pregnancy associated with the appearance of a circulating form of the leptin receptor. *J. Biol. Chem.* 272, 30546-30551.
[45] García M. D., Casanueva F. F., Dieguez C., Senarís R. M. (2000) Gestational profile of leptin messenger ribonucleic acid (mRNA) content in the placenta and adipose tissue in the rat, and regulation of the mRNA levels of the leptin receptor subtypes in the hypothalamus during pregnancy and lactation. *Biol. Reprod.* 62, 698-703.
[46] Seeber R. M., Smith J. T., Waddell B. J. (2002) Plasma leptin-binding activity and hypothalamic leptin receptor expression during pregnancy and lactation in the rat. *Biol. Reprod.* 66, 1762-1767.
[47] Trujillo M., Spuch L., Carro C., Senaris R. (2011). Hyperphagia and central mechanisms for leptin resistance during pregnancy. *Endocrinol*ogy 152, 1355-1365.
[48] Ladyman S. R., Grattan D. R. (2005) Suppression of leptin receptor messenger ribonucleic acid and leptin responsiveness in the ventromedial nucleus of the hypothalamus during pregnancy in the rat. *Endocrinology* 146, 3868-3874.
[49] Ladyman S. R., Grattan D. R. (2004) Region-specific reduction in leptininduced phosphorylation of signal transducer and activator of transcription-3 (STAT3) in the rat hypothalamus is associated with leptin resistance during pregnancy. *Endocrinology* 145, 3704-3711.
[50] García M. C., López M., Gualillo O., Seoane L. M., Diéguez C., Senarís R. M. (2003) Hypothalamic levels of NPY, MCH, and prepro-orexin mRNA during pregnancy and lactation in the rat: role of prolactin. *FASEB J.* 17, 1392-1400.

[51] Vickers M. H., Breier B. H., Cutfield W. S., Hofman P. L., Gluckman P. D. (2000). Fetal origin of hyperphagia, obesity, and hypertension and postnatal amplification by hpercaloric nutrition. *Am. J. Physiol. Endocrinol. Metab.* 279, E83–E87.

[52] Vickers M. H., Breier B. H., McCarthy D., Gluckman P. D. (2003). Sedentary behavior during postnatal life is determined by the prenatal environment and exacerbated by postnatal hypercaloric nutrition. *Am. J. Physiol. Regul. Integr. Comp. Physiol.* 285, R271-R273.

[53] Bouret S. G., Simerly R. B. (2004) Minireview: Leptin and development of hypothalamic feeding circuits. *Endocrinology* 145, 2621–2626.

[54] Jaquet D., Leger J., Leby-Marchal C., Oury J. F. (1998) Czernichow P: Ontogeny of leptin in human fetuses and newborns: effect of intrauterine growth retardation on serum leptin concentrations. *J. Clin. Endocrinol. Metab.* 83, 1243-1246.

[55] Ye Z-W., Wu X-M., Jiang J-G. (2009). Expression changes of angiotensin II pathways and bioactive mediators during human preadipocytes-visceral differentiation. *Metabolism* 58, 1288-1296.

[56] Bernard S. J., Yuen I., McMillen C., Symonds M. E., Owens P. C. (1999). Abundance of leptin m _ in fetal adipose tissue is related to fetal body weight. *J. Endocrinol.* 163, R1-R4.

[57] Martos-Moreno G. A., Barrios V., Saenz de Pipaon M., Pozo J., Dorronsoro I., Martinez-Biarge M., Quero J., Argente J. (2009). Influence of prematurity and growth restriction on the adipokine profile, igf1, and ghrelin levels in cord blood: relationship with glucose metabolism. *Eur. J. Endocrinol.* 161, 381-389.

[58] Mantzoros C. S., Rifas-Shiman S. L., Williams C. J., Fargnoli J. L., Kelesidis T., Gillman M. W. (2009). Cord blood leptin and adiponectin as predictors of adiposity in children at 3 years of age: a prospective cohort study. *Pediatrics* 123, 682-689.

[59] Bouret S. G., Draper S. J., Simerly R. B. (2004). Trophic action of leptin on hypothalamic neurons that regulate feeding. *Science* 304, 108-110.

[60] Reilly M. P., Iqbal N., Schutta M., et al. (2004). Plasma Leptin Levels Are Associated with Coronary Atherosclerosis in Type 2 Diabetes. *J. Clin. End. Metab.* 89, 3872-3878.

[61] Despres J. P. (2006) Lemieux I. Abdominal obesity and metabolic syndrome. *Nature* 444, 881-887.

[62] Hotamisligil G. S., Shargill N. S., Spiegelman B. M. (1993). Adipose expression of tumor necrosis factor-alpha:direct role in obesity-linked insulin resistance. *Science* 259, 87-91.

[63] Hotamisligil G. S., Peraldi P., Budavari A., Ellis R., White M. F., Spiegelman B. M. (1996). IRS-1-mediated inhibition of insulin receptor tyrosine kinase activity in TNF-alpha and obesity induced insulin resistance. *Science* 271, 665–668.

[64] Kwon H., Pessin J. E. (2013). Adipokines mediate inflammation and insulin resistance. *Front Endocrinol.* 4, 71.

[65] Speakman J. R., Stubbs R. J., Mercer J. G. (2002). Does body mass play a role in the regulation of food intake? *Proc. Nutr. Soc.* 61, 473-87.

[66] Leibel R. L. (2002). The role of leptin in the control of body weight. *Nutr. Rev.* 60, S15-9.

[67] Frayn K. N., Karpe F., Fielding B. A., Macdonald I. A., Coppack S. W. (2003). Integrative physiology of human adipose tissue. *Int. J. Obes. Relat. Metab. Disord.* 27, 875-88.

[68] Koutkia P., Canavan B., Johnson M. L., DePaoli A., Grinspoon S. (2003). Characterization of leptin pulse dynamics and relationship to fat mass, growth hormone, cortisol, and insulin. *Am. J. Physiol. Endocrinol. Metab.* 285, E372-9.
[69] Margetic S., Gazzola C., Pegg G. G., Hill R. A. (2002). Leptin: a review of its peripheral actions and interactions. *Int. J. Obes. Relat. Metab. Disord.* 26, 1407-33.
[70] Gale S. M., Castracane V. D., Mantzoros C. S. (2004). Energy homeostasis, obesity and eating disorders: recent advances in endocrinology. *J. Nutr.* 134, 295-8.
[71] Kursawe R., Caprio S., Giannini C., Narayan D., Lin A., D'adamo E., et al.(2013). Decreased transcription of ChREBP -alpha/beta isoforms in abdominal subcutaneous adipose tissue of obese adolescents with prediabetes or early type 2 diabetes: associations with insulin resistance and hyperglycemia. *Diabetes* 62, 837–844.
[72] Merchant A. T., Anand S. S., Vuksan V., Jacobs R., Davis B., Teo K , Yusuf S , SHARE, SHARE-AP Investigators. (2005). Protein intake is inversely associated with abdominal obesity in a multi-ethnic population. *J. Nutr.* 135, 1196-1201.
[73] Aasum E., Hafstad A. D., Severson D. L., Larsen T. S. (2003). Age-dependent changes in metabolism, contractile function, and ischemic sensitivity in hearts from db/db mice. *Diabetes* 52, 434-441
[74] Tönjes A., Fasshauer M., Kratzsch J., Stumvoll M., Blüher M. (2010). Adipokine Pattern in subjects with impaired fasting glucose and impaired glucose tolerance in comparison to normal glucose tolerance and diabetes. *PLoS ONE* 5, ID e13911
[75] Haas P., Straub R. H., Bedoui S., Nave H. (2008). Peripheral but not central leptin treatment increases numbers of circulating NK cells, granulocytes and specific monocyte subpopulations in non-endotoxaemic lean and obese LEW-rats. *Regul. Pept.* 151, 26-34.
[76] Kwon H., Pessin J. E. (2013). Adipokines mediate inflammation and insulin resistance. *Front. Endocrinol.* 71, 1-13.
[77] Gainsford T., Wilson T. A., Metcalf D., Handman E., Macfarlane C., et al. (1996) Leptin can induce proliferation, differentiation, and functional activation of hemopoietic cells. *Proc. Natl. Acad. Sci.* 93, 14564-14568.
[78] Allefi S., Petrai I., Bertolani C., Parola M., Colombatto S., Novo E., et al. (2005). Upregulation of proinflammatory and proangiogenic cytokines by leptin in human hepatic stellate cells. *Hepatology* 42, 1339-1348.
[79] Lo C. K., Lam Q. L., Yang M., Ko K. H., Sun I., Ma R., Wang S., Xu H., Tam S., Wu C. Y., Zheng B. J., Lu L.(2009). Leptin signaling protects NK cells from apoptosis during development in mouse bone marrow. *Cell Mol. Immunol.* 6, 353-360.
[80] Martin-Romero C., Santos-Alvarez J., Goberna R., Sánchez-Margalet V. (2000). Human Leptin enhances activation and proliferation of human circulating T lymphocytes. *Cell Immunol.* 199, 15-24.
[81] Mattu H.S., Randeva H.S. (2013). Role of adipokines in cardiovascular disease. *J. Endocrinol.* 216, T17-T36.
[82] Rutkowski J. M., Davis K. E., Scherer P. E. (2009). Mechanisms of obesity and related pathologies: the macro-and microcirculation of adipose tissue. *FEBS J.* 276, 5738-5746.
[83] Beltowsky J. (2006). Leptin and atherosclerosis. *Atherosclerosis* 189, 47-60.
[84] Dong F., Zhang X., Ren J. (2006). Leptin regulates cardiomyocytes contractile function through endothelin-1 receptor-NADPH oxidase pathway. *Hypertension* 47, 222-229.

[85] Palanivel R., Eguchi M., Shuralyova I., Coe I., Sweeney G. (2006). Distinct effects of short and long-term leptin treatment on glucose and fatty acid uptake and metabolism in HL-1 cardiomyocytes. *Metabolism* 55, 1067-1075.

[86] Madani S., De Girolamo S., Munoz D. M., Li R. K., Sweeney G. (2006). Direct effects of leptin on size and extracellular matriz components of human pediatric ventricular myocytes. *Cardiovascular Res.* 69, 716-725.

[87] Beltowski J. (2006). Role of leptin in blood pressure regulation and arterial hypertension. *J. Hypertens.* 24, 789-801.

[88] Momin A. U., Melikian N., Shah A. M., Grieve D. J., Wheatcroft S. B., John L., Gamel A., Desaj J. B., Nelson T., Driver C., et al. (2006). Leptin is an endothelial-independent vasodilator in humans with coronary artery diseases evidence for tissue specificity of leptin resistance. *Eur. Heart J.* 27, 2294-2299.

Sympathetic Nervous System

Several studies have shown that leptin influences the sympathetic nervous system (SNS) and ultimately, regulates bone metabolism [5, 8, 9] via this efferent neural pathway. Takeda et al. (2002) examined dopamine β-hydrolase (*Dbh*) deficient mice, a model that impairs sympathetic nervous function by blocking the production of norepinephrine and epinephrine, and found that these mice had a similar, although less severe cancellous bone phenotype to the leptin deficient *ob/ob* mice [5]. The supplementation of leptin into the hypothalamus of *Dbh* deficient mice resulted in no change in the bone mass of these mice, despite reduced mass of gonadal fat pads [5]. This demonstrated that leptin can affect bone mass via the SNS, however, these signals are independent from those regulating body weight.

Further investigation of the leptin-SNS signalling pathway revealed the role of β2-adrenergic receptors in primary mouse osteoblasts [5]. Treatments involving the β-adrenergic receptor agonist, isoproterenol, and the β-adrenergic receptor antagonist, propranolol, confirmed that these receptors on mouse and human osteoblasts were functional [5]. β2-adrenergic receptor deficient ($Adrb2^{-/-}$) mice had increases in cancellous bone mass, similar to *ob/ob* mice, as well as WTmice receiving a β-blocker [8, 10], suggesting leptin deficiency may regulate osteoblast activity through inhibition of adrenergic signalling. The administration of leptin directly into the brain by icv infusion did not alter cancellous bone mass in $Adrb2^{-/-}$ mice [8], suggesting a central axis for this effect. In support of this, transplantation of bone marrow cells from $Adrb2^{-/-}$ mice into irradiated WT mice increased bone formation [8]. Thus, the β2-adrenergic receptor is a crucial part of the leptin-SNS signalling cascade at the bone interface, particularly affecting osteoblasts.

Bone resorption is increased in response to alterations in the leptin-SNS signalling pathway. This also appears to result from central and peripheral actions. In the hypothalamus, leptin deficiency reduces the expression of the neuropeptide CART ('cocaine amphetamine regulated transcript'), promoting bone resorption [8]. In contrast, local β2-adrenergic receptor signalling, results in increased RANKL expression from osteoblast progenitor cells. Thus, RANKL expression was found to be lower on *Adrb2* deficient osteoblasts in comparison to WT osteoblasts [8, 10]. When WT osteoblasts were treated with a β2-adrenergic agonist, isoproterenol, and co-cultured with WT bone marrow monocytes (BMMs), this resulted in an increase in osteoclastogenesis [8]. In comparison, *Adrb2* deficient osteoblasts co-cultured with WT BMMs did not alter osteoclastogenesis [8]. Thus, leptin signalling from the brain via the SNS acts on osteoblasts to influence RANKL expression and subsequently osteoclast differentiation and cancellous bone resorption.

Neuropeptide Y

The adipokine leptin circulates in the blood and crosses the blood-brain barrier to bind to the leptin receptors present in the hypothalamus. In the arcuate nucleus, leptin binding results in the downstream suppression of the appetite and energy regulator, neuropeptide Y (NPY), and consequently, *ob/ob* mice have markedly increased expression of NPY in the hypothalamus [11]. NPY has been demonstrated to have a strong influence on cortical and cancellous bone mass in both NPY deficient ($NPY^{-/-}$) and specific Y receptor deficient mice, as well as following arcuate-specific over expression (12). NPY binds to a group of G-protein coupled receptors known as Y receptors: Y1, Y2, Y4, Y5 and y6 [13]. These Y receptors also bind to and mediate the actions of peptide YY (PYY) and pancreatic polypeptide (PP) [13]. These receptors have been demonstrated to be present in both mice and humans; however, y6 in humans is anon-functional truncated version [13]. NPY has a similar pharmacological affinity for the Y receptors as PYY with the greatest affinity for Y2, followed by Y1, Y5 and the least affinity for Y4 [13].

NPY deficient ($NPY^{-/-}$) mice have increased cancellous and cortical bone mass due to increases in bone formation rate, resulting from greater mineral apposition rate [14]. NPY deficiency has a generalised effect on the skeleton as both the distal femoral metaphysis and the fourth lumbar vertebra displaying a similar high bone mass phenotype [14]. Recently, Wong et al. (2013) produced dual NPY and leptin deficient ($NPY^{-/-}$*ob/ob*) mice to investigate the role of NPY in leptin-mediated signalling to bone [15]. $NPY^{-/-}$*ob/ob* mice displayed greater whole body, femoral and vertebral BMD compared to *ob/ob* mice [15]. These changes in BMD were the result of increased cortical bone formation rate [15]. Indeed, the loss of NPY from *ob/ob* mice corrected their reduced bone density and cortical bone formation rates to values comparable to wild type, suggesting a fundamental role for NPY in the cortical bone changes in leptin deficiency. These results are consistent with NPY's role to inhibit bone formation, and the high central expression of NPY in *ob/ob* mice. Although the $NPY^{-/-}$*ob/ob* mice had slightly lower body weights than the *ob/ob* mice, these mice had higher BMD [15], indicating thatthe leptin-NPY pathway regulates cortical bone mass independent of any potential effects of weight bearing. Interestingly, no changes in cancellous bone were observed between the $NPY^{-/-}$*ob/ob*and *ob/ob* mice, suggesting that the leptin-NPY pathway functions independently of the leptin-SNS adrenergic axis. Thus the elevation in NPY expression produced by deficient leptin signalling in *ob/ob* produces the reduction in cortical bone mass evident in *ob/ob*, while reduction of adrenergic signalling produces the increase in cancellous bone volume in these mice. This complex, envelope-specific regulation of bone turnover by leptin deficiency is consistent with the skeletal response to calorie deprivation evident in wild type mice [16].

To investigate the centralised nature of the leptin-NPY pathway's effect on bone, a recombinant adenovirus-associated virus (AAV-) that increases NPY expression (AAV-NPY) was introduced solely into the arcuate nucleus of WT mice [14]. This led to increases in body weight through gains in white adipose tissue mass, however, despite this increase in weight, cortical bone formation was significantly reduced (up to 7-fold) [14]. These results are consistent with the role of elevated NPY as marker of starvation; thus, triggering elevated food intake and inhibition of non-essential processes such as bone formation. Hence AAV-NPY mice represent a phenocopy of the *ob/ob* mouse, again reinforcing the importance of NPY to leptin deficient phenotype. Baldock et al. (2009) also administered AAV-NPY into the hypothalamus of $NPY^{-/-}$ mice to determine whether this central leptin-NPY pathway was solely responsible for the bone effects [14]. AAV-NPY injected mice had higher body weights and adiposity than their AAV-empty injected counterparts. [14]. However, the bone phenotype was only partially restored with the re-introduction of hypothalamic NPY [14], suggesting that other NPY pathways acting independent of the hypothalamus are involved in regulating bone (i.e. Y1 signalling present on osteoblasts) [17, 18]. Indeed, osteoblasts express leptin receptors, NPY receptor (Y1R) and produce NPY [19], similar to the neurons of the arcuate nucleus on the hypothalamus. However, the extent to which osteoblastic activity may be modulated by circulating leptin levels is unknown. It has been demonstrated that specific elevation of NPY in osteoblasts is capable of altering bone mass [20].

Thus, in summary, the leptin-NPY pathway is a powerful regulator of bone mass. Increased NPY levels are overall detrimental to both cancellous and cortical bone. Hypothalamic NPY signalling is a critical component of the regulation of bone by leptin, most prominently in cortical bone, reducing bone mass in leptin-deficient states. However, an increase in cancellous bone is present in *ob/ob* mice suggesting that the adrenergic pathway is more dominant in the regulation of cancellous bone than NPY signalling. Together the central pathways regulated by leptin appear to account for the complicated bone phenotype found in *ob/ob* and *db/db* mice. However, peripheral, osteoblastic processes are also important in the control of bone cell function by NPY.

Peripheral Effects of Leptin

Although the central signalling pathways have profound effects on bone, the nature of the peripheral effects of leptin and their contribution to the bone phenotype has been less clear. Adipocytes are predominantly located within the fat pads and thus, mainly affect the body via leptin dissemination in the blood. Additionally, adipocytes are also present within the bone marrow and leptin secretion may directly influence the bone microenvironment.

Leptin and Bone Cells

Ducy et al. (2000) were unable to detect the presence of leptin receptors in primary osteoblasts using RT-PCR or any direct response of leptin on *ex vivo* osteoblastic cultures [1]. However, subsequent studies have since confirmed the presence of leptin receptors in both rodent and human osteoblasts [21-26]. *Ex vivo* cultures of osteoblasts in the presence of leptin resulted in increased cell proliferation [25], increased differentiation via GSK-3β and the WNT pathway [27], increased mineralisation [26], and a reduction in the *Bax-α*/*Bcl-2* mRNA ratio, which is indicative of an anti-apoptotic effect [26]. A recent study by Zhang et al., (2013) analysed the differences between primary osteoblasts and osteoblasts that had been transfected with Ob-RbsiRNAto block leptin signalling [28]. They found that there was a decrease in expression in the transfected cells for genes associated with bone mineralisation and ossification; and complementary to this, increased gene expression in osteoblast differentiation and bone resorption [28]. A range of genes associated with osteoblasts were altered by the Ob-Rb siRNA such as alkaline phosphatase, osteomodulin, interleukin-6 (IL-6), transforming growth factor β receptor 2, and beta-catenin [28]. Whilst subcutaneous administration of leptin increased bone formationin *ob/ob* mice [29]. Therefore, the direct action of leptin on osteoblasts promotes bone formation both *ex vivo* and *in vivo*. This response is consistent with the reduction in bone mass and bone formation in cortical bone of *ob/ob* mice, but remains in contrast to the increase in cancellous bone volume evident in these mice. As mentioned above, the greater cancellous bone volume of *ob/ob* is consistent with starvation models in mice [16]. At present our understanding of the basis for the contrasting envelope-specific actions of leptin on bone mass remains elusive, however, it does indicate that at reduced leptin concentrations, the central, stimulatory effects on cancellous bone predominate, while at high concentrations, the direct effects may become increasingly important. However, the effect of leptin insensitivity, known to occur in regions of the hypothalamus during obesity [30], remains poorly defined. This aspect, particularly in long term obese individuals requires greater evaluation.

Leptin signalling also influences osteoclastogenesis and osteoclast activity, particular by altering the signalling between osteoblasts and osteoclasts. Decreased RANKL expression and increased expression of osteoprotegerin (OPG) and IL-6were present after exposure of osteoblast cultures to leptin [26, 31]. OPG is a decoy receptor for receptor activator of nuclear factor kappa B ligand (RANKL), which is promotes the differentiation of osteoclast precursors into mature osteoclasts. In agreement with the results from *ex vivo* cultures, Hamrick et al. (2005) noted that *ob/ob* mice display a low number of osteoclasts, whilst subcutaneous delivery of10 μg/day leptin for 14 days in these mice increased osteoclast number in vertebral cancellous bone [32]. This trend was accompanied by a non-significant increase in osteoblast surface as well [32]. Interestingly, the direct effects of leptin on osteoblasts and osteoclasts promote bone formation; therefore, these direct effects oppose the previously described central pathways. Thus, understandably the influence of leptin directly on bone has been rather controversial due to the nature of opposing effects between the pathways.

Influence of Leptin on MSC Differentiation

Mesenchymal stem cells (MSCs) are present in the bone marrow stroma. These cells have the potential to differentiate into osteogenic, adipogenic, chondrogenic and marrow stromal lineages [33]. Leptin receptor binding on MSCs was increased after 24hrs of either adipogenic or osteoblastic differentiation suggesting that there may be factors within the differentiation media that regulate leptin membrane receptors [33]. Similarly, Scheller et al. (2010) demonstrated that leptin could have multiple peripheral roles depending on the differentiation state of the MSC using leptin receptor conditional knockouts in MSCs and osteoblasts [34].

In addition to leptin stimulating osteoblast differentiation, leptin treatment also inhibits adipogenesis by phosphorylating and thus inactivating peroxisome proliferator-activated receptors (PPARγ) [33, 35, 36]. Yu et al. (2012) determined that PPARγ inhibits adipogenesis; however, found that knockdowns of PPARγ had no effect on osteogenesis [37]. Therefore, it is possible that leptin is influential in regulating MSC differentiation and controls the other downstream pathways associated with differentiation such as those regulating PPARγ.

The cAMP/PKA/CREB pathway is also implicated in enhancing adipogenesis and decreasing osteogenesis [38]. In MSCs, PKA stimulators decrease leptin synthesis and secretion [38]. The activation of PKA and subsequent repression of leptin has been shown to the decrease osteogenesis and the RANKL:OPG ratio, thus, in turn also decreasing osteoclastogenesis [38]. Therefore, leptin can have multiple effects on MSCs by altering leptin receptor binding, affecting differentiation or by affecting osteoblastic-osteoclastic signals.

COMPLEXITIES OF LEPTIN SIGNALLING TO BONE

In the presence of diverse and multiple leptin signalling pathways, the debate as to whether the leptin primarily acts peripherally or centrally has been contentious [1, 29, 34, 39, 40]. The central pathways clearly have profound effects with the adrenergic pathway accounting for changes in cancellous bone and the leptin-NPY pathway contributing to the effects on cortical bone mass. Importantly, these have been most overtly demonstrated in the absence of leptin, when starvation signals are active and energy conservation predominates, including a reduction in bone production and mass. In contrast to the central effects, the peripheral effects of leptin on the bone microenvironment are more consistent with leptin excess, and thus obesity, is consistent with bone anabolism. Thus, in order to appreciate the relevance of these pathways, a context-dependent paradigm is required. However, the vast majority of studies conducted on central leptin signalling, have not been associated with starvation, but rather activation of central starvation pathways and the ensuing peripheral obesity. Similarly, the majority of the studies examining leptin signalling pathways have been conducted in cell culture models or rodent models, where exogenous leptin supply has a marked effect on energy homeostasis; reducing weight and fat mass very rapidly. Thus studying these pathways in more physiological circumstances remains problematic.

In addition to the issues surrounding appropriate models for studying leptin biology, the fundamental dynamics of leptin signalling adds a further level of complexity, associated with leptin insensitivity. As serum leptin levels increase, the activity of the signalling pathway reduces, such that some regions, notably the arcuate nucleus, display greatly attenuated leptin responses during obesity [41]. This has also been demonstrated for bone, where 4-fold and 300-fold elevations of circulating leptin levels (via transgenic mouse models) produced similar changes cancellous bone volume [42]. Indeed, this insensitivity lies at the centre of the failure of leptin-based therapeutics to reduce obesity. The extent to which these processes occur in the osteoblastic leptin receptors remains to be defined.

Further work is still required to confirm the role of leptin on bone in humans. Studies analysing associations between leptin and bone have produced mixed results with either a positive or no association [43-47]. It has been observed that congenitally leptin deficient children do not have the skeletal changes such as short stature that have been described in *ob/ob* mice [48]. This suggests that differences in leptin signalling may be present between rodent and humans. However, the peripheral effects of leptin between rodent and human osteoblasts examined in cell culture are consistent demonstrating that leptin directly promotes bone formation [27, 49].

CONCLUSION

The study of leptin and its regulation of bone homeostasis has opened up previously unpredicted regulatory associations between the skeleton and other organ systems. As such, they have been a great success in broadening our appreciation of the biology of bone and its inter-connections throughout the body. Both central and peripheral leptin signalling have varied effects on bone metabolism. The utilisation of rodent and cell culture models and clinical studies have emphasised that there are multiple pathways regulating the actions and effects of leptin. The importance of leptin to bone is becoming increasingly relevant in light of the ever increasing obesity rates in contemporary society. The magnitude of the changes in obesity rates makes a thorough and systematic understanding of these leptin/bone interactions critical in our efforts to deal with these now common metabolic disturbances, not only in adults but also children.

REFERENCES

[1] Ducy P, Amling M, Takeda S, Priemel M, Schilling AF, Beil FT, et al. Leptin inhibits bone formation through a hypothalamic relay: a central control of bone mass. *Cell.* 2000; 100(2):197-207. Epub 2000/02/05.

[2] Baldock PA, Allison S, McDonald MM, Sainsbury A, Enriquez RF, Little DG, et al. Hypothalamic regulation of cortical bone mass: opposing activity of Y2 receptor and leptin pathways. *Journal of bone and mineral research: the official Journal of the American Society for Bone and Mineral Research.* 2006; 21(10):1600-7. Epub 2006/09/26.

[3] Baldock PA, Sainsbury A, Allison S, Lin EJ, Couzens M, Boey D, et al. Hypothalamic control of bone formation: distinct actions of leptin and y2 receptor pathways. *Journal of bone and mineral research: the official Journal of the American Society for Bone and Mineral Research.* 2005; 20(10):1851-7. Epub 2005/09/15.

[4] Hamrick MW, Pennington C, Newton D, Xie D, Isales C. Leptin deficiency produces contrasting phenotypes in bones of the limb and spine. *Bone.* 2004; 34(3):376-83. Epub 2004/03/09.

[5] Takeda S, Elefteriou F, Levasseur R, Liu X, Zhao L, Parker KL, et al. Leptin regulates bone formation via the sympathetic nervous system. *Cell.* 2002; 111(3):305-17. Epub 2002/11/07.

[6] Tartaglia LA, Dembski M, Weng X, Deng N, Culpepper J, Devos R, et al. Identification and expression cloning of a leptin receptor, *OB-R. Cell.* 1995; 83(7):1263-71.

[7] Fei H, Okano HJ, Li C, Lee GH, Zhao C, Darnell R, et al. Anatomic localization of alternatively spliced leptin receptors (Ob-R) in mouse brain and other tissues. *Proc. Natl. Acad. Sci. U S A.* 1997; 94(13):7001-5. Epub 1997/06/24.

[8] Elefteriou F, Ahn JD, Takeda S, Starbuck M, Yang X, Liu X, et al. Leptin regulation of bone resorption by the sympathetic nervous system and CART. *Nature.* 2005; 434(7032):514-20. Epub 2005/02/23.

[9] Hamrick MW, Ferrari SL. Leptin and the sympathetic connection of fat to bone. *Osteoporosis international: a Journal established as result of cooperation between the European Foundation for Osteoporosis and the National Osteoporosis Foundation of the USA.* 2008; 19(7):905-12. Epub 2007/10/10.

[10] Pierroz DD, Bonnet N, Bianchi EN, Bouxsein ML, Baldock PA, Rizzoli R, et al. Deletion of beta-adrenergic receptor 1, 2, or both leads to different bone phenotypes and response to mechanical stimulation. *Journal of bone and mineral research: the official Journal of the American Society for Bone and Mineral Research.* 2012; 27(6):1252-62. Epub 2012/03/13.

[11] Wilding JP, Gilbey SG, Bailey CJ, Batt RA, Williams G, Ghatei MA, et al. Increased neuropeptide-Y messenger ribonucleic acid (mRNA) and decreased neurotensin mRNA in the hypothalamus of the obese (ob/ob) mouse. *Endocrinology*. 1993; 132(5):1939-44. Epub 1993/05/01.

[12] Driessler F, Baldock PA. Hypothalamic regulation of bone. *Journal of molecular endocrinology*. 2010; 45(4):175-81. Epub 2010/07/28.

[13] Bjurholm A. Neuroendocrine peptides in bone. *International orthopaedics*. 1991; 15(4):325-9. Epub 1991/01/01.

[14] Baldock PA, Lee NJ, Driessler F, Lin S, Allison S, Stehrer B, et al. Neuropeptide Y knockout mice reveal a central role of NPY in the coordination of bone mass to body weight. *PLoS One*. 2009; 4(12):e8415. Epub 2009/12/23.

[15] Wong IP, Nguyen AD, Khor EC, Enriquez RF, Eisman JA, Sainsbury A, et al. Neuropeptide Y is a critical modulator of leptin's regulation of cortical bone. *Journal of bone and mineral research: the official Journal of the American Society for Bone and Mineral Research*. 2013; 28(4):886-98. Epub 2012/10/10.

[16] Hamrick MW, Ding KH, Ponnala S, Ferrari SL, Isales CM. Caloric restriction decreases cortical bone mass but spares trabecular bone in the mouse skeleton: implications for the regulation of bone mass by body weight. *J. Bone Miner. Res*. 2008; 23(6):870-8. Epub 2008/04/26.

[17] Lee NJ, Nguyen AD, Enriquez RF, Doyle KL, Sainsbury A, Baldock PA, et al. Osteoblast specific Y1 receptor deletion enhances bone mass. *Bone*. 2011; 48(3):461-7. Epub 2010/11/03.

[18] Sousa DM, Baldock PA, Enriquez RF, Zhang L, Sainsbury A, Lamghari M, et al. Neuropeptide Y Y1 receptor antagonism increases bone mass in mice. *Bone*. 2012; 51(1):8-16. Epub 2012/04/10.

[19] Igwe JC, Jiang X, Paic F, Ma L, Adams DJ, Baldock PA, et al. Neuropeptide Y is expressed by osteocytes and can inhibit osteoblastic activity. *Journal of cellular biochemistry*. 2009; 108(3):621-30. Epub 2009/08/12.

[20] Matic I, Matthews BG, Kizivat T, Igwe JC, Marijanovic I, Ruohonen ST, et al. Bone-specific overexpression of NPY modulates osteogenesis. *Journal of musculoskeletal & neuronal interactions*. 2012; 12(4):209-18. Epub 2012/12/01.

[21] Cornish J, Callon KE, Bava U, Lin C, Naot D, Hill BL, et al. Leptin directly regulates bone cell function in vitro and reduces bone fragility in vivo. *The Journal of endocrinology*. 2002; 175(2):405-15. Epub 2002/11/14.

[22] Lee YJ, Park JH, Ju SK, You KH, Ko JS, Kim HM. Leptin receptor isoform expression in rat osteoblasts and their functional analysis. *FEBS letters*. 2002; 528(1-3):43-7. Epub 2002/09/26.

[23] Steppan CM, Crawford DT, Chidsey-Frink KL, Ke H, Swick AG. Leptin is a potent stimulator of bone growth in ob/ob mice. *Regulatory peptides*. 2000; 92(1-3):73-8. Epub 2000/10/12.

[24] Reseland JE, Syversen U, Bakke I, Qvigstad G, Eide LG, Hjertner O, et al. Leptin is expressed in and secreted from primary cultures of human osteoblasts and promotes bone mineralization. *Journal of bone and mineral research: the official Journal of the American Society for Bone and Mineral Research*. 2001; 16(8):1426-33. Epub 2001/08/14.

[25] Iwamoto I, Fujino T, Douchi T. The leptin receptor in human osteoblasts and the direct effect of leptin on bone metabolism. *Gynecological endocrinology: the official Journal of the International Society of Gynecological Endocrinology.* 2004; 19(2):97-104. Epub 2004/12/31.

[26] Gordeladze JO, Drevon CA, Syversen U, Reseland JE. Leptin stimulates human osteoblastic cell proliferation, de novo collagen synthesis, and mineralization: Impact on differentiation markers, apoptosis, and osteoclastic signaling. *Journal of cellular biochemistry.* 2002; 85(4):825-36. Epub 2002/04/23.

[27] Zeadin MG, Butcher MK, Shaughnessy SG, Werstuck GH. Leptin promotes osteoblast differentiation and mineralization of primary cultures of vascular smooth muscle cells by inhibiting glycogen synthase kinase (GSK)-3beta. *Biochemical and biophysical research communications.* 2012; 425(4):924-30. Epub 2012/08/22.

[28] Zhang J, Li T, Xu L, Li W, Cheng M, Zhuang J, et al. Leptin promotes ossification through multiple ways of bone metabolism in osteoblast: a pilot study. *Gynecological endocrinology : the official Journal of the International Society of Gynecological Endocrinology.* 2013; 29(8):758-62. Epub 2013/05/28.

[29] Turner RT, Kalra SP, Wong CP, Philbrick KA, Lindenmaier LB, Boghossian S, et al. Peripheral leptin regulates bone formation. *Journal of bone and mineral research : the official Journal of the American Society for Bone and Mineral Research.* 2013; 28(1):22-34. Epub 2012/08/14.

[30] Myers MG, Cowley MA, Munzberg H. Mechanisms of leptin action and leptin resistance. *Annual review of physiology.* 2008; 70:537-56. Epub 2007/10/17.

[31] Lamghari M, Tavares L, Camboa N, Barbosa MA. Leptin effect on RANKL and OPG expression in MC3T3-E1 osteoblasts. *Journal of cellular biochemistry.* 2006; 98(5): 1123-9. Epub 2006/02/16.

[32] Hamrick MW, Della-Fera MA, Choi YH, Pennington C, Hartzell D, Baile CA. Leptin treatment induces loss of bone marrow adipocytes and increases bone formation in leptin-deficient ob/ob mice. *Journal of bone and mineral research: the official Journal of the American Society for Bone and Mineral Research.* 2005; 20(6):994-1001. Epub 2005/05/11.

[33] Hess R, Pino AM, Rios S, Fernandez M, Rodriguez JP. High affinity leptin receptors are present in human mesenchymal stem cells (MSCs) derived from control and osteoporotic donors. *Journal of cellular biochemistry.* 2005; 94(1):50-7. Epub 2004/11/02.

[34] Scheller EL, Song J, Dishowitz MI, Soki FN, Hankenson KD, Krebsbach PH. Leptin functions peripherally to regulate differentiation of mesenchymal progenitor cells. *Stem cells.* 2010; 28(6):1071-80. Epub 2010/05/28.

[35] Thomas T, Gori F, Khosla S, Jensen MD, Burguera B, Riggs BL. Leptin acts on human marrow stromal cells to enhance differentiation to osteoblasts and to inhibit differentiation to adipocytes. *Endocrinology.* 1999; 140(4):1630-8. Epub 1999/03/31.

[36] Astudillo P, Rios S, Pastenes L, Pino AM, Rodriguez JP. Increased adipogenesis of osteoporotic human-mesenchymal stem cells (MSCs) characterizes by impaired leptin action. *Journal of cellular biochemistry.* 2008; 103(4):1054-65. Epub 2007/11/02.

[37] Yu WH, Li FG, Chen XY, Li JT, Wu YH, Huang LH, et al. PPARgamma suppression inhibits adipogenesis but does not promote osteogenesis of human mesenchymal stem

cells. *The international journal of biochemistry & cell biology*. 2012; 44(2):377-84. Epub 2011/11/29.

[38] Yang DC, Tsay HJ, Lin SY, Chiou SH, Li MJ, Chang TJ, et al. cAMP/PKA regulates osteogenesis, adipogenesis and ratio of RANKL/OPG mRNA expression in mesenchymal stem cells by suppressing leptin. *PLoS ONE*. 2008; 3(2):e1540. Epub 2008/02/07.

[39] Bartell SM, Rayalam S, Ambati S, Gaddam DR, Hartzell DL, Hamrick M, et al. Central (ICV) leptin injection increases bone formation, bone mineral density, muscle mass, serum IGF-1, and the expression of osteogenic genes in leptin-deficient ob/ob mice. *Journal of bone and mineral research: the official Journal of the American Society for Bone and Mineral Research*. 2011; 26(8):1710-20. Epub 2011/04/27.

[40] Williams GA, Callon KE, Watson M, Costa JL, Ding Y, Dickinson M, et al. Skeletal phenotype of the leptin receptor-deficient db/db mouse. *Journal of bone and mineral research: the official Journal of the American Society for Bone and Mineral Research*. 2011; 26(8):1698-709. Epub 2011/02/18.

[41] Enriori PJ, Evans AE, Sinnayah P, Cowley MA. Leptin resistance and obesity. *Obesity*. 2006; 14 Suppl 5:254S-8S. Epub 2006/10/06.

[42] Elefteriou F, Takeda S, Ebihara K, Magre J, Patano N, Kim CA, et al. Serum leptin level is a regulator of bone mass. *Proc. Natl. Acad. Sci. U S A*. 2004; 101(9):3258-63. Epub 2004/02/24.

[43] Ahmadi F, Salari S, Maziar S, Esfahanian F, Khazaeipour Z, Ranjbarnovin N. Relationship between serum leptin levels and bone mineral density and bone metabolic markers in patients on hemodialysis. *Saudi Journal of kidney diseases and transplantation: an official publication of the Saudi Center for Organ Transplantation, Saudi Arabia*. 2013; 24(1):41-7. Epub 2013/01/29.

[44] Zhao HY, Bi YF, Ma LY, Zhao L, Wang TG, Zhang LZ, et al. The effects of bisphenol A (BPA) exposure on fat mass and serum leptin concentrations have no impact on bone mineral densities in non-obese premenopausal women. *Clinical biochemistry*. 2012; 45(18):1602-6. Epub 2012/09/18.

[45] Thomas T, Burguera B, Melton LJ, 3rd, Atkinson EJ, O'Fallon WM, Riggs BL, et al. Role of serum leptin, insulin, and estrogen levels as potential mediators of the relationship between fat mass and bone mineral density in men versus women. *Bone*. 2001; 29(2):114-20. Epub 2001/08/15.

[46] Morcov C, Vulpoi C, Branisteanu D. Correlation between adiponectin, leptin, insulin growth factor-1 and bone mineral density in pre and postmenopausal women. *Revista medico-chirurgicala a Societatii de Medici si Naturalisti din Iasi*. 2012; 116(3):785-9. Epub 2013/01/01.

[47] Parm AL, Jurimae J, Saar M, Parna K, Tillmann V, Maasalu K, et al. Bone mineralization in rhythmic gymnasts before puberty: no longitudinal associations with adipocytokine and ghrelin levels. *Hormone research in paediatrics*. 2012; 77(6):369-75. Epub 2012/06/13.

[48] Farooqi IS, Jebb SA, Langmack G, Lawrence E, Cheetham CH, Prentice AM, et al. Effects of recombinant leptin therapy in a child with congenital leptin deficiency. *The New England Journal of medicine*. 1999; 341(12):879-84. Epub 1999/09/16.

[49] Kim JM, Choi JS, Kim YH, Jin SH, Lim S, Jang HJ, et al. An activator of the cAMP/PKA/CREB pathway promotes osteogenesis from human mesenchymal stem cells. *Journal of cellular physiology*. 2013; 228(3):617-26. Epub 2012/08/14.

In: Leptin: Biosynthesis, Functions and Clinical Significance ISBN: 978-1-62948-801-1
Editor: Edward L. Blum

Chapter 10

THE PHYSIOLOGICAL ROLES OF LEPTIN IN THE ORAL AND MAXILLOFACIAL REGION: PROMOTIVE EFFECTS ON MUCOSAL WOUND HEALING AND TOOTH DEVELOPMENT

Reiko Tokuyama and Kazuhito Satomura
Department of Oral Medicine and Stomatology,
Second Department of Oral and Maxillofacial Surgery,
School of Dental Medicine, Tsurumi University, Japan

ABSTRACT

Leptin, a 16 kDa circulating anti-obesity hormone, is a product of the obese (*ob*) gene. This molecule has been known to exhibit many physiological actions on body weight homeostasis, lipid metabolism, hematopoiesis, thermogenesis, ovarian function, and angiogenesis. Recently, leptin was reported to exist in saliva. However, its function in oral cavity remains to be elucidated. In this chapter, the physiological roles of leptin in oral and maxillofacial region are discussed, especially by focusing on the leptin's effects on wound healing of oral mucosa, and tooth development.

Immunohistochemical analysis revealed leptin receptor (Ob-R) was expressed in spinous cells and granular cells of human and rabbit gingival epithelium. In addition, locally administered leptin induced more rapid healing of chemical burn wounds artificially created in gingiva by enhancing the migration of oral mucosal epithelial cells and stimulating angiogenesis in connective tissue beneath the wounded area.

A topical administration of leptin also promoted the healing of chemical burn wounds created on the back skin of mice accelerating the angiogenesis in the subcutaneous connective tissue beneath the ulcer and the cell migration of skin keratinocytes. These findings strongly suggest that leptin could be a potent and promising medicine to promote the wound healing in mucosa and skin.

On the other hand, another immunohistochemical study revealed that leptin was expressed in two major tooth-forming cells in tooth germs: ameloblasts (enamel-forming cells) and odontoblasts (dentin-forming cells). More interestingly, dental papilla cells in the vicinity of odontoblastic layer expressed much more leptin. In addition, more CD31-positive vascular endothelial cells were distributed in this area. Judging from the previous study that leptin has an angiogenic effect, these findings strongly suggest the possibility that ameloblasts, odontoblasts and some dental papilla cells are recruiting the blood vessels into tooth germs by secreting leptin to ensure the immaculate tooth development.

In summary, leptin, a multi-functional molecule not only as a systemic hormone but also as a local growth factor, plays important physiological roles in oral and maxillofacial region.

BACKGROUND

Leptin, a 16 kDa non-glycosylated polypeptide anti-obesity hormone of 146 amino acids, is a product of the obese (*ob*) gene [1]. Although it was reported that leptin is mainly produced by adipose tissue [1], recent studies have demonstrated that this molecule is produced by some other tissues such as placenta [2], stomach [3], skeletal muscles [4], brain and pituitary gland [5, 6]. Leptin is also known to exhibit a variety of physiological actions on body weight homeostasis [7], lipid metabolism [8], hematopoiesis [9], thermogenesis [10], ovarian function [11], bone formation [12, 13], angiogenesis [14, 15] and wound healing [16-18].

On the other hand, leptin receptor is expressed in various tissues such as hypothalamus [19, 20], adipose tissue [21], skeletal muscle [22], hepatocytes [21, 23], and so on. These multifunctionality of leptin and wide distribution of its receptor suggest that leptin plays a variety of physiological roles not only as an systemic hormone but also as an local growth factor.

Interestingly, it was recently reported that leptin exists in human saliva [24], but physiological role of leptin in oral cavity remains to be elucidated. In this chapter, the possible physiological roles of leptin in oral and maxillofacial region will be discussed, especially by focusing on leptin's influence on wound healing of oral mucosa/skin and tooth development.

A. EFFECT OF LEPTIN ON THE WOUND HEALING OF ORAL MUCOSA

1. Localization of Leptin Receptor in Human/Rabbit Oral Mucosa

An immunohistochemical analysis using anti-leptin receptor antibody revealed that leptin receptor was expressed in spinous/granular cells of epithelial tissue and vascular endothelial cell of subepithelial connective tissue of oral mucosa of human and rabbit (Figure 1). These facts suggest that oral mucosal epithelial cells and vascular endothelial cells are target of leptin.

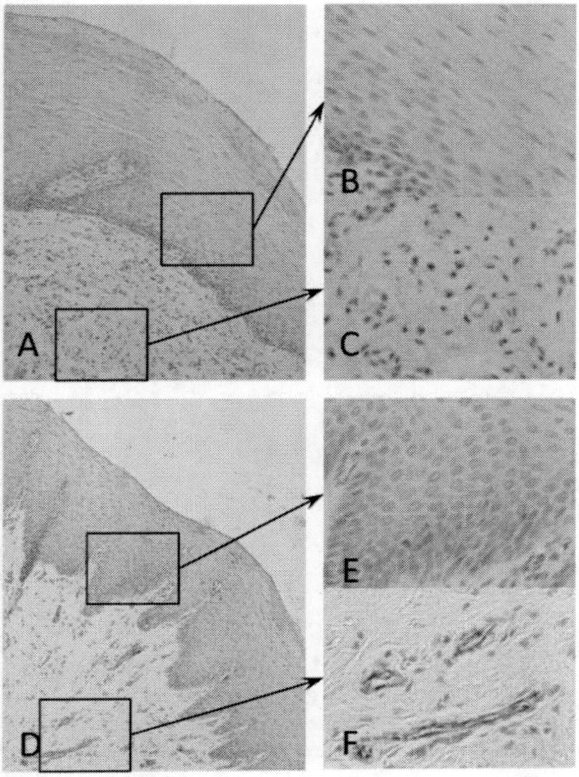

Figure 1. Immunohistochemical localization of leptin receptor in normal human and rabbit oral mucosa. (A-C) human, (D-F) rabbit. (B, C, E and F) leptin. Leptin receptor was expressed in spinous/granular cells of epithelial tissue (B and E) and vascular endothelial cells of subepithelial connective tissue (C and F) of oral mucosa of human and rabbit.

2. Effect of Leptin on the Wound Healing of Oral Mucosa

To elucidate the effect of leptin on wound healing of oral mucosa, rabbit oral mucosa chemical burn model was used. In brief, pieces (5×5 mm) of filter paper soaked with 50% acetic acid were attached for 2 minites onto mandibular gingiva of Japanese white rabbits (2.5-3.0 kg, male) to produce chemical burns. Ten μl solution of 100 ng/ml leptin or phosphate-buffered saline (PBS) (as a control) was mixed in Cellmatrix® (type I collagen, Nitta Gelatin Inc., Osaka, Japan) and topically applied on wound everyday. The size of ulcer was measured on day 6 and day 13 after burn formation, and the gingival tissue around the wound was obtained for histological analysis. In addition, body weight (BW), aspartate aminotransferase (AST), alanine aminotransferase (ALT) and blood sugar level (BS) were also measured for the detection of adverse effects. These experiments showed that wound areas were significantly decreased in leptin-treated group compared with control group (Figure 2). In addition, the duration required for complete healing of ulcer was shortened in leptin-treated group (Figure 3). The levels of BW, AST, ALT or BS were not affected through experiment period, showing that topically-administered leptin had no systemic adverse effects.

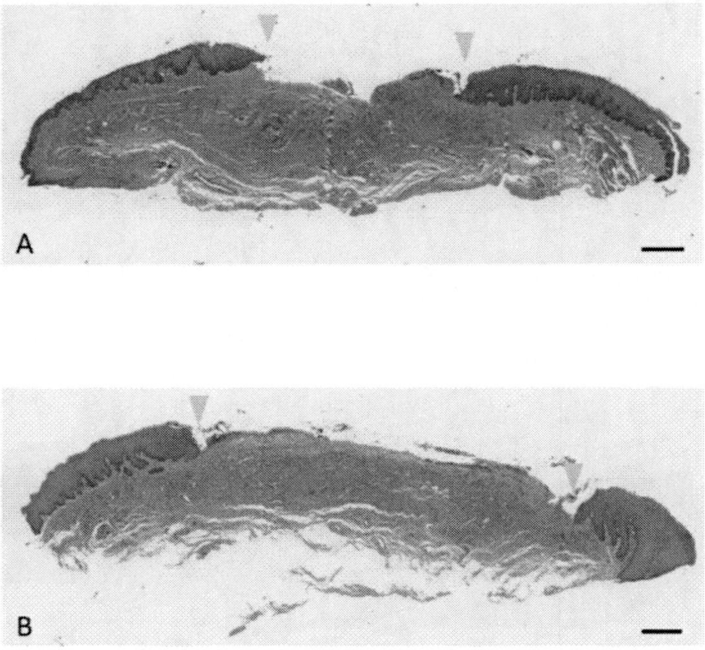

Figure 2. Histological finding of wound repair of gingiva at day 6 after initial wounding in leptin-treated and control group. (A) leptin. (B) control. Spaces between arrow heads show ulcerative area without epithelium. Wound heal is significantly enhanced in leptin-treated group. H-E staining. Bars : 500 μm.

3. Mechanism of the Promotive Effect of Leptin on the Wound Healing of Oral Mucosa

To elucidate the mechanism underlying leptin's promotive effect on oral mucosal wound healing, some cell biological assays were performed using human oral mucosal epithelial cell line (RT7) and human gingival fibroblastic cell line (GT1) (generous gifts from Prof. Nobuyuki Kamata, Hiroshima University, Japan).

RT-PCR analysis showed the expression of leptin receptor in both RT7 cells and GT1 cells.

The cell proliferation assay using RT7 cells and GT1 cells revealed that the proliferation of these cells was not affected with leptin at any concentrations examined (0, 0.1, 1 and 10 ng/ml).

Semi-quantitative RT-PCR analysis was performed to examine whether leptin has any influence on differentiation and/or function of oral mucosa. As a result, leptin had no apparent effect on the expression of mRNA encoding *Keratin 4*, *Keratin 10* and *Transglutaminase I* in RT7 cells; *fibronectin*, *laminin* and *type IV collagen* in GT1 cells.

Next, to examine the effect of leptin on cell migration, scratch assay using RT7 cells was performed. This assay showed that leptin promoted the migration of RT7 cells (Figure 4).

Moreover, immunohistochemical analysis of gingival tissues beneath the ulcer using anti-CD31 (a marker of endothelial cells [25-28]) antibody showed that more blood vessels distributed in the connective tissue beneath the ulcer in leptin-treated group compared with control group (Figure 5).

Taken together, from these findings, leptin was proven to promote the wound healing of oral mucosa by accelerating epithelial cell migration and enhancing angiogenesis around wounded area.

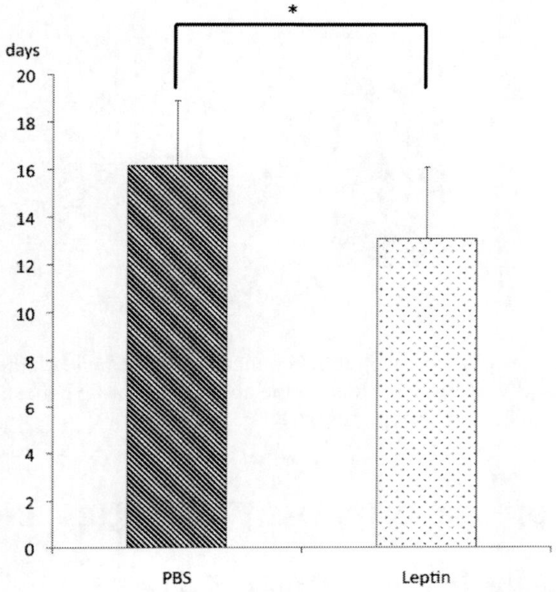

Figure 3. Period until the healing of rabbit gingiva. The duration required for complete healing of ulcer was shortened in leptin-treated group. *P<0.05

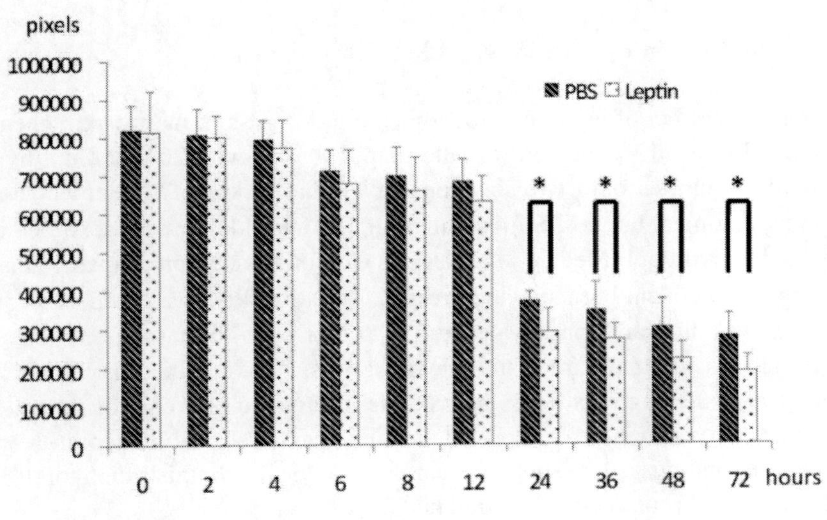

Figure 4. Effect of leptin on the migration of RT7 cells. The areas without cells were calculated. The area without cells decreased significantly in leptin-treated group from 24 to 72 hours after wounding. *P<0.05

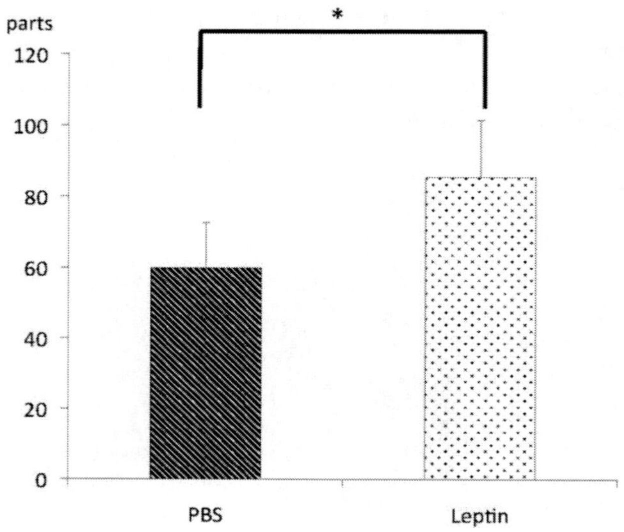

Figure 5. Number of blood vessels in subepithelial connective tissue beneath the ulcer. At 6 days after initial wounding, more blood vessels distributed in the connective tissue beneath the ulcer in leptin-treated group compared with control group. *P<0.01.

B. Effect of Leptin on the Wound Healing of Skin

1. Localization of Leptin in Human/Mouse Skin

Another immunohistochemical analysis showed that leptin receptor was expressed in keratinocytes and fibroblasts and vascular endothelial cells in the skin of human and mice.

2. The Effect of Leptin on the Wound Healing of Skin

To elucidate the effect of leptin on wound healing of the skin, mouse skin chemical burn model was used. Pieces (12 × 12 mm) of filter paper soaked with 20% sodium hypochlorite was attached for 5 minites onto two locations of the back skin of ICR mice (6-week-old, male) to produce chemical burns. Ten μl solution of 100 ng/ml leptin was absorbed in 12 × 12 mm bio-absorbable hydrogel (MedGel®, MeDGEL Corporation, Kyoto, Japan). This hydrogel was attached to the chemical burn site and dressed. Ten μl of PBS was used as a control. The size of the ulcer was measured on day 4 and day 8 after burn formation, and the skin tissue around the wound was obtained for histological analysis. As a result, at day 4, no significant difference in wound healing was noted between leptin-treated and control group. At day 8, however, significantly enhanced re-epithelialization was observed in leptin-treated group (Figure 6). These findings suggested that single and local administration of leptin using bioabsorbable hydrogel promoted the wound healing of skin.

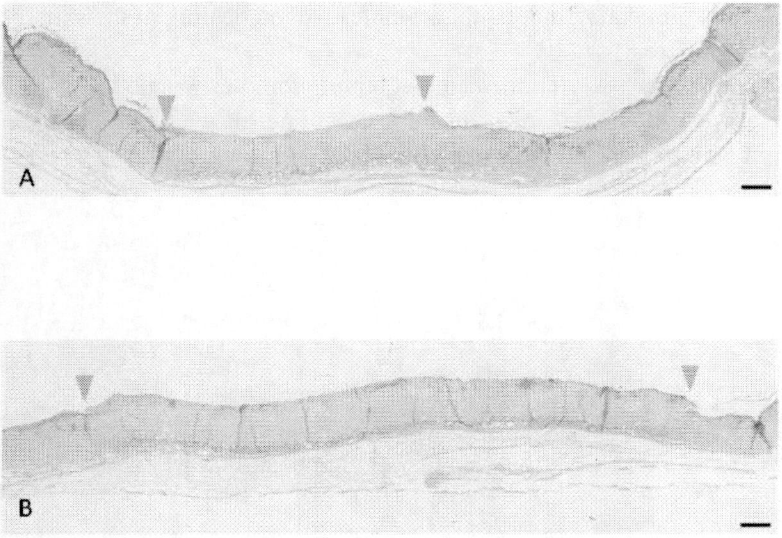

Figure 6. Histological findings of wound repair of skin at day 8 after initial wounding in leptin-treated and control group. (A) leptin. (B) control. Spaces between arrow heads show ulcerative area without epithelium. Wound heal is significantly enhanced in leptin-treated group. H-E staining. Bars : 500 μm.

3. Mechanism of the Promotive Effect of Leptin on the Wound Healing of Skin

To elucidate how topically administered leptin could promote wound healing, the influences of leptin on the proliferation, differentiation and migration of human skin fibroblasts (HSB cells) and human skin keratinocytes (HSK cells) (Takara Bio Inc., Shiga, Japan) were investigated using the above-mentioned methods.

RT-PCR analysis revealed the expression of leptin receptor in both HSB cells and HSK cells. The cell proliferation assay for HSB cells and HSK cells showed that the proliferation of these cells was not affected with leptin at any concentrations examined between 0 and 10 ng/ml. Semi-quantitative RT-PCR analysis showed that leptin had no significant effects on mRNA expression of keratinocyte- and fibroblast-related genes including *laminin*, *fibronectin*, *type I*, *II* and *IV collagen*.

Next, to examine the effect of leptin on cell migration of human keratinocytes, scratch assay using HSK cells was performed. As a result, the significant effect was not observed during initial 8 hours. However, the area without cells decreased significantly in leptin-treated group compared with control group from 12 to 48 hours after scratching (Figure 7). This result demonstrated that leptin promotes the cell migration of human keratinocytes.

Moreover, we elucidated whether leptin accelerates the angiogenesis in the connective tissues beneath the wound in the skin as well as oral mucosa by histological analysis. The localization of blood vessels was analyzed by immunohistochemistry by using anti-CD31 antibody. As a result, at day 4 after initial wounding, no significant difference on the number of CD31-positive cells was detected between leptin-treated and control group. However, at day 8 after initial wounding, the number of CD31-positive cells significantly increased in leptin-treated group, indicating that leptin promotes wound healing of the skin by accelerating the angiogenesis (Figure 8).

From these findings, it was confirmed that leptin promotes wound healing of the skin and the oral mucosa by a similar mechanism: promoting of epithelial cell migration and enhancing angiogenesis beneath the wound.

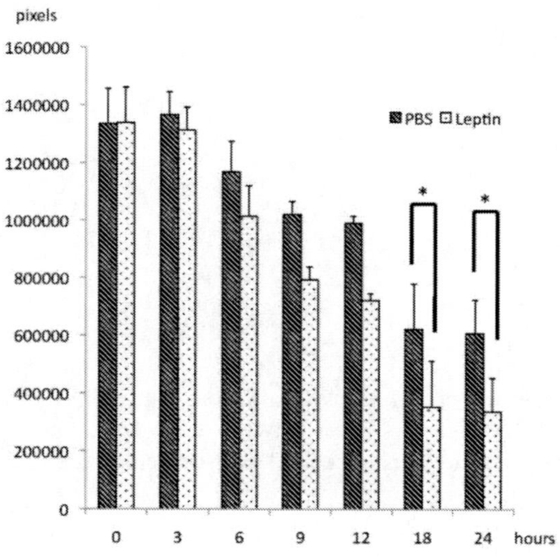

Figure 7. Effect of leptin on the migration of human skin keratinocytes. The areas without cells were calculated. The area without cells decreased significantly in leptin-treated group from 18 to 24 hours after wounding. *P<0.05.

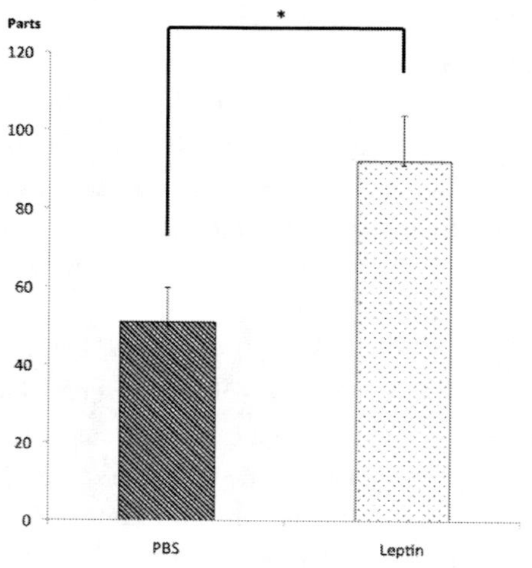

Figure 8. Number of vascular endothelial cells in subepithelial connective tissue beneath the ulcer. At 8 days after initial wounding, more vascular endothelial cells distributed in the connective tissue beneath the ulcer in leptin-treated group compared with control group. *P<0.05.

C. Leptin Regulates the Angiogenesis in Tooth Germ

1. Tooth Development

Tooth development is a dynamic process in which complex tooth morphogenesis proceeds through epithelial-mesenchymal interaction [29]. In the bell stage of tooth development, some dental papilla cells adjacent to the inner enamel epithelium differentiate into odontoblasts and start secreting the dentin matrix. Concurrent with these events, inner enamel epithelial cells differentiate into ameloblasts and secrete the enamel matrix [30, 31]. In the process of matrix formation, ameloblasts and odontoblasts are considered to be regulated not only by local growth factors, but also by systemic hormones such as growth hormone and melatonin [32]. Moreover, for sufficient matrix proteins to be made, it seems to be critical for ameloblasts and odontoblasts to be supplied with rich nutritious materials. This suggests that ameloblasts and/or odontoblasts could express some factors to induce angiogenesis around themselves in order to obtain nutrients and to receive systemic signals. Thus, we immunohistochemically examined the expression of leptin, which has an angiogenic activity, in rat and human tooth germs.

2. Localization of Leptin in Tooth Germs

An immunohistochemical analysis was performed to examine the expression of leptin in incisors and molars in the mandible of 3-day-old rats.

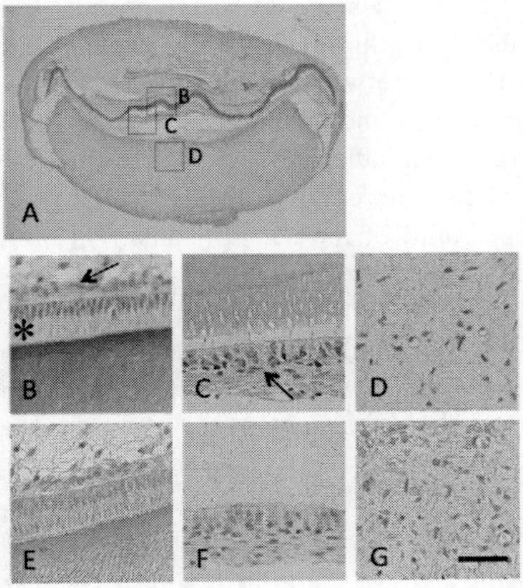

Figure 9. General histology of a human tooth germ (A) stained with hematoxylin and eosin. (B) Ameloblasts (asterisk), stratum intermedium cells (arrow), and enamel, (C) odontoblasts (arrow), (D) dental papilla cells. (E-G) Immunohistochemical localization of leptin in human tooth germ (AEC and hematoxylin). Leptin was expressed in ameloblasts (E), atratum intermedium cells (E), odontoblasts (F) and dental papilla cells (G). Bar is 10 μm. (Referred from Ide S et al. Leptin and vascular endothelial growth factor regulate angiogenesis in tooth germs. Histochem Cell Biol, 135:281-292, 2011.).

In this stage of development, the formation of enamel and dentin was observed in both incisors and molars. Histologically, ameloblasts, odontoblasts, stratum intermedium and osteoblasts were positive for leptin. Another immunohistochemical analysis was performed to examine leptin expression in tooth germs of human mandibular third molars. In the late bell stage, tooth crown formation had begun and some dentin and enamel tissues were noted in the area where the cups would later be formed. In these areas, ameloblasts, odontoblasts, stratum indermedium, stellate reticulum, enamel and dentin could be histologically recognized. Immunohistochemical analysis revealed that leptin was intensely expressed in the ameloblasts, stratum intermedium cells and odontoblasts; and some dental papilla cells were also noted to be slightly positive for leptin (Figure 9).

3. Distribution of Blood Vessels in Human Dental Papillae

To date, no direct evidence has been available to indicate that leptin expressed in ameloblasts and odontoblasts induce angiogenesis in tooth germs. Therefore, we investigated the distribution of blood vessels in human tooth germs by immunohistochemical analysis for CD31 which is endothelial cell marker [25-28]. The dental papillae of the human tooth germs were divided into three portions: upper, middle and lower thirds along the axis from the odontoblastic layer to the dental sac layer. Twenty fields (425 μm × 320 μm each) for each portion in the three sections were arbitrarily selected and the number of CD31-positive cells was counted; and the percentage of CD31-positive cells in the nucleated cell population were calculated for each portion. As a result, a considerable number of CD31-positive cells were observed in the upper third of the dental papilla, while only a few CD31-positive cells were noted in the lower third. The parcentage of CD31-positive cells in the nucleated cell population was 15.0% in the upper third, 6.3% in the middle third, and 1.3% in the lower third, respectively (Figure 10). There was a statistically significant difference in the CD31-positive cell rate between the upper and middle, and upper and lower thirds. No significant difference was found between the middle and lower third. Briefly, immunohistochemical and histometric analysis showed that more CD31-positive cells, presumably endothelial cells, were distributed in the upper third of the dental papilla. On the other hand, in the dental papillae, the total number of nucleated cells except for endothelial cells was 526.8 ± 31.4/field in the upper third, 235.8 ± 8.1/field in the middle third, and 145.0 ± 17.3/field in lower third, respectively (Figure 11). There was a statistically significant difference in the number of nucleated cells between the upper and middle, upper and lower, and middle and lower thirds. This showed that the cell density of the upper third was much higher than any other thirds.

4. Distribution of Leptin-Positive Cells in Human Dental Papilla

The distribution of leptin-positive cells in human dental papilla was examined. In the dental papilla, the total number of leptin-positive cells was 493.2 ± 21.8/field in the upper third, 220.8 ± 8.5/field in the middle third, and 131.3 ± 8.0/field in lower third, respectively (Figure 12 A-D).

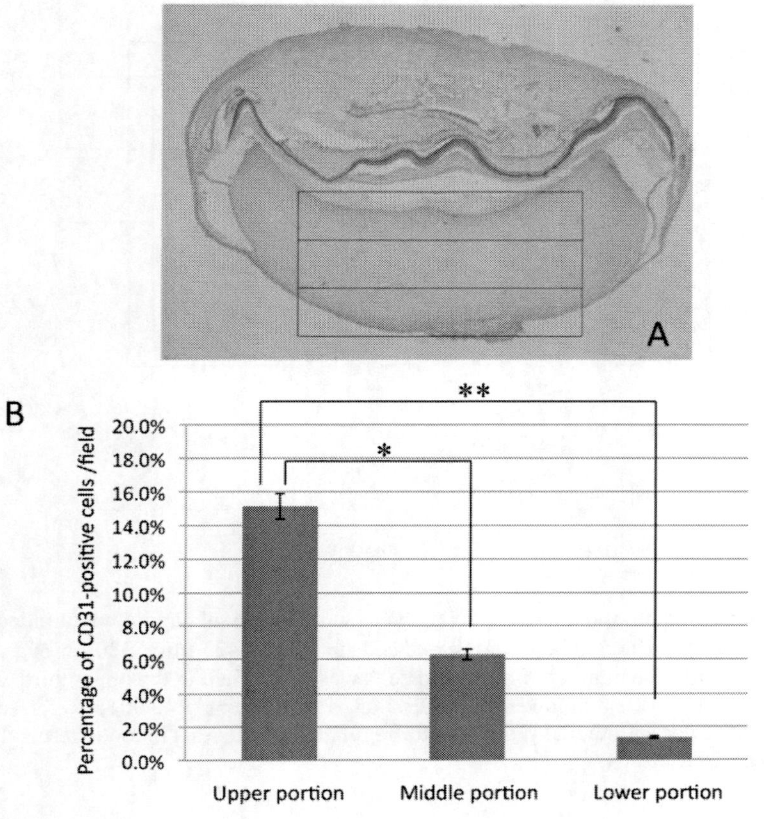

Figure 10. (A) Diagram of segmentalized dental papilla of human tooth germ. The dental papilla was divided into thirds: upper, middle and lower. The number of CD31-positive or CD34-positive cells was counted in each third. The percentage of CD31-positive cells was 15.0% in the upper third, 6.3% in the middle third and 1.3% in the lower third (B). *$P<0.05$, **$P<0.01$, ***$P<0.001$. (Referred from Ide S et al. Leptin and vascular endothelial growth factor regulate angiogenesis in tooth germs. Histochem Cell Biol, 135:281-292, 2011.).

There was a statistically significant difference in the number of leptin-positive cells between the upper and middle, upper and lower, and middle and lower thirds. The parcentage of leptin-positive cells in the nucleated cell population was 93.6% in the upper third, 93.2% in the middle third, and 92.0% in the lower third, respectively (Figure 12 E). No significant difference was found in the leptin-positive cell rate among the upper, middle and lower thirds. Briefly, the immunohistochemical analysis of leptin expression in dental papilla tissues revealed that almost same proportion of cells was positive for leptin in any three portions. In other words, although the parcentage of leptin-positive cells is consistent throughout the dental pulp, there are statistically much more leptin-positive cells exist in the upper third of dental papillae. These results strongly suggested that the cell density in the dental pulp may influence the gradient of leptin, and that this leptin gradient in dental papilla tissue may induce the angiogenesis through recruiting endothelial cells deep into the tooth germs and branching the vessels [33].

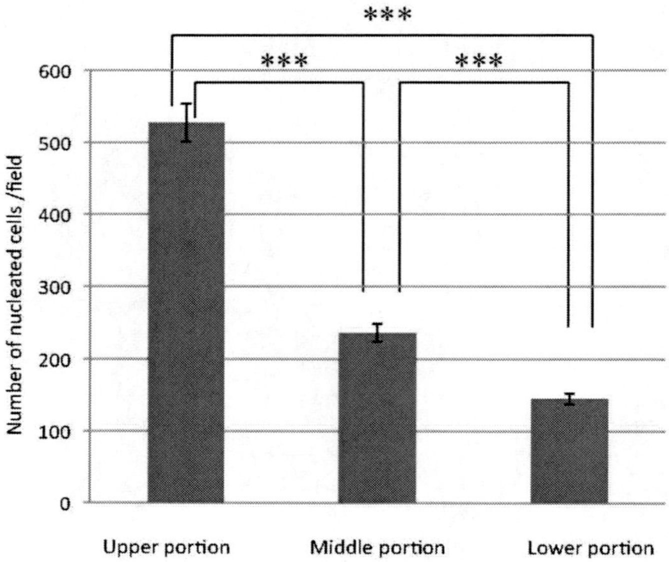

Figure 11. Photomicrograph of human dental papilla tissue. The dental papilla was divided into thirds: upper, middle and lower. The number of nucleated cells in a field (425 μm × 320 μm) was counted arbitrarily in each third. The number of nucleated cells was 526.8/field in the upper third, 235.8/field in the middle third and 145.0/field in lower third. *P<0.05, **P<0.01, ***P<0.001. (Referred from Ide S et al. Leptin and vascular endothelial growth factor regulate angiogenesis in tooth germs. Histochem Cell Biol, 135:281-292, 2011.).

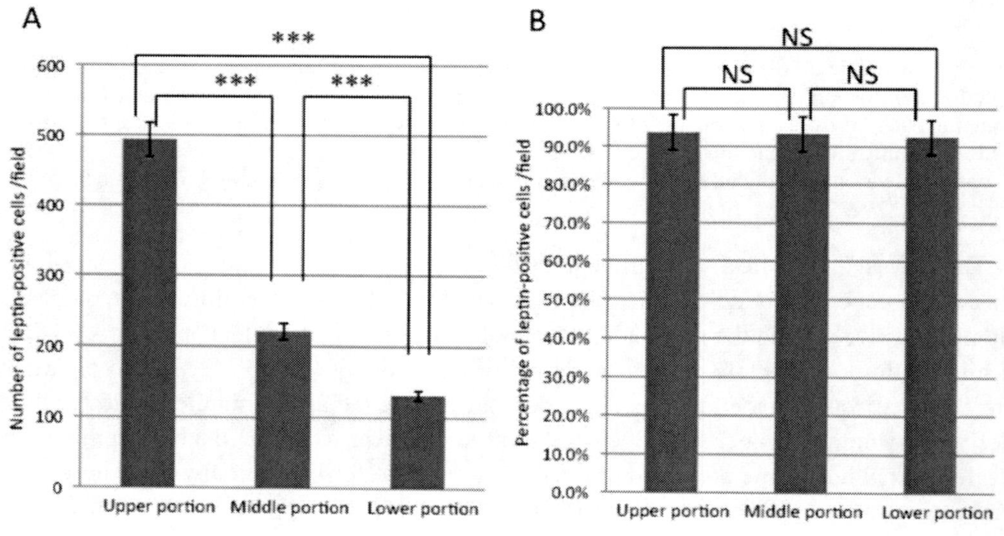

Figure 12. Immunohistochemical localization of leptin in human dental papilla. The dental papilla was divided into third: upper, middle and lower. The number of leptin-positive cells was 493.2 in the upper third, 220.8 in the middle third and 131.3 in the lower third (A). The percentage of leptin-positive cells in the nucleated cell population was 93.6% in the upper third, 93.2% in the middle third and 92.0% in the lower third (B). *P<0.05, **P<0.01, ***P<0.001. (Referred from Ide S et al. Leptin and vascular endothelial growth factor regulate angiogenesis in tooth germs. Histochem Cell Biol, 135:281-292, 2011.).

Conclusion

Leptin is capable of promoting wound healing of oral mucosa and skin by influencing epithelial cell migration and angiogenesis in the connective tissue beneath the wound. This fact strongly suggests the possible and promising usefulness of leptin as a new wound healing-promoting drug. Moreover, it is also suggested that leptin may be useful for treatment and/or prevention of abnormal condition in oral cavity such as lichen planus, intractable stomatitis occurred with radiotherapy and/or chemotherapy against head and neck cancers. In addition, the findings presented in this chapter suggested that leptin expressed by ameloblasts and odontoblasts is involved in tooth development by inducing angiogenesis in tooth germs. Taken together, leptin is proven to play physiological roles in oral and maxillofacial region as well as other tissues and organs not only as a systemic hormone but also as a local growth factor.

References

[1] Zhang Y, Proenca R, Maffei M, Barone M, Leopold L & Friedman JM. (1994). Positional cloning of the mouse obese gene and its human homologue. *Nature,* 372, 425-432.

[2] Masuzaki H, Ogawa Y, Sagawa N, Hosoda K, Matsumoto T, Mise H, Nishimura H, Yoshimasa Y, Tanaka I, Mori T & Nakao K. (1997). Nonadipose tissue production of leptin: leptin as a novel placenta-derived hormone in humans. *Nat. Med.,* 3, 1029-1033.

[3] Bado A, Levasseur S, Attoub S, Kermorgant S, Laigneau JP, Bortoluzzi MN, Moizo L, Lehy T, Guerre-Millo M, Marchand-Brustel YL & Lewin MJM. (1998). The stomach is a source of leptin. *Nature,* 394, 790-793.

[4] Wang J, Liu R, Hawkins M, Barzilai N & Rossetti L. (1998). A nutrient-sensing pathway regulates leotin gene expression in muscle and fat. *Nature,* 393, 684-688.

[5] Jin L, Burguera BG, Couse ME, Scheithauer BW, Lamsan J, Eberhardt NL, Kulig E & Lloyd RV. (1999). Leptin and leptin receptor expression in normal and neoplastic human pituitary: evidence of a regulatory role for leptin on pituitary cell proliferation. *J. Clin. Endocrinol. Metab.,* 84, 2903-2911.

[6] Morash B, Li A, Murphy PR, Wilkinson M & Ur E. (1999). Leptin gene expression in the brain and pituitary gland. *Endocrinology,* 140, 5995-5998.

[7] Friedman JM & Halaas JL. (1998). Leptin and the regulation of body weight in mammals. *Nature,* 395, 763-770.

[8] Bryson JM, Phuyal JL, Swan V & Caterson ID. (1999). Leptin has acute effects on glucose and lipid metabolism in both lean and gold thioglucose-obese mice. *Am. J. Physiol.,* 277, E417-E422.

[9] Gainford T, Willson TA, Metcalf D, Handman E, McFarlane C, Ng A, Nicola NA, Alexander WS & Hilton DJ. (1996). Leptin can induce proliferation, differentiation, and functional activation of hematopoietic cells. *Proc. Natl. Acad. Sci. USA,* 93, 14564-14568.

[10] Hwa JJ, Ghibaudi L, Compton D, Fawzi AB & Strader CD. (1996). Intracerebroventricular injection of leptin increases thermogenesis and mobilizes fat metabolism in ob/ob mice. *Horm. Metab. Res.,* 8, 659-663.
[11] Spicer LJ & Francisco CC. (1997). The adipose obese gene product, leptin evidence of a direct inhibitory role in ovarian function. *Endocrinology,* 138, 3374-3379.
[12] Ducy P, Amling M, Takeda S, Priemel M, Schilling AF, Beil FT, Shen J, Vinson C, Rueger JM & Karsenty G. (2000). Leptin inhibits bone formation through a hypothalamic relay: a central control of bone mass. *Cell,* 100, 197-207.
[13] Kume K, Satomura K, Nishisho S, Kitaoka E, Yamanouchi K, Tobiume S & Nagayama M. (2002). Potential role of leptin in endochondral ossification. *J. Histochem. Cytochem.,* 50, 150-169.
[14] Bouloumie A, Drexler HCA, Lafontan M & Busse R. (1998). Leptin, the product of ob gene, promotes angiogenesis. *Circ. Res.,* 83, 1059-1066.
[15] Sierra-Honigmann MR, Nath AK, Murakami C, Garcia-Cardena G, Papapetropoulos A, Sessa WC, Madge LA, Schechner JS, Schwabb MB, Polverini PJ & Flores-Riveros JR. (1998). Biological action of leptin as an angiogenic factor. *Science,* 281, 1683-1686.
[16] Frank S, Stallmeyer B, Kampfer H, Kolb N & Pfeilschifter J. (2000). Leptin enhances wound re-epithelialization and constitutes a direct function of leptin in skin repair. *J. Clin. Invest.,* 106, 501-509.
[17] Murad A, Nath AK, Cha ST, Demir E, Flores-Riveros J & Sierra-Honigmann M. (2003). Leptin is an autocrine-paracrine regulator of wound healing. *FASEB J.,* 17, 1895-1897.
[18] Stallmeyer B, Kampfer H, Podda M, Kaufman R, Pfeilschifter J & Frank S. (2001). A novel keratinocyte mitogen: regulation of leptin and its functional receptor in skin repair. *J. Invest. Dermatol.,* 117, 98-105.
[19] Fei H, Okano J H, LiC, Lee GH, Zhao C, Darneli R & Friedman JM. (1997). Anatomic localization of alternatively spliced leptin receptors (Ob-R) in mouse brain and other tissues. *Proc. Natl. Acad. Sci. USA,* 94, 7001-7005.
[20] Mercer JG, Hoggard N, Williams LM, Lawrence CB, Hannah LT & Trayhurn P. (1996). Localization of leptin receptor mRNA and the long form splice variant (Ob-R) in mouse hypothalamus and adjacent brain regions by in situ hybridization. *FEBS Lett,* 387, 113-116.
[21] Matteis RD, Dashtipour K, Ognibene A & Cinti S. (1998). Localization of leptin receptor splice variants in mouse peripheral tissues by immunohitochemistry. *Proc. Nutr. Soc.,* 57, 441-448.
[22] Guerra B, Santana A, Fuentes T, Guerra SD, Socorro AC, Dorado C & Calbet JAL. (2007). Leptin receptor in human skeletal muscle. *J. Appl. Physiol.,* 102, 1786-1792.
[23] Cohen P, Yang G, Yu X, Soukas AA, Wolfish CS, Friedman JM & Li C. (2005). Induction of leptin receptor expression in the liver by leptin and food deprivation. *J. Biol. Chem.,* 280, 10034-10039.
[24] Groschl M, Rauh M, Wagner R, Neuhuber W, Metzler M, Tamguney G, Zenk J, Schoof E, Dorr HG, Blum WF, Rascher W & Dotsch J. (2001). Identification of leptin in human saliva. *J. Clin. Endocrinol. Metab.,* 86, 5234-5239.
[25] Parums DV, Cordell JL, Micklem K, Heryet AR, Gatter KC & Mason DY. (1990). JC70: a new monoclonal antibody that detects vascular endothelium associated antigen on routinely processed tissue sections. *J. Clin. Pathol.,* 43, 752-757.

[26] Deyoung BR, Swanson PE, Argenyi ZB, Ritter JH, Fitzgibbon JF, Stahl DJ, Hoover W & Wick MR. (1995). CD31 immunoreactivity in mesenchymal neoplasms of the skin and subcutis: report of 145 cases and review of putative immunohistologic markers of endothelial differentiation. *J. Cutan. Pathol.,* 22, 215-222.

[27] Newman PJ, Berndt MC, Gorski J, White GC 2nd, Lyman S, Paddock C & Muller WA. (1990). PECAM-1 (CD31) cloning and relation to adhesion molecules of the immunoglobulin gene superfamily. *Science,* 247, 1219-1222.

[28] Delisser HM, Newman PJ & Albelda SM. (1994). Molecular and functional aspects of PECAM-1/CD31. *Immunol. Today,* 15, 490-495.

[29] Thesleff I & Mikkola M. (2002). The role of growth factors in tooth development. *Int. Rev. Cytol.,* 217, 93-135.

[30] Ten Cate AR. (1994). Oral histology. 4th edn. Mosby, St. Louis, pp 58-80.

[31] Nait Lechguer A, Kuchler-Bopp S, Hu B, Haikel Y & lesot H. (2008). Vascularization of engineered teeth. *J. Dent. Res.,* 12, 1138-1143.

[32] Kumasaka S, Shimozuma M, Kawamoto T, Mishima K, Tokuyama R, Kamiya Y, Davaadorj P, Saito I & Satomura K. (2002). Possible involvement of melatonin in tooth development: expression of melatonin 1a receptor in human and mouse tooth germs. *Histochem. Cell Biol.,* 133, 577-584.

[33] Ide S, Tokuyama R, Davaadorj P, Shimozuma M, Kumasaka S, Tatehara S & Satomura K. (2011). Leptin and vascular endothelial growth factor regulate angiogenesis in tooth germ. *Histochem. Cell Biol.,* 135, 281-292.

In: Leptin: Biosynthesis, Functions and Clinical Significance ISBN: 978-1-62948-801-1
Editor: Edward L. Blum

Chapter 11

RESPIRATORY RESPONSES TO MICROINJECTIONS OF LEPTIN INTO THE PRE-BÖTZINGER COMPLEX OF THE RAT

Alexey N. Inyushkin*[*] *and Elena M. Inyushkina
Department of Human and Animal Physiology, Samara State University, Russian Federation

ABSTRACT

In recent studies dealing with the central control of respiration, we reported that a pleiotropic hormone mainly produced by white adipose tissue, leptin has a substantial dose-dependent excitatory effect on breathing when it is microinjected into the nucleus of the solitary tract. The present study was undertaken to assess the characteristics of the respiratory effects induced by action of leptin in the pre-Bötzinger complex, a region primarily involved in respiratory rhythm generation both *in vitro* and *in vivo*. Therefore, the respiratory responses to unilateral microinjections (200 nl) of 0.1 nM, 10 nM and 1 μM leptin into the pre-Bötzinger complex were investigated in urethane anesthetized, spontaneously breathing Wistar rats. No changes in respiration were induced by 0.1 nM leptin microinjections. At higher (10 nM and 1 μM) concentrations leptin microinjections into the pre-Bötzinger complex elicited a dose-related increase in respiratory minute volume with the highest concentration resulting in an increase from 77.2 ± 3.2 to 95.5 ± 4.9 ml/min ($p<0.001$: Holm-Sidak test). This increase was due primarily to an elevation in respiratory frequency from 64.4 ± 2.7 to 82.3 ± 4.6 breaths/min ($p<0.001$: Holm-Sidak test) without obvious changes in tidal volume or peak amplitude of diaphragm or external intercostal muscles integrated EMG. The elevation in respiratory rate was largely a result of a significant decrease in expiratory duration in a dose-related fashion, whereas inspiratory duration was not significantly altered.

The time course of respiratory facilitatory effect of leptin was characterized by a moderately rapid onset and long duration. Excitation was observed within 3 min after microinjection with a peak effect occurring at approximately 20 min after administration. In general, the effect was over within 50 min.

[*] Corresponding author: ainyushkin@mail.ru.

To our knowledge, these results are the first to indicate that leptin causes respiratory stimulation by a direct action on the pre-Bötzinger complex. Taken together with our previous data, these results suggest that leptin may be involved in matching ventilation to metabolic requirements to stimulate ventilation. Further studies will require identifying central mechanisms by which activation of leptin receptors alters the respiratory control.

INTRODUCTION

The discovery of anorexigenic hormone leptin [13] was a landmark event in modern physiology. During last two decades, hypothalamic mechanisms underlying the inhibitory effect of leptin on appetite, food intake and energy expenditure have been studied in detail [3, 4, 28, 40, 50, 51, 61]. Adipose tissue is the primary source of leptin and most obese people have elevated circulating leptin concentrations, increased O_2 consumption and production of CO_2. To maintain homeostasis of arterial acid-base status and $PaCO_2$, corresponding increase in alveolar ventilation is necessary, however there is a subset of obese individuals in a condition termed obesity hypoventilation syndrome [1, 10, 37, 46] suffer from hypoventilation and substantial elevation in $PaCO_2$. These obese individuals are characterized by a failure of the high leptin levels to suppress appetite, food intake and to increase energy expenditure, which is generally attributed to a resistance to leptin [1, 10, 40]. Most people with obesity hypoventilation syndrome suffer from obstructive sleep apnea characterized by episodes of apnea during the night, interrupted sleep and excessive daytime sleepness.

The suggestion about leptin as an important contributor in the physiological linkage between metabolism and ventilation is supported by studies in rodents. For example, studies conducted in ob/ob mice having a mutation in the gene responsible for production of leptin (ob gene) and lack of functional leptin have shown that these markedly obese mice chronically hypoventilate with an increase in $PaCO_2 > 45$ mm Hg [41, 42, 47]. A consequent marked decrease in ventilatory chemosensitivity to hypercapnea associated with hypoventilation was found in these animals as a reduction of the correlation slope between minute ventilation and $PaCO_2$, and i.v. or i.c.v. administration of leptin restored normal ventilation and chemosensitivity [5, 41].

Previous studies in rats are in consistent with the concept of the involvement of leptin in respiratory control mechanisms. It is known that obese rats with recessive mutations of leptin receptor (Koletsky or Zucker rats) exhibit abnormalities of breathing pattern and a blunted ventilatory response to hypercapnia [12, 56], though exist the evidence of minor role for leptin receptor in a heritability of respiratory frequency in Zucker rats [25]. Interestingly, the stimulatory effects of leptin replacement in leptin-deficient mice on baseline ventilation were independent of weight, metabolism and food intake [41, 42]. Also central action of leptin replacement in leptin-deficient mice in modulating the chemorespiratory response to hypercapnia was independent of leptin-induced weight loss [5].

In our previous study it was shown that microinjections of leptin directly into the "respiratory" area of the solitary tract nucleus (NTS) produce a substantial dose-dependent respiratory stimulation, primarily manifested as an increase in tidal volume and magnitude of integrated activity of the inspiratory muscles without significant changes in respiratory rate or duration of the respiratory phases [23, 24]. The respiratory stimulant effect of leptin on tidal volume, at least in part, was attributed to an inhibition of the Breuer-Hering inflation reflex as well as to an increase in ventilatory response to CO_2 stimulation of central chemoreceptors located in the NTS [24].

Another potential site of leptin action within the brain stem could be on pre-Bötzinger complex (pre-BötC) located in the rostral ventrolateral medulla. The pre-BötC first on the basis of *in vitro* studies has been postulated to be essential for respiratory rhythm generation in neonatal mammals [8, 49, 53]. Later the pre-BötC has been demonstrated to play an important role in the generation and modulation of respiratory rhythm in adult animals *in vivo* [48, 54]. The pre-BötC contains neurons constituting the minimal essential network (kernel) for respiratory rhythmogenesis [26, 27, 33, 49, 58], producing rhythmic bursts of neuronal activity that resemble various patterns of inspiration such as eupneic inspiration, gasps, and sighs [30]. Modulation of the pre-BötC network likely involves regulation of multiple aspects including the modulation of membrane properties and synaptic interactions [14, 26, 30, 45, 58]. It has been demonstrated that the pre-BötC is a site of action for many various peptide modulators of respiration including substance P, opioids, TRH, somatostatin, adenosine [2, 6, 17, 22, 38, 43, 60]. The current study was conducted to test a hypothesis that local administration of leptin into the pre-BötC in adult rats would lead to a modulation of respiratory rhythm. We now extend our previous findings supporting the hypothesis and showing that stimulant respiratory effect of intravenous [9] or intracerebroventricular [5] leptin could be attributed in part to modulatory action on local rhythm generating network of the pre-BötC.

METHODS

Experimental protocol was approved by Commission on Biological Ethics of Samara State University, and all experiments were conducted in accordance with the Russian Code of Practice for the Care and Use of Animals for Scientific Purposes. Experiments were performed on twenty-four adult Wistar rats of both sexes weighting 200–260 g. Rats were anesthetized with urethane (1.5 g/kg i.p., in a volume of 3 ml/kg). Anaesthesia depth was monitored over experiment by ensuring that there was no response to noxious pinch. Supplemental doses of urethane were administered if required. A curved tracheal cannula was inserted at the level of the lower third of trachea. Animals were kept under spontaneous ventilation throughout the experiment. The animal was fixed in a stereotaxic apparatus with the head ventroflexed. The dorsal surface of the medulla was widely exposed by occipital craniotomy with the aid of a motoflex drill, and the dura and arachnoid membranes were removed. The posterior part of the cerebellum was retracted rostrally to provide access to the medulla.

An A&D DT-501 electrothermometer was used to monitor rectal temperature, which was maintained at 35.0 ± 0.5 °C by a heating pad.

Glass micropipettes with a tip diameter of 20–30 μm were used for pressure microinjection of leptin or artificial cerebrospinal fluid (control microinjections) [16, 31]. Leptin (Sigma, USA) or control solution were microinjected unilaterally with a MSh-1 microsyringe (Agat, Russia) into the area of the pre-Bötzinger complex: 1.5 mm rostral to the *obex*, 2.2 mm left to the midline, and 2.5 mm deep to the medullary surface [11]. Leptin was dissolved in artificial cerebrospinal fluid [36] to reach concentrations of 0.1 nM, 10 nM or 1 μM. Injection volume was 200 nl. Volume estimated by syringe scale and by observing the meniscus movement along a calibrated grid. Solutions were injected at a constant rate and injection durations were 3–5 s.

Respiratory parameters were assessed on spirograms and electromyograms (EMG) of the diaphragm and external intercostal muscles. The former were recorded using a miniature spirograph (Laboratory of Medical Equipment, Samara Aerospace University) connected with the tracheal cannula. The signal from the spirograph was then sampled at 500 Hz (1401Mikro, CED Ltd., Cambridge, UK) and recorded on computer using Spike2 software (v. 4, CED Ltd., Cambridge, UK). Spirograms were used to measure respiratory tidal volume (V_T, ml), inspiratory duration (T_I, s), expiratory duration (T_E, s) and total cycle duration (T_{TOT}, s). Respiratory rate (f, breaths/min) then calculated as 60 s / T_{TOT}, and respiratory minute volume (V_I, ml/min) determined as the product of V_T and f. EMG recordings were made using bipolar steel needle electrodes. EMG of the diaphragm was recorded via an incision in the anterior abdominal wall under rib cage on the right side. EMG of the external intercostal muscles was recorded in the sixth–eighth intercostal spaces. Electromiograms were amplified, band pass filtered (0.1–2 kHz), sampled at 10 kHz (1401Mikro, CED Ltd., Cambridge, UK) and recorded on computer using Spike2 software. Integrated EMG was obtained off-line using a full-wave rectifying and fourth-order Bessel filter. The amplitude of respiratory bursts on integrated EMG (in relative units) was used as a measure of the electric activity of the inspiratory muscles. Spirogram and EMG recorded continuously throughout the experiment, and baseline values of the respiratory parameters (averaging 30 s of data prior to the microinjection) were compared with those at 1, 2, 3, 4, 5, 6, 7, 8, 9, 10, 15, 20, 30, 40, 50, and 60 min after the microinjection.

At the end of each experiment the rat was killed (3 M KCl, i.v.), the brainstem was removed and placed in fixative (4% formaldehyde in saline) for 2 weeks. After that frozen serial sections (50 μm) were made in the frontal plane to verify the stereotaxically located microinjection sties (by track), according to atlas of Paxinos & Watson [44].

Data were analyzed statistically using SigmaStat (v. 3.1, Systat Software Inc., USA). Analysis of the responses to leptin microinjections was made by means of ANOVA for repeated measurements. If statistically significant changes were found, subsequent post-hoc comparisons were made with the initial values (before leptin administration) using the Holm-Sidak test. Kolmogorov-Smirnov test was used to decide if a sample comes from a population with normal distribution. All values are expressed as means ± standard error of the mean (SEM). Significance was indicated if $P<0.05$.

Results

Unilateral microinjection of leptin into the area of the pre-Bötzinger complex caused a dose-related stimulation of respiration. Injection of 0.1 nM leptin (n=6) did not produce statistically significant changes of breathing pattern or EMG of the inspiratory muscles. The representative example of the effects of 0.1 nM leptin is shown in Figure 1. Since such concentration of leptin did not evoke respiratory responses, it was determined as subthreshold. Control microinjections of artificial cerebrospinal fluid into the area of the pre-Bötzinger complex (n=6) also did not cause any significant change in respiratory parameters.

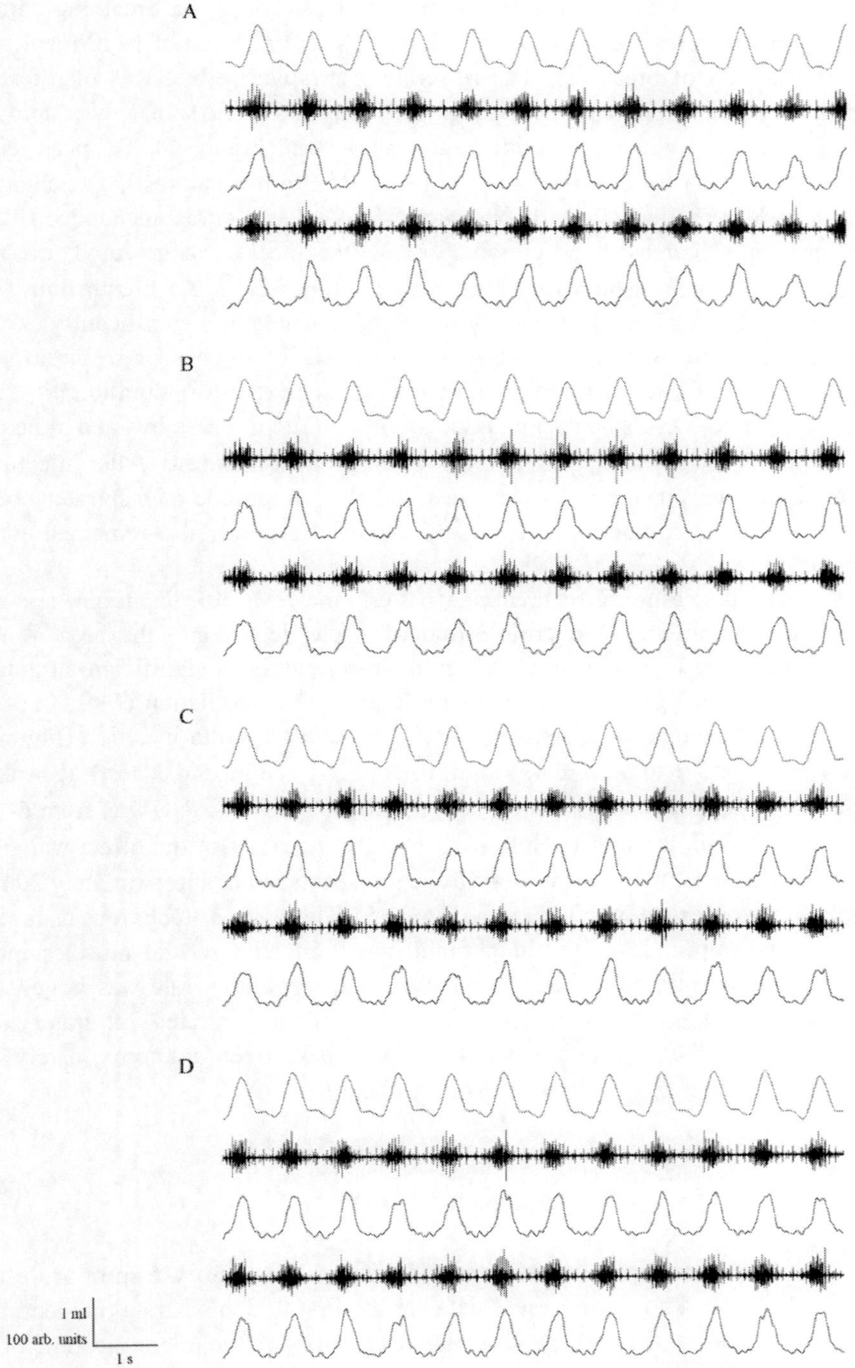

Figure 1. Respiratory response to microinjection of 0.1 nM leptin into the pre-BötC area. A: before leptin administration; B: 5 min, C: 20 min, D: 40 min after leptin administration. Trace fragments are presented, from top to bottom: spirogram, diaphragm EMG, integrated diaphragm EMG, external intercostal muscles EMG, integrated external intercostal muscles EMG. Calibration: 1 ml for spirogram, 100 arbitrary units for integrated EMG; the horizontal bar is 1 s.

The effects of unilateral microinjection of 10 nM leptin (n=6) on breathing pattern and EMG of inspiratory muscles are presented in Figure 2. Microinjection of 10 nM leptin caused a moderate stimulation of breathing. The respiratory stimulant effect was manifested as a progressive increase in ventilation (*P*<0.01: one way ANOVA) that was maximal at approximately 15 min following administration of leptin (Figure 3). At peak effect V_I increased from 64.3 ± 2.8 to 73.1 ± 2.9 ml/min (*P*<0.01: Holm-Sidak test). The change in V_I was caused by an increase in f (*P*<0.01: one way ANOVA) as V_T was unchanged (Figure 3). The respiratory rate increased progressively and the peak change in f occurred at approximately 15 min when f increased from 61.2 ± 2.8 to 72.4 ± 3.5 breaths/min (*P*<0.01: Holm-Sidak test). The respiratory frequency remained elevated and significantly exceeded a baseline value for up to 30 min post-injection. Analysis of indices of respiratory timing revealed a reduction of T_{TOT} as a result of shortening of T_E. Expiratory duration progressively shortened (*P*<0.05: one way ANOVA) in association with the increase in f and at peak effect T_E reduced from 0.72 ± 0.04 to 0.59 ± 0.04 s (*P*<0.01: Holm-Sidak test). After injection of 10 nM leptin no significant change in T_I was observed. The amplitude of respiratory bursts on integrated EMG of the diaphragm and external intercostal muscles also remained unaffected by 10 nM leptin.

Figure 4 shows the response of breathing pattern and EMG of diaphragm and external intercostal muscles to unilateral microinjection of 1 μM leptin into the area of the pre-Bötzinger complex. The injection of 1 μM leptin (n=6) caused a significant stimulation of respiratory activity inducing a progressive increase in minute ventilation (*P*<0.001: one way ANOVA) that became maximal at approximately 20 min after leptin injection (Figure 5). V_I increased from 77.2 ± 3.2 to 95.5 ± 4.9 ml/min (*P*<0.001: Holm-Sidak test) at peak effect. The increase in V_I was due to an elevation in f (*P*<0.001: one way ANOVA) from 64.4 ± 2.7 to 82.3 ± 4.6 breaths/min (*P*<0.001: Holm-Sidak test). The onset of the effect was observed within 3 min, the peak change in respiratory frequency occurred at approximately 20 min and a complete recovery observed within 50 min (Figure 5). There were no obvious changes in V_T (Figure 5) or peak amplitude of the diaphragm or external intercostal muscles integrated EMG after 1 μM leptin microinjection. The elevation in respiratory rate was largely a result of a significant shortening of T_E, whereas T_I was not significantly altered. Expiratory duration progressively reduced (*P*<0.001: one way ANOVA) at peak effect (at approximately 20 min) from 0.70 ± 0.04 to 0.54 ± 0.05 s (*P*<0.01: Holm-Sidak test).

CONCLUSION

The present results confirm the previously described stimulatory respiratory effects of leptin [9, 23, 24]. To our knowledge, these data are the first to demonstrate that leptin acts in the pre-BötC of anaesthetised rats to stimulate respiration. After microinjection of leptin, respiratory minute volume was increased primarily as a result of large increases in respiratory frequency rather than in tidal volume. No consistent changes in peak amplitude of the diaphragm or external intercostal muscles integrated EMG were seen. A significant shortening of expiratory duration was seen, whereas inspiratory duration was not changed. The effective concentration range of leptin in the injected solution was 10 nM to 10 μM, whereas 0.1 nM leptin did not evoke respiratory responses.

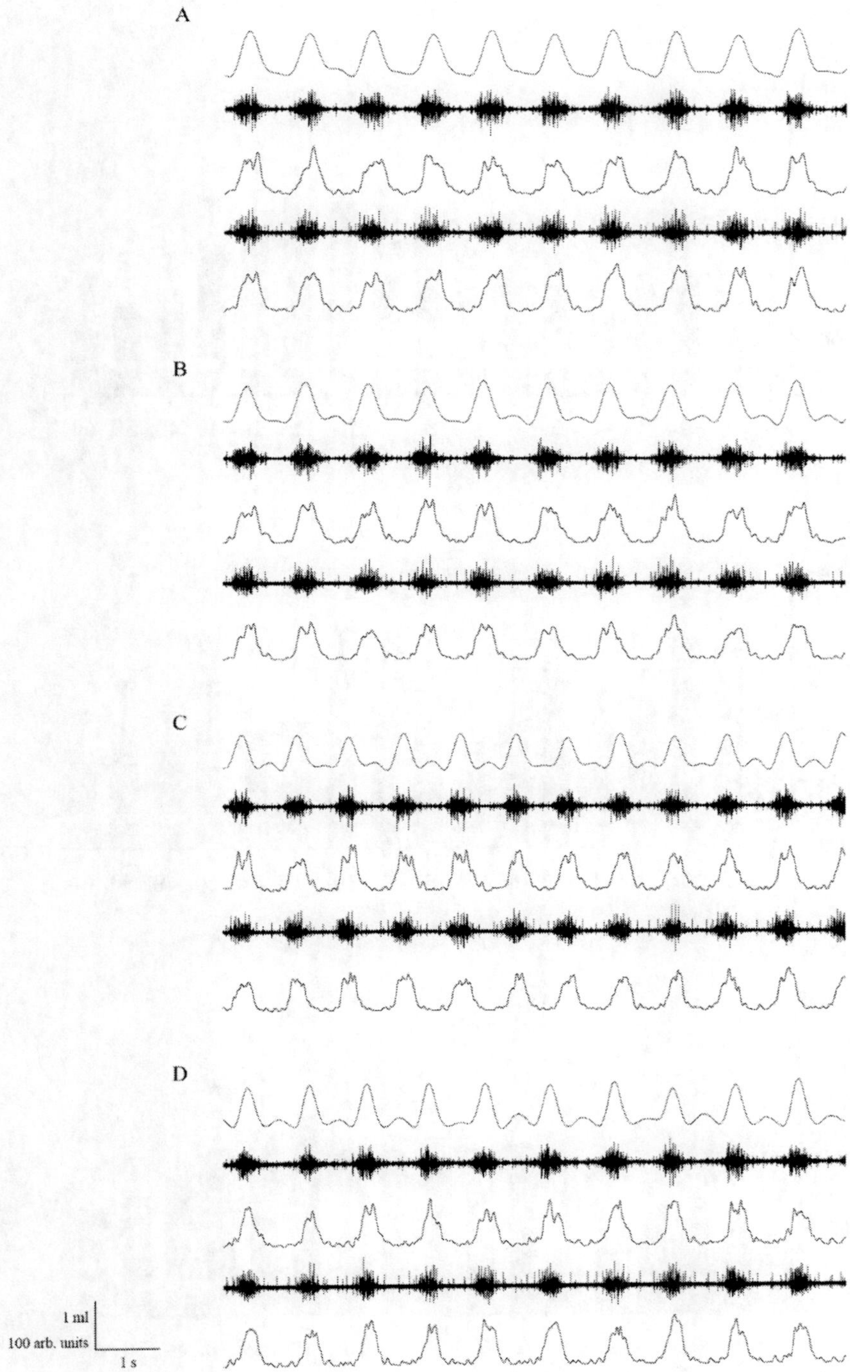

Figure 2. Respiratory response to microinjection of 10 nM leptin into the pre-BötC area. A: baseline state; B: 5 min, C: 20 min, D: 40 min after leptin administration. Trace fragments are presented, from top to bottom: spirogram, diaphragm EMG, integrated diaphragm EMG, external intercostal muscles EMG, integrated external intercostal muscles EMG. Calibration: 1 ml for spirogram, 100 arbitrary units for integrated EMG; the horizontal bar is 1 s.

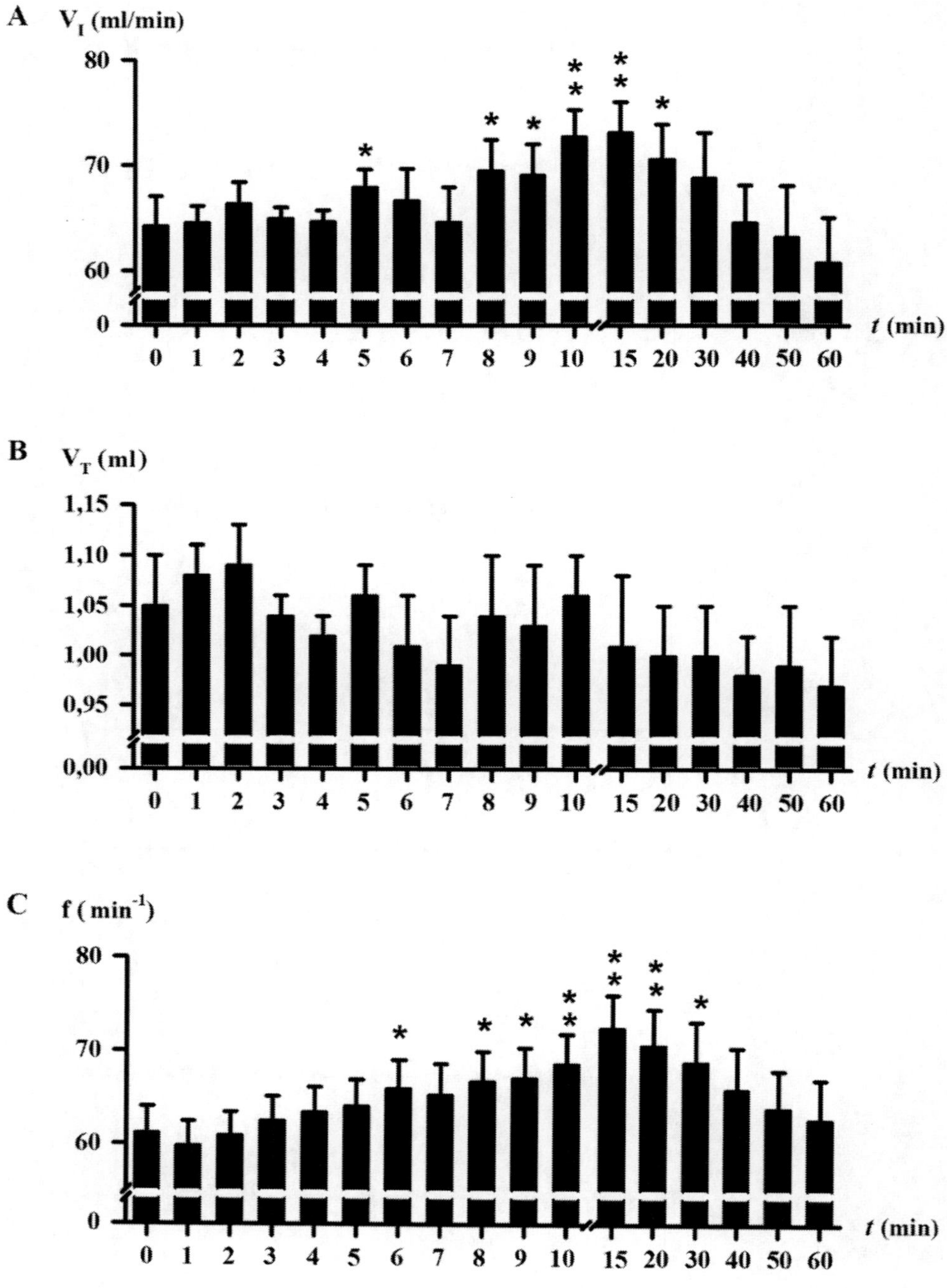

Figure 3. Minute ventilation (A), tidal volume (B) and respiratory frequency (C) at baseline (0) and at different time points (1 to 60 min) after 10 nM leptin administration into the pre-BötC area (n = 6). Note the increase in minute ventilation and respiratory frequency, $*P < 0.05$, $**P < 0.01$.

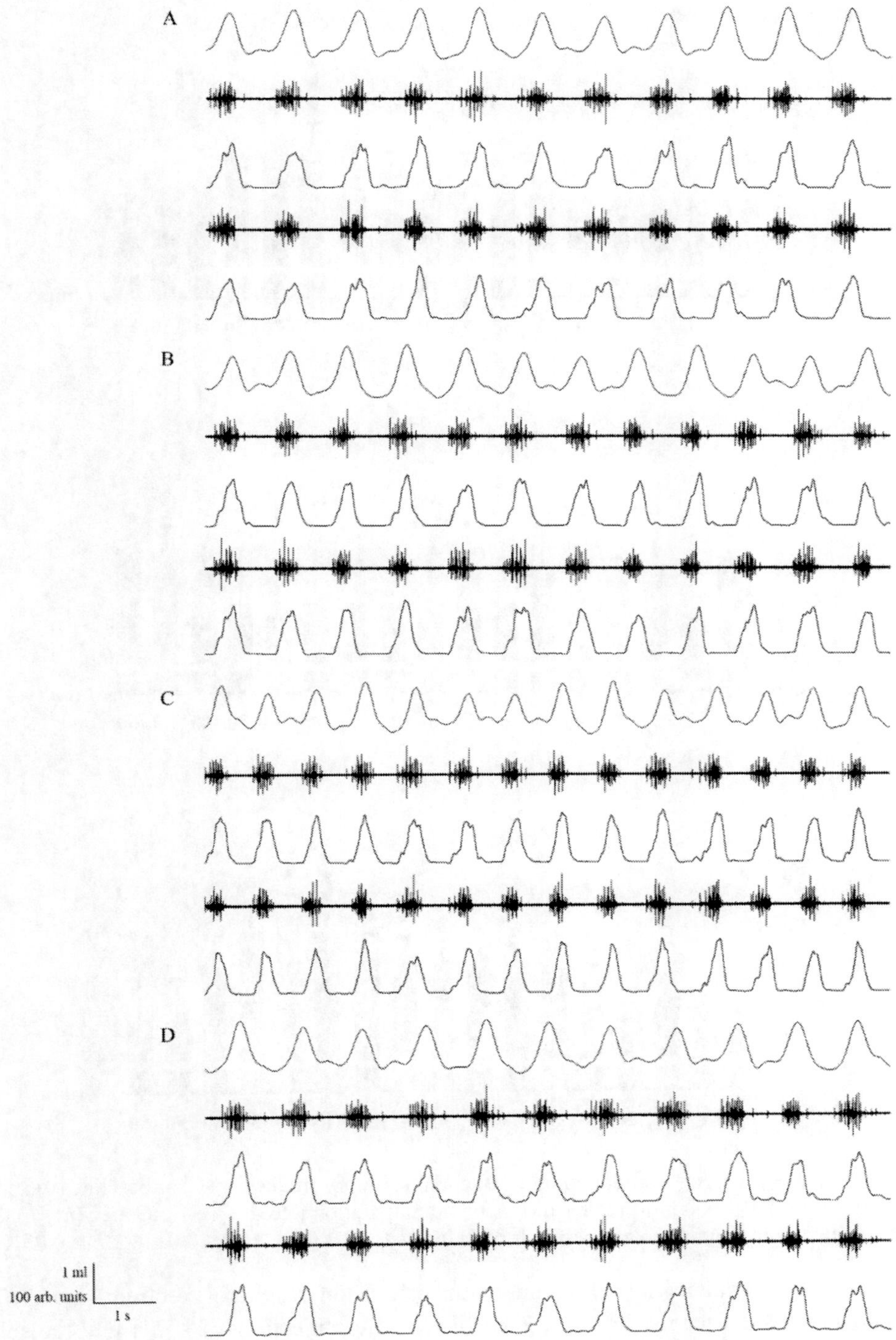

Figure 4. Respiratory response to microinjection of 1 μM leptin into the pre-BötC area. A: baseline state; B: 5 min, C: 20 min, D: 40 min after leptin administration. Trace fragments are presented, from top to bottom: spirogram, diaphragm EMG, integrated diaphragm EMG, external intercostal muscles EMG, integrated external intercostal muscles EMG. Calibration: 1 ml for spirogram, 100 arbitrary units for integrated EMG; the horizontal bar is 1 s.

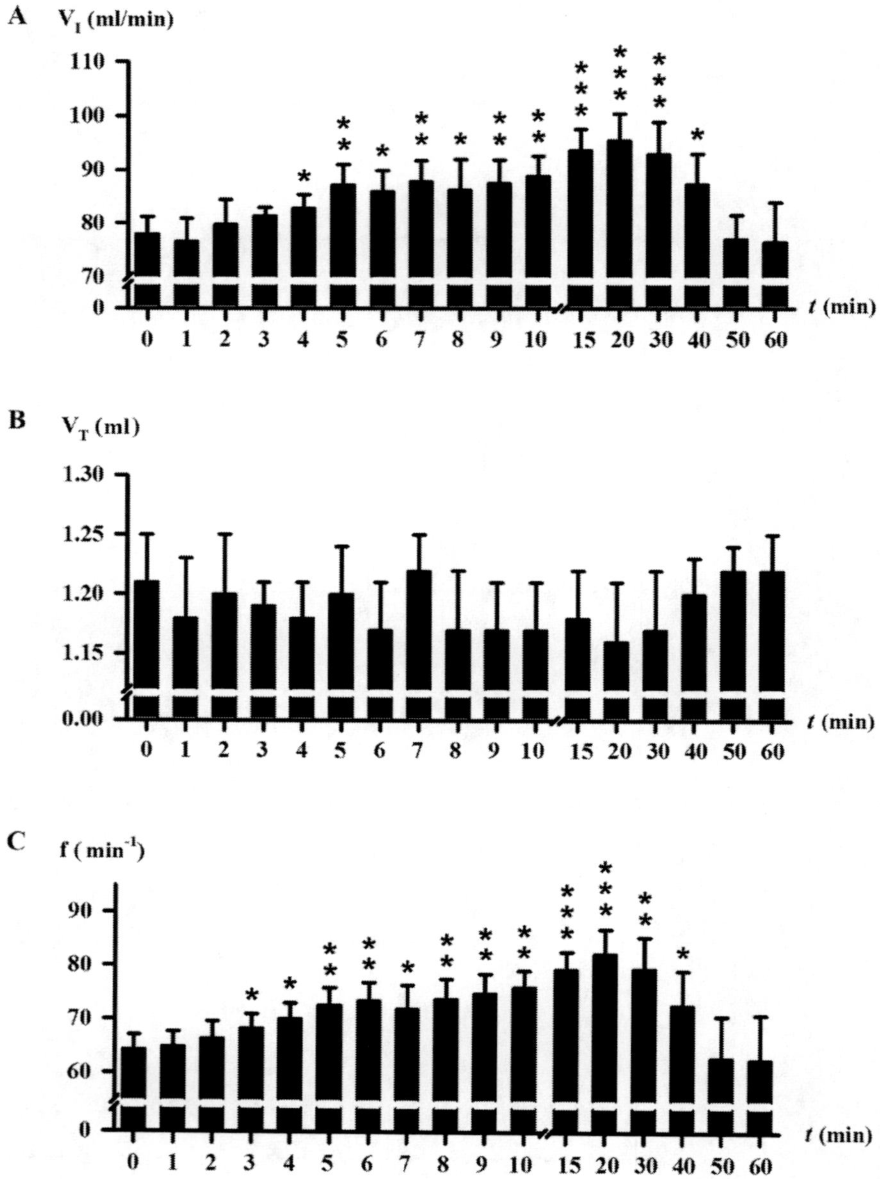

Figure 5. Minute ventilation (A), tidal volume (B) and respiratory frequency (C) at baseline (0) and at different time points (1 to 60 min) after 1 μM leptin administration into the pre-BötC area (n = 6). Note the increase in minute ventilation and respiratory frequency, $*P < 0.05$, $**P < 0.01$, $***P < 0.001$.

However, the results with stimulant leptin effects on respiratory activity are different from those observed after i.v. infusion [9] or direct microinjections [23, 24] into the solitary tract nucleus. Unlike the present data, after i.v. infusion or local administration of leptin into the solitary tract nucleus the respiratory stimulation was manifested mainly as an increase in tidal volume or its neural equivalent, the peak amplitude of integrated phrenic nerve discharge. This indicates that the characteristic of the stimulant respiratory effect of leptin depends not only on its peculiar biochemical properties, but also on the functional specificity of the pre-BötC, primarily involved in mechanisms of respiratory rhythmogenesis. The present data together with the results of our previous study [23, 24] suggest the existence of several rather than one site for leptin action within the medullary respiratory network. The pre-BötC was shown to be a site of action for many various peptide modulators of respiration including substance P, opioids, TRH, somatostatin, adenosine [2, 6, 17, 22, 38, 43, 60]. The present results indicate that leptin is likely to be involved in modulation of respiratory rhythmogenesis via the pre-BötC.

To confirm a possible involvement of endogenous leptin in physiological modulation of the pre-BötC neuronal network, the data concerning the presence of leptin receptors and their mRNA in the area of interest have to be taken into account. One form of leptin receptor, Ob-Rb, has been demonstrated in various brain regions [7, 34, 35]. This form of the receptor has a consensus amino acid sequence involved in the activation of Janus kinase-signal transducer and activator of transcription (JAK-STAT) tyrosine kinases [15, 29] and activates STAT protein [15, 20, 32, 61]. There is substantial evidence for presence of functionally significant leptin receptors and their mRNA in the rodent hindbrain [18, 19, 35], however, their high level was found in the solitary tract nucleus rather than in the ventrolateral brain stem where the pre-BötC is located. Though the present results do not match the distribution pattern of leptin receptors in the brain stem, we cannot rule out a role for the pre-BötC in mediation the respiratory stimulant effect of leptin. Further studies of leptin receptor distribution in the ventrolateral brain stem with special attention focused on the pre-BötC area potentially could help to explain results of the present study.

Cellular mechanisms of leptin action on elements of the medullary respiratory network have not been studied so far, but works performed both *in vitro* and *in vivo* demonstrated direct effects of leptin on membrane potential, spike frequency, spike coding, shape of spikes, ATP-sensitive potassium channels and Ca^{2+} signaling of hypothalamic neurons [21, 39, 52, 55, 57, 59].

Similar mechanisms may potentially underlay the stimulant respiratory action of leptin on components of the respiratory network including the pre-BötC.

In conclusion, the study provides the first evidence that leptin can exert a stimulant respiratory effect after local administration into the pre-BötC, playing an important role in respiratory rhythm generation. Taken together with our previous data, these results suggest that leptin may be involved in matching ventilation to metabolic requirements to stimulate ventilation via the pre-BötC.

References

[1] Al Dabal, L. & BaHammam, A. S. (2009). Obesity hypoventilation syndrome. *Ann. Thorac. Med.* 4, 41–49.

[2] Ballanyi, K., Panaitesku, B. & Ruangkittisakul A. (2010). Indirect opioid actions on inspiratory pre-Bötzinger complex neurons in newborn rat brainstem slices. *Adv. Exp. Biol. Med.* 669, 75–79.

[3] Banks, A. S., Davis, S. M., Bates, S.H. & Myers, M. G. Jr. (2000). Activation of downstream signals by the long form of the leptin receptor. *J. Biol. Chem.* 275, 14563–14572.

[4] Banks, W. A. (2004). The many lives of leptin. *Peptides*. 25, 331–338.

[5] Bassi, M., Giusti, H., Leite, C. M., Anselmo-Franci, J. A., do Carmo, J. M., da Silva, A. A., Hall, J. E., Colombari, I. & Glass, M. L. (2012). Central leptin replacement enhances chemorespiratory responses in leptin-deficient mice independent of changes in body weight. *Pflugers Arch*. 464, 145–153.

[6] Ben-Mabrouk, F. & Tryba, A. K. (2010). Substance P modulation of TRPC3⁄ 7 channels improves respiratory rhythm regularity and ICAN-dependent pacemaker activity. *Eur. J. Neurosci*. 31, 1219–1232.

[7] Burguera, B., Couce, M. E., Long, J., Lamsam, J., Laakso, K., Jensen, M. D., Parisi, J. E. & Lloyd, R. V. (2000). The long form of the leptin receptor (OB-Rb) is widely expressed in the human brain. *Neuroendocrinology*. 71, 187–195.

[8] Butera, R., Rinzel, J. & Smith, J. C. (1999). Models of respiratory rhythm generation in the pre-Bötzinger complex. I. Bursting pacemaker neurons. *J. Neurophysiol*. 81, 382–397.

[9] Chang, Z., Ballou, E., Jiao, W., McKenna K. E., Morrison, S. F. & McCrimmon, D. R. (2013). Systemic leptin produces a long-lasting increase in respiratory motor output in rats. *Front. Physiol*. 4, 16.

[10] Chau, E. H., Lam, D., Wong, J., Mokhlesi, B. & Chung, F. (2012). Obesity hypoventilation syndrome: a review of epidemiology, pathophysiology, and preoperative considerations. *Anesthesiol*. 117, 188–205.

[11] Chitravanshi, V. C. & Sapru, H. N. (1999). Phrenic nerve responses to chemical stimulation of the subregions of ventral medullary respiratory neuronal group in the rat. *Brain Res*. 821, 443–460.

[12] Farkas, G. A. & Schlenker, E. H. (1994). Pulmonary ventilation and mechanics in morbidly obese Zucker rats. *Am. J. Respir. Crit. Care Med*. 150, 356–362.

[13] Friedman, J. M. (2010). A tale of two hormones. *Nat. Med*. 16, 1100–1106.

[14] Funk, G. D., Smith, J. C. & Feldman, J. L. (1993). Generation and transmission of respiratory oscillations in medullary slices: role of excitatory amino acids. *J. Neurophysiol*. 70, 1497–1515.

[15] Ghilardi, N., Ziegler, S., Wiestner, A., Stoffel, R., Heim, M. H. & Skoda, R. C. (1996). Defective STAT signaling by the leptin receptor in diabetic mice. *Proc. Natl. Acad. Sci. USA*. 93, 6231–6235.

[16] Goodchild, A. K., Dampney, R. A. L. & Bandler, R. (1982). A method for evoking physiological responses by stimulation of cell bodies, but not axons of passage, within localized regions of the central nervous system. *J. Neurosci. Methods*. 6, 351–363.

[17] Greer, J. J., al-Zubaidy, Z. & Carter, J. E. (1996). Thyrotropin-releasing hormone stimulates perinatal rat respiration *in vitro*. *Am. J. Physiol*. 271, R1160–R1164.

[18] Grill, H. J., Schwartz, M. W., Kaplan, J. M., Foxhall, J. S., Breininger, J. & Baskin, D. G. (2002). Evidence that the caudal brainstem is a target for the inhibitory effect of leptin on food intake. *Endocrinology*. 143, 239–246.

[19] Hosoi, T., Kawagishi, T., Okuma, Y., Tanaka, J. & Nomura, Y. (2002). Brain stem is a direct target for leptin's action in the central nervous system. *Endocrinology*. 143, 3498 –3504.

[20] Hubschle, T., Thom, E., Watson, A., Roth, J., Klaus, S. & Meyerhof, W. (2001). Leptin induced nuclear translocation of STAT3 immunoreactivity in hypothalamic nuclei involved in body weight regulation. *J. Neurosci*. 21, 2413–2424.

[21] Inyushkin, A. N., Bhumbra, G. S. & Dyball, R. E. J. (2009). Leptin modulates spike coding in the rat suprachiasmatic nucleus. *J. Neuroendocrinol*. 21, 705–714.

[22] Inyushkin, A. N., Merkulova, N. A. & Chepurnov, S. A. (1999). The pre-Bötzinger complex participates in generating the respiratory effects of thyroliberin. *Neurosci. Behav. Physiol*. 29, 321–326.

[23] Inyushkin, A. N., Inyushkina, E. M. & Merkulova, N. A. (2009). Respiratory responses to microinjections of leptin into the solitary tract nucleus. *Neurosci. Behav. Physiol*. 39, 231–240.

[24] Inyushkina, E. M., Merkulova, N. A. & Inyushkin, A. N. (2010). Mechanisms of the respiratory activity of leptin at the level of the solitary tract nucleus. *Neurosci. Behav. Physiol*. 40, 707–713.

[25] Iyengar, S. K., Stein, C. M., Russo, K., Erokwu, B. O. & Strohl, K. P. (2004). The fa leptin receptor mutation and the heritability of respiratory frequency in a Brown Norway and Zucker intercross. *J. Appl. Physiol*. 97, 811–820.

[26] Koizumi, H., Koshiya, N., Chia, J. X., Cao F., Nugent, J., Zhang, R. & Smith, J. C. (2013). Structural-functional properties of identified excitatory and inhibitory interneurons within pre- Bötzinger complex respiratory microcircuits. *J. Neurosci*. 33, 2994 –3009.

[27] Koshiya, N. & Smith, J. C. (1999). Neuronal pacemaker for breathing visualized *in vitro*. *Nature*. 400, 360 –363.

[28] Kloek, C., Haq, A. K., Dunn, S. L., Lavery, H. J., Banks, A. S. & Myers, M. G. Jr. (2002). Regulation of Jak kinases by intracellular leptin receptor sequences. *J. Biol. Chem*. 277, 41547–41555.

[29] Lee, G. H., Proenca, R., Montez, J. M., Carroll, K. M., Darvishzadeh, J. G., Lee, J. I. & Friedman, J. M. (1996). Abnormal splicing of the leptin receptor in diabetic mice. *Nature*. 379, 632–635.

[30] Lieske, S. P., Thoby-Brisson, M., Telgkamp, P. & Ramirez, J. M. (2000). Reconfiguration of the neural network controlling multiple breathing patterns: eupnea, sighs and gasps. *Nat. Neurosci*. 3, 600–607.

[31] Lipski, J., Bellingham, M. C., West, M. J. & Pilowsky, P. (1988). Limitations of the technique of pressure microinjection of excitatory amino acids for evoking responses from localized regions of the CNS. *J. Neurosci. Methods*. 26, 169–179.

[32] McCowen, K. C., Chow, J. C. & Smith, R. J. (1998). Leptin signaling in the hypothalamus of normal rats *in vivo*. Endocrinology. 139, 4442–4447.

[33] McCrimmon, D. R., Ramirez J. M., Alford, S. & Zuperku E. J. (2000). Unraveling the mechanisms for respiratory rhythm generation. *BioEssays* 22, 6–9.

[34] Mercer, J. G., Hoggard, N., Williams, L. M., Lawrence, C. B., Hannah, L. T. & Trayhurn, P. (1996). Localization of leptin receptor mRNA and the long form splice variant (Ob-Rb) in mouse hypothalamus and adjacent brain regions by in situ hybridization. *FEBS Lett*. 387, 113–116.

[35] Mercer, J. H., Moar, K. M. & Hoggard, N. (1998). Localization of leptin receptor (Ob-R) messenger ribonucleic acid in the rodent hindbrain. *Endocrinology*. 139, 29 –34.

[36] Mitchell, R. A., Loeschcke, H. H. & Massion, N. H. (1963). Respiratory responses mediated through superficial chemosensitive areas on the medulla. *J. Appl. Physiol*. 18, 523–533.

[37] Mokhlesi, B. (2010). Obesity hypoventilation syndrome: a state-of-the-art review. *Respir. Care*. 55, 1347–1362.

[38] Montandon, G., Qin, W., Liu, H., Ren, J., Greer, J. J., & Horner, R. L. (2011). PreBötzinger complex neurokinin-1 receptor-expressing neurons mediate opioid-induced respiratory depression. *J. Neurosci*. 31, 1292–1301.

[39] Muroya, S., Funahashi, H., Yamanaka, A., Kohno, D., Uramura, K., Nambu, T., Shibahara, M., Kuramochi, M., Takigawa, M., Yanagisawa, M., Sakurai, T., Shioda, S. & Yada, T. (2004). Orexins (hypocretins) directly interact with neuropeptide Y, POMC and glucose-responsive neurons to regulate Ca^{2+} signaling in a reciprocal manner to leptin: orexigenic neuronal pathways in the mediobasal hypothalamus. *Eur. J. Neurosci*. 19, 1524–1534.

[40] Myers, M. G., Cowley, M. A., & Munzberg H. (2008). Mechanisms of leptin action and leptin resistance. *Annu. Rev. Physiol*. 70, 537–556.

[41] O'Donnell, C. P., Schaub, S. D., Haines, A. S., Berkowitz, D. I., Tankersley, C. G., Schwartz, A. R. & Smith P. L. (1999). Leptin prevents respiratory depression in obesity. *Amer. J. Respir. Crit. Care Med*. 159, 1477–1484.

[42] O'Donnell, C. P., Tankersley, C. G., Polotsky, V. Y., C. G., Schwartz, A. R. & Smith P. L. (2000). Leptin, obesity and respiratory function. *Respirat. Physiol*. 119, 173–180.

[43] Pantaleo, T., Mutolo, D., Cinelli, E. & Bongianni, F. (2011). Respiratory responses to somatostatin microinjections into the Bötzinger complex and the pre-Bötzinger complex of the rabbit. *Neurosci. Lett*. 498, 26–30.

[44] Paxinos, G. & Watson, C. (1998). The rat brain in stereotaxic coordinates. Fourth edition. San Diego, CA: Academic Press.

[45] Pena, F., Parkis, M. A., Tryba, A. K. & Ramirez, J. M. (2004). Differential contribution of pacemaker properties to the generation of respiratory rhythms during normoxia and hypoxia. *Neuron*. 43, 105–117.

[46] Piper, A. J. & Grunstein, R. R. (2011). Obesity hypoventilation syndrome: mechanisms and management. *Am. J. Respir. Crit. Care Med*. 183, 292–298.

[47] Polotsky, V. Y., Smaldone, M. C., Scharf, M. T., Li, J., Tankersley, C. G., Smith, P. L., Schwartz, A. R. & O'Donnell, C.P. (2004). Impact of interrupted leptin pathways on respiratory control. *J. Appl. Physiol*. 96, 991–998.

[48] Ramirez, J. M., Schwarzacher, S. W., Pierrefiche, O. & Olivera, B. M. (1998). Selective lesion of the cat pre-Bötzinger complex in vivo eliminates breathing but not gasping. *J. Physiol*. 507, 895–907.

[49] Rekling, J. C. & Feldman, J. L. (1998). PreBötzinger complex and pacemaker neurons: hypothesized site and kernel for respiratory rhythm generation. *Annu. Rev. Physiol*. 60, 385–405.

[50] Sahu, A. (2004). Leptin signaling in the hypothalamus: emphasis on energy homeostasis and leptin resistance. *Front. Neuroendocrinol*. 24, 225–253.

[51] Schwartz, M. W., Woods, S. C., Porte, D. Jr., Seeley, R. J. & Baskin, D. G. (2000). Central nervous system control of food intake. *Nature*. 404, 661–671.

[52] Shiraishi, T., Sasaki, K., Niijima, A. & Oomura Y. (1999). Leptin effects on feedingrelated hypothalamic and peripheral neuronal activities in normal and obese rats. *Nutrition*. 15, 576–579.

[53] Smith, J., Ellenberger, H., Ballanyi, K., Richter, D. & Feldman, J. (1991). Pre-Bötzinger complex: a brainstem region that may generate respiratory rhythm in mammals. *Science*. 254, 726–729.

[54] Solomon, I. C., Edelman, N. H. & Neubauer, J. A. (1999). Patterns of phrenic motor output evoked by chemical stimulation of neurons located in the pre-Bötzinger complex *in vivo*. *J. Neurophysiol*. 81, 1150–1161.

[55] Spanswick, D., Smith, M. A., Groppi, V. E., Logan, S. D. & Ashford, M. L. J. (1997). Leptin inhibits hypothalamic neurons by activation of ATP-sensitive potassium channels. *Nature*. 390, 521–525.

[56] Strohl, K. P. & Thomas, A. J. (2001). Ventilatory behavior and metabolism in two strains of obese rats. *Respir. Physiol*. 124, 85–93.

[57] Takahashi, K. A. & Cone, R. D. (2005). Fasting induces a large, leptin-dependent increase in the intrinsic action potential frequency of orexigenic arcuate nucleus neuropeptide Y / agouti-related protein neurons. *Endocrinology*. 146, 1043–1047.

[58] Thoby-Brisson, M. & Ramirez, J. M. (2001). Identification of two types of inspiratory pacemaker neurons in the isolated respiratory neural network of mice. *J. Neurophysiol*. 86, 104–112.

[59] Traebert, M., Riediger, T., Whitebread, S., Scharrer, E. & Schmid, H. A. (2002). Ghrelin acts on leptin-responsive neurones in the rat arcuate nucleus. *J. Neuroendocrinol*. 14, 580–586.

[60] VanDam, R. J., Shields, E. J. & Kelty, J. D. (2008). Rhythm generation by the pre-Bötzinger complex in medullary slice and island preparations: effects of adenosine A1 receptor activation. *BMC Neurosci*. 9, 95.

[61] Vaisse, C., Halaas, J. L., Horvath, C. M., Darnell, J. E. Jr., Stoffel, M., & Friedman, J. M. (1996). Leptin activation of Stat3 in the hypothalamus of wild-type and ob/ob mice but not db/db mice. *Nat. Genet*. 14, 95–97.

In: Leptin: Biosynthesis, Functions and Clinical Significance ISBN: 978-1-62948-801-1
Editor: Edward L. Blum

Chapter 12

LEPTIN AS A REPRODUCTIVE MODULATOR: AN ECO-PHYSIOLOGICAL APPROACH

Elena Bukovetzky [*] ***and Abraham Haim*** [†]
Haifa University, Research Fields: Environmental Biology and Endocrinology, Israel

ABSTRACT

The survival of a species in an unpredictable ecosystem as the desert depends among others on the adaptation of its reproductive system, in terms of matching reproductive activity with water and food availability in the habitat, and halting it when these are limited. Integration of the various environmental cues will eventually determine which populations will be able to breed at an appropriate time thus surviving as a species in xeric environments. Osmotic stress was noted as an effective internal signal for reducing reproductive activity in desert-adapted *Acomys* populations.

In the basis of our study lies the assumption that a possible mechanism by which dietary salinity causes an osmotic stress, which affects reproduction in desert adapted common spiny mice *Acomys cahirinus* in association with osmoregulatory hormones; vasopressin and aldosterone. As leptin regulates energy intake, it seemed of great interest to assess its role in reproduction of desert adapted rodents, inhabiting an unpredictable environment.

For a long time energy source storage seemed as the only role of WAT, apart from providing thermal and mechanical insulation. For now WAT in our understanding is a highly dynamic, endocrine tissue, being involved in a wide range of physiological and metabolic processes far beyond the paradigm of fuel storage.

White adipocytes secrete several major hormones, protein signals and factors, most notably is the peptide hormone leptin. Circulating leptin levels serve as a signal for the state of body energy repletion to body cells most importantly the central nervous system (CNS) where it suppresses food intake and permits energy expenditure. In addition to its metabolic effects, leptin is well known as a modulator of reproduction.

The results of our studies show an involvement of leptin in metabolism and regulation of reproductive function in rodents. We tested desert and mesic adapted *A.*

[*] Corresponding author: Elena Bukovetzky, Ph.D. research fields: environmental biology and endocrinology. E-mail: dvorkinae@yahoo.com; daele2008@gmail.com.

[†] E-mail: ahaim@haifa.research.ac.il.

cahirinus for investigating the role of leptin as a modulator of reproductive pathways in *Acomys* populations from two different ecosystems.

Our data and those of previous studies including the desert adapted golden spiny mouse, reported on a massive reduction of body mass in salinity treated (ST)-mice, under short and long day photoperiod conditions for males and females, coupled with a colossal reduction of WAT, leading to a complete absence of the tissue in 85% of ST-mice. ST caused a significant ($p < 0.05$) decrease in serum leptin levels in both, LD- and SD-acclimated desert-adapted A. cahirinus females, compared with their control groups.

In general, by using the reverse transcriptase polymerase chain reaction (RT-PCR) method, we detected a significant increase in expression levels of mRNA receptor genes for leptin (Ob-RT) in testis and WAT of ST-treated mice. High gene expression levels of leptin (Ob-Rt) mRNA receptors were noted in ovaries of SD-ST desert-adapted females ($p < 0.05$), while in the testes high gene expression levels were noted only in LD-ST desert-adapted individuals ($p < 0.05$), compared with their controls.

Our results on endocrine and molecular levels are of importance for the proposed idea that, in desert rodents, reproduction is being controlled not only by water availability but, also by the amount of energy resources. Such rodents show that the hormone leptin, which regulates energy storage through its receptors presented on the gonads, or on WAT or hypothalamus, is involved in regulation of desert-adapted rodents' reproduction.

INTRODUCTION

White adipose tissue (WAT) is the main site of energy storage in mammals, substrate being deposited as triacylglycerols at a high energy density. For long time energy storage was seen as essentially the only role of WAT, apart from providing thermal and mechanical insulation. For now, to our understanding WAT is seen as a highly dynamic, endocrine organ, being involved in a wide range of physiological and metabolic processes far beyond the paradigm of fuel storage [1].

White adipocytes secrete leptin together with a diverse range of other hormones, protein signals and factors. Leptin (from the Greek *leptos*, meaning thin) is a non-glycosylated polypeptide with a molecular mass of approximately 16 kDa, encoded by the *ob* gene and achieves hormonal status by virtue of its secretion into the bloodstream (*Obese Gene*; [2]). The primary effects of leptin involve the mobilization of lipolytic pathways of energy expenditure as it signals to the hypothalamus that energy sufficiency has been met [3].

The leptin gene is highly conserved across species where the mouse protein exhibits 83% homology with that of human [2]. Leptin mRNA levels are variable in different WAT depots, suggesting that there are site-specific variations in the expression of the leptin gene. The concentration of leptin circulating in the bloodstream depends primarily on the amount of the protein stored in body fat deposits, and this relationship presents a positive correlation [4]. The concentration of leptin circulating in the blood is two to three times higher in females than in males. Additionally, in females synthesis of leptin in relation to body mass is not only approximately 75% higher, but leptin is also much more easily released from WAT [5]. High levels of endogenous leptin, associated with excess body fat, are responsible for the earlier occurrence of first menstruation in girls who are overweight compared with lean girls at the same age [6]. It has been suggested that these observed differences may be partly due to the impact of sex hormones.

Nutritional status has a definitely impact on the concentration of leptin in the blood. Undernutrition, or even short-term restriction of access to food, results in a significant reduction in leptin concentrations in ruminants [7], rodents [8] and humans [9].

It is generally accepted that there is a close relationship between reproductive processes and nutritional status [10]. Malnutrition has a negative impact on reproductive processes, ranging from a reduction in libido to negative effects on pregnancy (implantation disorders, increased fetal resorption, and abortion) and the inhibition of ovulation. Exogenous leptin accelerates entry into a period of sexual maturity of female rodents, including mice [11] and rats [12]. Pregnancy and lactation are important factors that determine the amount of leptin in the bloodstream. Interestingly, hyperleptinemia occurring during pregnancy is not associated with a reduction in food intake, which suggests that this state induces a kind of leptin resistance [13].

In linking energy homeostasis to feeding behavior and procreative functions, leptin plays a crucial role in the regulation of reproductive processes, acting at all levels of the gonadotropic axis. The effects of leptin on gonadotropin-releasing hormone (GnRH) are mediated through inter-neuronal pathways involving neuropeptide-Y, proopiomelanocortin and kisspeptin. Furthermore, leptin regulates reproductive function by altering the sensitivity of the pituitary gland to GnRH and acting at the ovary level to regulate follicular and luteal steroidogenesis. Thus leptin serves as a putative signal that links metabolic status with the reproductive axis [14]. The multitude of organs in which the presence of leptin receptors has been identified confirms the pleiotropic character of leptin's action. For example, leptin exhibits direct action within the peripheral sites of the reproductive axis, the ovary, including inhibition of estradiol secretion from ovarian follicles [15], thus participating in the regulation of the growth and maturation of this organ

In the last decade, many factors affecting the appetite and energy expenditure have been described. It has been shown that the effects of many of these factors are dependent on photoperiod [16]. The pineal hormone melatonin (MLT), which is a signal for light/dark daily cycles and for seasonal changes in photoperiod, resulting in functionally and anatomically modulation of numerous interactions linked with adaption to seasonal changes in food intake according to annual environmental changes.

Melatonin can affect WAT also through sympathetic innervations [17]. In addition to the indirect effects of MLT, which occurs through the nervous system, MLT may directly modulate the activity of WAT *via* the endocrine system by acting on specific receptors on membranes of adipocytes [18].

Available evidence indicates that MLT regulates the reproductive function in seasonal mammals through its inhibitory action at various levels of the hypothalamic–pituitary–gonadal (HPG) axis. The pulls-style secretion of GnRH, from a small number of neurons in the hypothalamus, controls luteinizing hormone (LH) and follicle-stimulating hormone (FSH) secretion, which, in turn, regulates the functional activity of gonads [19, 20]. Seasonal leptin resistance allows sheep to live in a changing climate and store energy that they will be able to utilize in periods of reduced food availability [21]. Changes during the year related to leptin sensitivity have been observed in other seasonal animal species. In Siberian hamsters, the potency of exogenous leptin in reducing food intake is significantly more marked in periods of short days than during long days [22, 23]. These observations provide an insight into the phenomenon of seasonal changes in sensitivity to leptin, not only in relation to the regulation of food intake, but also related to the modifying effects of season on other leptin-induced responses.

Survival of a species in unpredictable ecosystems necessitates the adaptation of the reproductive system, in terms of matching reproductive activity with water and energy sources availability, and halting it when these are limited [24]. Integration of the various environmental cues will eventually determine which species will be able to breed at the right time and to survive in xeric environments. Previous results demonstrated the rather unexpected finding that matured adipocytes do express genes of specific receptors of hypothalamic VP, in all three receptor subtypes V-1A, V1-B and V-2 [1, 25]. Thus, WAT involvement in reproduction of desert adapted rodents is not only through secreted leptin [26] but also as a source for water supply. In addition, we reported a massive reduction of W_b in ST-mice, under short and long photoperiods for males and females, coupled with a colossal reduction of WAT, leading to a complete absence in 85% of ST-mice [27, 28]. Based on previous results describing the importance of water / food availability as a proximal and photoperiod as an initial cue for successful breeding was suggested. The aim of this was to strengthen the idea of leptin as a modulator of reproduction of *Acomys* populations.

Methods

Studied mice were recruited from a desert adapted laboratory colony of desert- and mesic-adapted *A. cahirinus* maintained at Oranim campus, University of Haifa. Desert adapted mice in the colony are descendants of individuals originally captured on the western Dead Sea shores while those of the mesic population were captured on Mount Carmel. All tested mice, at the beginning of acclimation, were adults, aged four months. In the colony, mice were maintained at an ambient temperature of 26 ± 2 °C under a photoperiod regime of 12L: 12D. In order to avoid bias results related to W_b, both SD and LD acclimated groups had a similar average W_b (34-36 ± 3 g) at the beginning of experiments. Ethical clearance for the use of animals was provided by The Ethical Committee, University of Haifa [27].

Acclimation to Increasing Salinity under Different Photoperiod Regimes

36 individuals (18 females and 18 males) were acclimated to SD conditions (8L: 16D) while 26 individuals (12 females and 14 males) were acclimated to LD (16L: 8D) inside a controlled environmental cabinet (158x77x74 cm; Meditest 600/1300, Austria) for three weeks. Lights were on between 07:00 and 15:00h for SD-mice and between 07:00 and 23:00h for LD-mice. Mice were kept individually, in separate plastic cages (35x25x15 cm). Dry food (rat pellet, Koffolk, Israel) and 2% agar gel (20g of dry agar dissolved in 1000ml of deionized water) as a sole water source were provided *ad libitum*. W_b was recorded to the nearest 0.1g using a digital balance (Sartorius 5500, Germany). Room temperature was set at the mice lower critical point of 28 ± 1^0C [29]. After three weeks of acclimation, salinity treated (ST) mice (n=9 and 7 in SD and LD acclimated groups, respectively) were challenged with a gradually increasing salinity (osmotic stress) that desert rodents may experience in the wild,

by dissolving increasing concentrations of NaCl into the agar (0.9%, 1.5%, 2.5%, and 5% NaCl dissolved in agar solution). Each salinity level was offered to the mice for two weeks. Altogether, the experiment lasted eight weeks. One group for each acclimation regime (n=9 and 7 in SD and LD acclimated mice, respectively) was set as a control group and was supplied with constant concentration of 0.9% NaCl in the agar through the whole experiment period [28].

Food Restriction (FR) Treatment Under Different Photoperiod Regimes

Twenty four *A. cahirinus* males were acclimated to short day (SD - 8L: 16D) while twenty six males were acclimated to long day (LD - 16L: 8D) inside a cabinet (158×77×74 cm) (Meditest 600/1300, Austria) for three weeks. Lights were on between 07:00 and 15:00h for SD; 07:00 and 23:00h for LD. Mice were kept in separate plastic cages (35×25×15 cm). Food (rat pellets, Koffolk, Israel) and 2% agar gel cubes (20 g of dry agar dissolved in 1000 ml of deionized water) as a source of water were provided *ad libitum*. Salinity concentration in the agar cubes was 0.9% NaCl for all studied groups. Mice were weighed to the nearest 0.1g using a digital balance (Sartorius 5500, Germany). Cabinet temperature was set at their lower critical point 28 ± 1^0C [29].

After three weeks of acclimation to SD or LD, mice from both photoperiods' acclimated groups were divided into sub-groups for the following treatments [32]:

1) Control group - *i.p* administrations of sterile saline solution (0.9% NaCl), n=6 for SD and n=6 for LD, acclimated mice.
2) Food restricted (Fr) group - mice were offered 75% of their 100% food intake, calculated from their average food intake at the last week of photoperiod acclimation, in addition sterile saline solution (0.9% NaCl) was administrated *i/p*, n=6 for SD and n=7 for LD, acclimated mice.

Melatonin (MLT) /Aldosterone (ALD) Treatments

Twenty eight individuals (14 females and 14 males) of mesic *A. cahirinus* were acclimated to LD (16L: 8D) inside a climatic cabinet (158x77x74 cm) (Meditest 600/1300, Austria) for three weeks. Lights were on between 07:00 and 23:00h. Cool fluorescent light with a dominant wave length of 470 nm and at an intensity of 450 lux, during photophase and red dim light (697 nm) of 25 lux during scotophase. (Animals were kept in separate plastic cages (35x25x15 cm). Food (rat pellets, Koffolk, Israel) and 2% agar gel (20 g of dry agar dissolved in 1000 ml of deionized water) as a source of water were provided *ad libitum*. W_b was recorded to the nearest 0.01g using a digital balance (Sartorius, 5500 Germany).

After three weeks of acclimation tested animals were injected with MLT solution (50μg/kg) or ALD solution (10mg/kg) (Sigma, Israel) for 21 days. The control group was injected only with saline solution (0.9% NaCl) also for 21 days.

Sacrificing Animals and Collecting Samples

Collecting Samples: At the end of experiments (After acclimation to the highest dietary salinity (5% NaCl), MLT, ALD, FR treatment) mice were anesthetized using *i.p.* cocktail injection of Ketamin (10mg/kg) and Rampoone (100mg/kg). All anesthetized mice were sacrificed by decapitation at 10:00h; three hours after lights were on. Blood samples were collected and centrifuged at 3000 rpm for 10 min, and serum was collected, stored at -20^0 C for sex hormones and leptin levels determination. WAT and gonads were removed and weighed. Organs masses were determined using an analytical scale (1907 MP8 Sartorius, Germany) and normalized to percent W_b. Organs were stored at -20^{0}C in RNA later (Beit Haemek, Israel) for RNA stability until further analysis.

Testosterone and progesterone detection: Serum was obtained from blood collected after mice decapitation. Testosterone and progesterone hormonal levels were measured using a commercial ELISA kit (Cayman chemical, USA) according **to manufacturer's** instructions. The assays were based on the competition between progesterone/testosterone and acetylcholinesterase (AChE) conjugate (progesterone/testosterone Tracer). The complex of antiserum- progesterone/testosterone binds to mouse monoclonal anti-rabbit IgG. The product of these enzymatic reactions determined spectrophotometrically, by ELISA reader (Power Wave XS, BioTek Gen 5) at a wavelength of 410nm.

Determination of Serum Leptin Levels: Serum leptin levels were measured by using a commercial ELISA (R&D System, USA) kit according **to manufacturer's** instructions. This assay employs the quantitative sandwich enzyme immunoassay technique. The product of these enzymatic reactions determined spectrophotometrically, by ELISA reader (Power Wave XS, BioTek Gen 5) at a wavelength of 450 nm.

Total RNA Extraction and Reverse Transcription: The reverse transcription-polymerase chain reaction (RT-PCR) has become a standard tool in quantification of gene expression analysis studies [30]. Total RNA was extracted from mice testis using RNeasy Mini Kit (Qiagen, Germany). For mRNA purification from testis and RNA extraction from WAT we used EZ-RNA kit (Biological Industries, Israel, Beit Haemek Ltd.). Isolated total RNA was quantified photometrically at a wavelength of 260 nm. Quality of RNA was verified by loading 1 μL of total RNA onto a RNA 6000 Nano Chip using the Nano Assay 600 Bioanalyzer (Agilent, Waldbronn, Germany) following the manufacturer's instructions. Single stranded cDNA was generated out of 0.5 μg total RNA using a High Capacity cDNA RT Kit (Applied Biosystems, UK). The obtained cDNA was stored (-20 °C) for further analysis.

Receptors Detection

The expression of leptin receptor was measured only in gonads (Ob-Rt: For reference we used NCBI sequence NM_146146.2). For reference housekeeping gene GAPDH (glyceraldehyde-3- phosphate dehydrogenase: NM_008084.2 as reference sequence) was used.

Primer Design and qRT-PCR Amplification: All primer sets on exon-exon junction site, were designed to have a T_m of approximately 60 °C, to have a GC content of approximately 50%, and to generate a PCR amplicone less than 150 bps. Finally, BLAST searchers were performed on primer pair sequences using the NCBI database to check for uniqueness. qRT - PCR (quantitative real-time reverse transcription-PCR) has become the benchmark for the detection and quantification of RNA targets. Quantitative real time PCR (qRT-PCR) was performed using SYBR Green technology [30]; primers were designed by Sigma, Israel. For the real-time PCR procedure, gene-specific primers and SYBR Green Real-Time PCR Master Mix (T Applied Biosystems, CA, USA) were used. Relative gene expression was detected by the ABI Prism 7000 Genetic Analyzer (Applied Biosystems, CA, USA). The relative expression (Relative quantification: RQ) of target gene (Ob-Rt gene), was normalized to the amount of GAPDH as housekeeping gene transcript in the same cDNA. RQ relates the PCR signal of the target transcript in a treatment group to that of another sample such as an untreated control. A melting curve analysis was performed to verify that a single PCR product was generated; negative controls, performed by omitting reverse transcriptase from the RT.

RESULTS

Gradually elevated ST caused a significant ($p<0.05$) decrease of serum leptin levels in both, LD- and SD-acclimated desert-adapted *A. cahirinus* females and males, compared with their control groups. Leptin levels in serum significantly ($p<0.05$) decreased in MLT-treated mesic LD-acclimated *A. cahirinus* females. However, leptin levels of mesic *A. cahirinus* males were affected only by ALD treatment, which caused a significant increase ($p<0.05$) in leptin serum levels, compared with their controls.

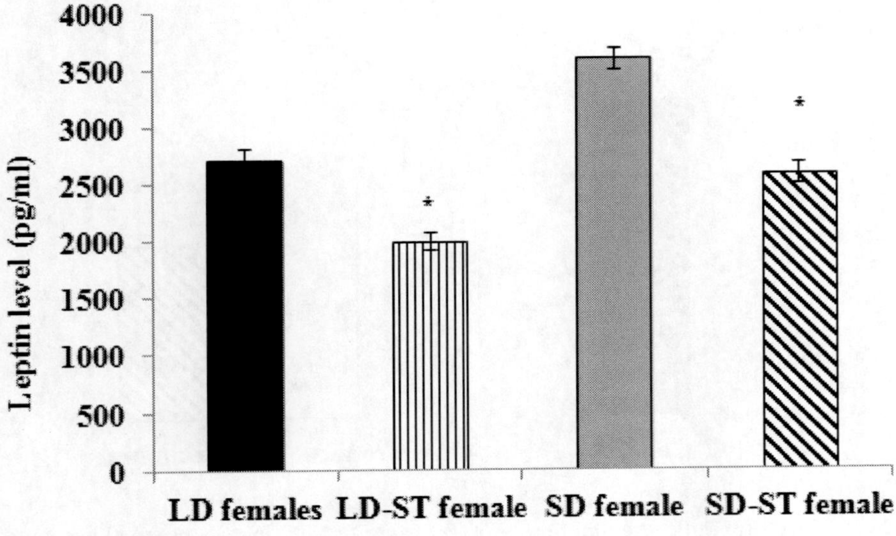

Figure 1A. Serum leptin levels (pg/ml) of desert-adapted *A. cahirinus* females, under LD- and SD-acclimation in response to ST, compared with control mice. Values of experimental groups are compared with those of their controls, n=7 in LD-acclimated groups and n=9 in SD-acclimated females. *A. cahirinus* females responded to ST by a significant (*$p<0.05$) decrease in leptin levels under both photoperiods compared with their controls.

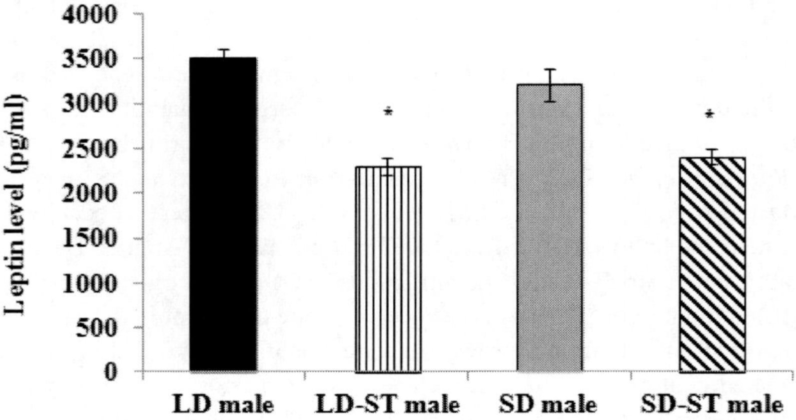

Figure 1B. Serum leptin levels (pg/ml) of *A. cahirinus* males, under LD- and SD-acclimation in response to ST, compared with control mice. Values of experimental group are compared with those of their controls, n=7 in LD-acclimated mice (both in experimental and control) and n=9 in SD-acclimated mice. ST to *A. cahirinus* males caused a significant (*$p<0.05$) decrease in leptin levels under both photoperiod regimes, compared with their controls.

High gene expression levels of leptin (Ob-Rt) mRNA receptors were noted in ovaries of SD-ST females ($p< 0.05$), while in testes, a significant ($p < 0.05$) increase in Ob-Rt expression was noted only in LD-ST individuals, compared with their controls. Ob-Rt testis expression levels of desert-adapted *A. cahirinus,* under LD, decreased significantly ($p<0.05$) as a results of food restriction.

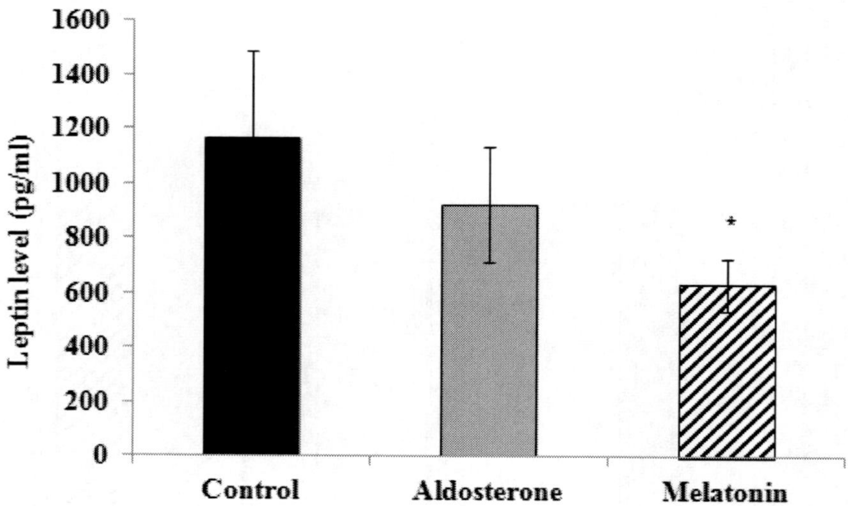

Figure 2A. Leptin levels (pg/ml) in serumof mesic *A. cahirinus* females in response to aldosterone (ALD) and melatonin (MLT) treatment, values of experimental groups are compared with those of their controls, n=7 in each group. Under MLT- treatment *A. cahirinus* serum leptin levels significantly (*$p<0.05$) decreased compared with their controls.

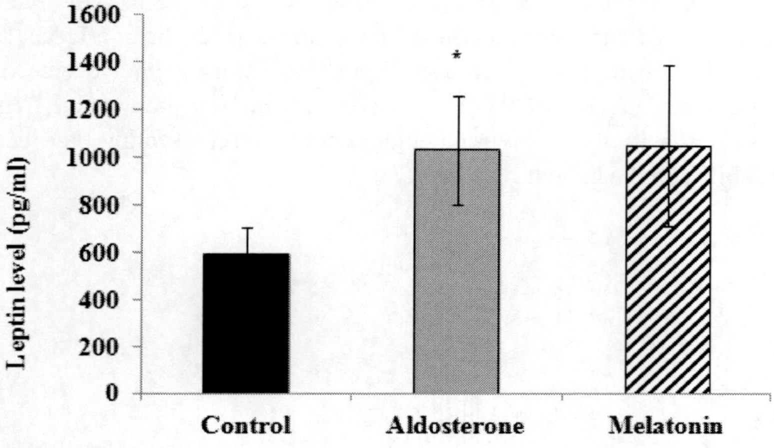

Figure 2B. Leptin serum levels (pg/ml) of mesic *A. cahirinus* males in response to aldosterone (ALD) and melatonin (MLT) treatments, values of experimental groups are compared with those of their controls, n=7 in each experimental group. ALD- treated *A. cahirinus* males significantly (*p<0.05) increased leptin serum levels, compared with their controls.

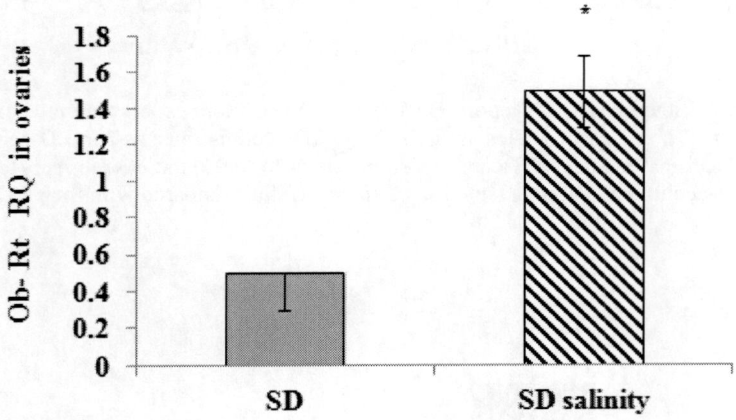

Figure 3A. Relative quantification (RQ) of leptin (Ob-Rt) receptors expression in ovaries of ST and control desert-adapted *A. cahirinus,* under SD, n=9 in each group. ST caused a significant (*p<0.05) increase in receptor expression levels in SD-desert-adapted *A. cahirinus* ovaries, compared with their SD-controls.

DISCUSSION

The metabolic status of an organism, which is defined in part by the availability of energy and nutrients to tissues, influences almost all biological functions, where among them, reproductive capacity is one of the most important [16]. Therefore, leptin acts as a critical link between WAT and the reproductive system, indicating whether adequate energy reserves are available for a successful reproductive function. In the basis of our study lies the suggestion that a possible mechanism by which environmental changes affects reproductive ability of *Acomys* populations can be associated with leptin [24, 27, 31], which has a direct effect through their receptors on the gonads or indirect effect *via* WAT [28,32]. In order to test this idea, our studies examined changes in leptin secretion levels as results of ST, MLT, and ALD, treatments. Quantification of leptin receptors expression by using the reverse transcriptase polymerase chain reaction (RT-PCR), on gonads expand our knowledge regarding the reproductive system sensitivity to environmental conditions representing day length (MLT), water/food availability in the habitat.

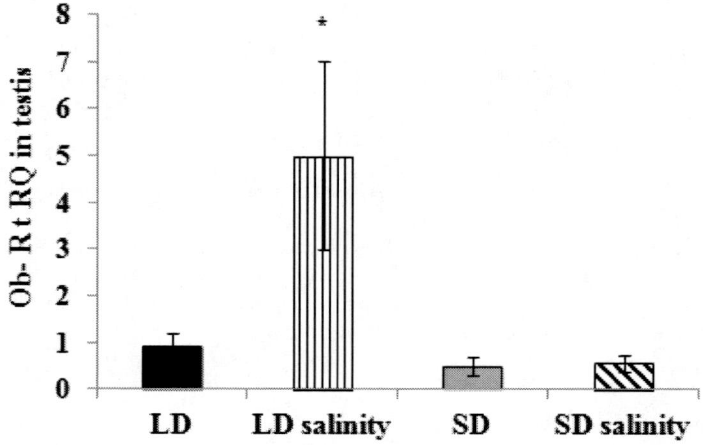

Figure 3B. Relative quantification (RQ) of leptin (Ob-Rt) mRNA receptors expression in testis of ST and control desert-adapted *A. cahirinus,* males, under LD and SD acclimations, n=7 in LD-acclimated groups and n=9 in SD-acclimated males. ST caused a significant (*p<0.05) increase in receptor expression levels of LD-acclimated desert-adapted *A. cahirinus* testis, compared with their LD-controls.

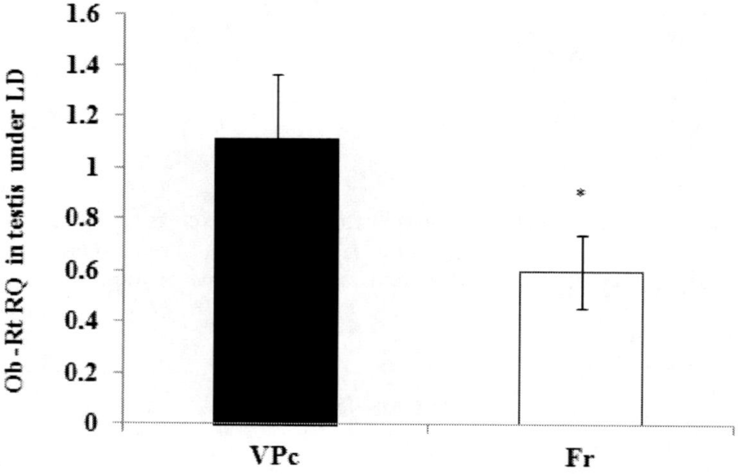

Figure 3C. Relative quantification (RQ) of leptin (Ob-Rt) mRNA receptors expression in testis of LD-acclimated food restricted (Fr) desert-adapted *A. cahirinus,* compared with their controls, n=7 in each group. Fr caused a significant (*p<0.05) decrease in receptor expression levels in testis of LD-acclimated desert-adapted *A. cahirinus*, compared with their LD-controls.

In rodents it is well established that leptin gene expression and plasma levels are proportional to total body WAT stores [33]. Leptin has been shown to promote sexual maturation in various rodent species and its role in reproduction has been investigated at various sites within the hypothalamo-pituitary-gonadal (HPG) axis [34]. Moreover, leptin concentration is higher in the luteal phase compared with the follicular phase of the ovarian cycle [13]. Leptin administration prevented the disruptive effects of acute food deprivation on reproductive function in cycling and lactating rat females suggesting that leptin levels contribute to the regulation of reproductive function [35].

The amount of body fat influences fertility, indicating a link between WAT amounts and the reproductive system [36]. It was suggested that high sodium chloride content diet could modulate leptin levels, independently of obesity. In accordance with this recently conceived concept regarding leptin physiology [37], rodents treated with a high salt diet were resistant to metabolic effects of leptin: as W_b, and adipose mass-reducing [38,39], but leptin's sympatho-excitatory actions still remains intact. A dramatically decrease in W_b and WAT mass in ST desert-adapted mice was noted [27]. Our data show a significant ($p<0.05$) decrease in serum leptin levels in desert-adapted rodents, in response to ST.

Exposure of ovariectomized adult ewes to LD-conditions for 4-6 weeks stimulated leptin expression and release from WAT, which its effect was independent of any change in the number of adipocytes or feed intake [40]. A similar effect of long days on leptin expression was previously reported in Siberian hamster (*Phodopus sungorus*) [41]. Diurnal variations in circulating leptin concentrations have also been reported in humans [42]. The role of MLT in leptin secretion is still poorly understood. Exogenous MLT reduced the blood levels of leptin in Siberian hamsters (*P. sungorus*) [43]. In Syrian hamsters (*Mesocricetus auratus*), high MLT blood levels were associated with a decrease in leptin concentrations, and the removal of the pineal gland resulted in an increases of leptin levels [44]. We reported that LD-acclimated desert-adapted *A. cahitrinus* were more sensitive to gradually increase in salinity [27, 28], while mesic *A. cahirinus* females, but not males responded to MLT-treatment by a decrease of leptin levels.

Expression of the *db* gene (*Diabetes Gene*), which encodes for a leptin receptor [45] has been confirmed within several organs and tissues as: pituitary [46], adipose tissue in sheep [47], on the granulosa, theca and interstitial cells of the ovary [48], in mice testis [49].

The results presented in this chapter and published in [28, 32] emphasize an Ob-Rt gene expression in the testis and ovaries of both, mesic and xeric *Acomys* populations. ST caused an increase in expression levels of Ob-Rt gene in SD-acclimated female ovaries and in LD-acclimated male testis of desert-adapted populations [28]. Food deprivation caused a significant decrease in the expression of this receptor, in the testis [32].

Therefore, our results on the endocrine and molecular levels are of importance for the proposed idea as they show that hormones regulating day length, water balance as well as energy storage (leptin) through their receptors presented on the gonads are involved in regulating of reproduction of *Acomys* populations. Future interventional studies involving leptin administration are expected to further clarify this role of leptin and may provide new insight and therapeutic options for the reproductive dysfunction associated with states of obesity evolving from a relative leptin deficiency or resistance.

REFERENCES

[1] Schaffler, A; Scholmerich, J; Buchler, C. The role of 'adipotropins' and the clinical importance of a potential hypothalamic-pituitary-adipose axis (2006). *Natural Clinical Practice. Endocrinology and Metabolism,* 2, 374-383.

[2] Zhang, Y; Proenca, R; Maffei, M; Barone, M; Leopold, L; Friedman, JM (1994). Positional cloning of the mouse obese gene and its human homologue. *Nature*, 372(6505), 425-432.

[3] Kershaw, E.E and. Flier, J.S. (2004). Adipose tissue as an endocrine organ. *The Journal of Clinical Endocrinology and Metabolism,* 89 (6), 2548-2556.

[4] Maffei, M; Halaas, J; Ravussin, E; Pratley, RE; Lee, GH; Zhang, Y; Fei, H; Kim, S; Lallone R; Ranganathan, S; Kern, PA; Friedman, JM (1995). Leptin levels in human and rodent: measurement of plasma leptin and ob RNA in obese and weight-reduced subjects. *Nature Medicine*, 1(11), 1155-1161.

[5] Licinio, J; Negrao, AB; Mantzoros, C; Kaklamani, V; Wong, M-L; Bongiorno, PB; Negro,P; Mulla, A; Veldhuis, J; Cearnal, L; Flier, J; Gold, P (1998). Sex differences in circulating human leptin pulse amplitude: clinical implications. *Journal of Clinical Endocrinology and Metabolism*, 83(11), 4140-4147.

[6] Jaruratanasirikul, S; Mo-Suwan, L; Lebel, L (1997). Growth pattern and age at menarche of obese girls in a transitional society. *Journal of Pediatric Endocrinology and Metabolism*, 10(5) 487-490.

[7] Amstalden, M; Garcia, MR; Williams, SW; Stanko, RL; Nizielski, SE; Morrison, CD; Keisler, DH; Williams, GL (2000). Leptin gene expression, circulating leptin, and luteinizing hormone pulsatility are acutely responsive to short-term fasting in prepubertal heifers: relationships to circulating insulin and insulin-like growth factor I. *Biology of Reproduction*, 63(1) pp. 127-133.

[8] Trayhurn, P; Thomas, MEA; Duncan, JS; Rayner, DV (1995). Effects of fasting and refeeding on *ob* gene expression in white adipose tissue of lean and obese (*ob/ob*) mice. *FEBS Letters*, 368(3) 488-490.

[9] Boden, G; Chen, X; Mazzoli, M; Ryan, I (1996). Effect of fasting on serum leptin in normal human subjects. *Journal of Clinical Endocrinology and Metabolism*, 81(9) 2419-2423.

[10] Sahu, A. (2003). Leptin signaling in the hypothalamus: emphasis on energy homeostasis and leptin resistance. *Frontiers in Neuroendocrinology*, 24(4) 225-253.

[11] Ahima, RS; Dusday, J; Flier, SN; Prabakaran, D; Flier, JS (1997). Leptin accelerates the onset of puberty in normal female mice. *Journal of Clinical investigation,* 99, 391-395.

[12] Cheung, CC; Thornton, JE;Kuijper, JL; Weigle, DS; Clifton, DK; Steiner, RA (1997). Leptin is metabolic gate for the onset of puberty in the female rat. *Endocrinology*, 138(2) 855-858.

[13] Popovic, V. & Casanueva, F. F. (2002) Leptin, nutrition and reproduction: new insights. *Hormones*, 1(4), 204-217.

[14] Hausman, DB; DiGirolamo, M; Bartness, TJ; Hausman, GJ; Martin, RJ (2001). The biology of white adipocyte proliferation. *Obesity Review*, 2, 239-254.

[15] Spicer, L.J & Francisco, C.C. (1997). The adipose obese gene product, leptin: evidence of a direct inhibitory role in ovarian function. *Endocrinology*, 138(8), 3374-3379.

[16] Szczesna, M & Zieba, A. (2011). Role of Leptin in the Reproduction and Metabolism: Focus on Regulation by Seasonality in Animals In book: *Update on Mechanisms of Hormone Action - Focus on Metabolism, Growth and Reproduction* book edited by Gianluca Aimaretti with Paolo Marzullo and Flavia Prodam: 2011, chapter 13.

[17] Adam, C.L & Mercer, J.G. (2004). Appetite regulation and seasonality: implications for obesity. *The Proceedings of the Nutrition Society*, 63(3), 413-419.

[18] Ng, T.B & Wong, C.M. (1986). Effects of pineal indoles and arginine vasotocin on lipolysis and lipogenesis in isolated adipocytes. *Journal of Pineal Research,* 3(1), 55-66.

[19] Glass, J.D& Knotts, L.K. (1987). A brain site for the antigonadal action of melatonin in the white-footed mouse (*Peromyscus leucopus*): involvement of the immunoreactive GnRH neuronal system. *Neuroendocrinology*, 46, 48-55.

[20] Kennaway, D.J and Rowe, S.A. (1995). Melatonin binding sites and their role in seasonal reproduction. *Journal Reproduction Fertility Suppl*, 49, 423-435.

[21] Digby, SN; Chadwick, MA; Blache, D (2011). Salt intake and reproductive function in sheep, *Animal*, 5 (8), 1207-1216.

[22] Atcha, Z; Cagampang, FR; Stirland, JA; Morris, ID; Brooks, AN; Ebling, FJ; Klingenspor,M; Loudon, AS (2000). Leptin acts on metabolism in a photoperiod-dependent manner, but has no effect on reproductive function in the seasonally breeding Siberian hamster (*Phodopus sungorus*). *Endocrinology*, 141(11), 4128-4135.

[23] Klingenspor, M; Niggemann, H; Heldmaier, G (2000). Modulation of leptin sensitivity by short photoperiod acclimation in the Djungarian hamster, *Phodopus sungorus. Journal of Comparative Physiology; Biochemical, Systemic, and Environmental Physiology,* 170(1) 37-43.

[24] Shanas, U & Haim, A. (2004). Diet salinity and vasopressin as reproduction modulators in the desert-dwelling golden spiny mouse (*Acomys russatus*). *Physiology and Behavior*, 81, 645-650.

[25] Schaffler, A; Binart, N; Scholmerich, J; Buchler, C. (2005). Hypothesis paper Brain talks with fat--evidence for a hypothalamic-pituitary-adipose axis? *Neuropeptides*, 39, 363-367.

[26] Friedman, J.M & Halaas, J.L. (1998). Leptin and the regulation of body weight in mammals. *Nature*, 395, 763–770.

[27] Bukovetzky, E; Schwimmer, H; Fares, F; Haim, A. (2012a). Photoperiodicity and increasing salinity as environmental cues for reproduction in desert adapted rodents. *Hormones and Behavior*, 61, 84-90

[28] Bukovetzky, E; Fares, F; Haim, A. (2012c). Metabolic and endocrine responses of desert-adapted Mice Reproductive System to Increased Salinity, *Journal of Life Sciences,* 6, 454-459.

[29] Weissenberg, S & Shkolnik, A. (1994). Metabolic rate and water economy in the desert and Mediterranean populations of the common spiny mouse (*Acomys cahirinus*) in Israel. Israeli *Journal of Zoology*, 40,135-143.

[30] Bustin, S.A (2002). Quantification of mRNA using real-time reverse transcription PCR (RT-PCR): Trends and problems. Journal of Molecular Endocrinology, 29, 23-39.

[31] Wube, T; Haim, A; Fares, F (2009). Effect of increased dietary salinity on the reproductive status and energy intake of xeric and mesic populations of the spiny mouse, *Acomys*, *Physiology and Behavior*, 2009, 122-127.

[32] Bukovetzky, E; Fares, F; Schwimmer H; Haim ,A (2012b) Reproductive and metabolic responses of desert adapted common spiny male mice (*Acomys cahirinus*) to vasopressin treatment. *Comparative Biochemistry and Physiology, Part A*, 162(4), 349-356.

[33] Hiraoka, J; Hosoda, K; Ogawa, Y; Ikeda, K; Nara, Y; Masuzaki, H(1997). Augmentation of obese (ob) gene expression and leptin secretion in obese spontaneously hypertensive rats (obese SHR or Koletsky rats), *Biochemistry Biophysics Research Community,* 231 , 582-285.

[34] Clarke, I.J & Henry, B.A. (1999). Leptin and reproduction, *Reviews of Reproduction*, 4 , 48-55.

[35] Abizaid, A; Kyriazis, D; Woodside, B. (2004). Effect of leptin administration on lactational infertility in food restricted rats depend on milk delivery. *Journal Physiology Regul. Integr. Comp. Physiol.*, 286, 217–225.

[36] Frisch, R.E (1990). The right weight: body fat, menarche and ovulation. *Bailliere's Clin. Obstet. Gynaecol.,* 4, 419–439.

[37] Mark, AL; Correia, ML; Rahmouni, K; Haynes, WG. (2002). Selective leptin resistance: A new concept in leptin physiology with cardiovascular implications, *Journal of Hypertension*, 20, 1245-1250.

[38] Levin, N; Nelson, C; Gurney, A; Vandlen, R; de Sauvage, F. (1996). Decreased food intake does not completely account for adiposity reduction after *ob* protein infusion. *Proceedings of the National Academy of Sciences of the United States of America,* 93 (4) , 1726-1730.

[39] Barzilai, N. Wang, J. Massilon, D. Vuguin, P. Hawkins, M. Rossetti, L. (1997). Leptin selectively decreases visceral adiposity and enhances insulin action. *The Journal of clinical investigation,* 100 (12) , 3105-3110.

[40] Bocquier, F; Bonnet, M; Faulconnier, Y; Guerre-Millo, M; Martin, P; Chilliard, Y (1998). Effects of photoperiod and feeding level on perirenal adipose tissue metabolic activity and leptin synthesis in the ovariectomized ewe. *Reproduction, Nutrition, Development,* 38(5), 489-498.

[41] Klingenspor, M; Dickopp, A; Heldmaier, G; Klaus, S (1996). Short photoperiod reduces leptin gene expression in white and brown adipose tissue of *Djungarian hamsters. FEBS Letters*, 399(3), 290-294.

[42] Licinio, J; Negrao, AB; Mantzoros, C; Kaklamani, V; Wong, M; Bongiorno, PB; Mull, A; Cearnal, L; Veldhuis, JD; Flier, JS; McCann, SM; Gold, PW (1998b). Synchronicity of frequently sampled 24-h concentrations of circulating leptin, luteinizing hormone, and estradiol in healthy women. *Proceedings of the National Academy of Sciences of the United States of America,* 95(5), 2541-2546.

[43] Korhonen, T; Mustonen, AM; Nieminen, P; Saarela, S (2008). Effects of cold exposure, exogenous melatonin and short-day treatment on the weight-regulation and body temperature of the Siberian hamster (*Phodopus sungorus*). *Regulatory Peptides,* 149(1-3), 60-66.

[44] Gunduz, B. (2002). Daily rhythm in serum melatonin and leptin levels in the Syrian hamster (*Mesocricetus auratus*). Comparative Biochemistry and Physiology. *Part A, Molecular and Integrative Physiology*, 132(2), 393-401.

[45] Tartaglia, LA; Dembski, M; Weng, X; Den, N; Culpepper, J; Devos, R; Richards, GJ; Campfield, LA; Clark, FT; Deeds, J; Muir, C; Skaner, S; Moriarty, A; Moore, KJ; Smutko, JS; Mays, GG; Woolf, EA; Monero, CA; Tepper, RI (1995). Identification and expression cloning of a leptin receptor, *OB-R. Cell*, 83(7), 1263-1271.

[46] Iqbal, J; Pompolo, S; Considine, RV; Clarke, IJ (2000). Localization of leptin receptor-like immunoreactivity in the corticotropes, somatotropes, and gonadotropes in the ovine anterior pituitary. *Endocrinology*, 141(4) 1515-1520.

[47] Dyer, CJ; Simmons, JM; Matteri, RL; Keisler, DH (1997). Leptin receptor mRNA is expressed in ewe anterior pituitary and adipose tissues and is differentially expressed in hypothalamic regions of well-fed and feed-restricted ewes. *Domestic Animal Endocrinology*, 14(2), 119-128.

[48] Karlsson, C; Lindell, K; Svensson, E; Bergh, C; Lind, P; Billig, H; Carlsson, LM; Carlsson, B (1997). Expression of functional leptin receptors in human ovary. *Journal of Clinical Endocrinology & Metabolism,* 82 (12), 4144-4148.

[49] Caprio, M; Isidori, AM; Carta, AR; Moretti, C ; Dufau, ML; Fabbri A (1999). Expression of leptin receptors in rodents Leydig cells. *Endocrinology*, 140(11), 4939-4947.

INDEX

A

access, 159, 175
accounting, 135
acetic acid, 143
acetylcholine, 63
acetylcholinesterase, 178
acid, 4, 5, 9, 13, 15, 64, 65, 67, 75, 76, 81, 100, 119, 127, 158
acidic, 63, 67, 71
acrosome, 86, 95, 108
ACTH, 90
action potential, 171
active transport, 64
acylation, 92
adaptation, xi, 58, 106, 115, 173, 176
adenosine, 3, 18, 106, 159, 167, 171
adenovirus, 132
adhesion, 52, 155
adipocyte, 34, 36, 46, 106, 118, 124, 130, 184
adiponectin, 2, 14, 30, 46, 53, 54, 97, 105, 119, 120, 125, 139
adipose tissue, vii, viii, ix, x, xi, 2, 8, 17, 18, 23, 33, 34, 40, 45, 47, 48, 50, 51, 54, 55, 56, 59, 61, 62, 73, 83, 89, 92, 101, 107, 112, 113, 115, 116, 117, 118, 122, 124, 125, 126, 129, 132, 142, 157, 174, 183, 184, 186, 187
adiposity, viii, ix, 45, 47, 48, 58, 79, 97, 104, 105, 111, 117, 118, 125, 132, 186
adiposity signal, viii, ix, 45, 47, 111
adjustment, 53
adolescents, 46, 51, 53, 54, 55, 59, 93, 105, 106, 115, 117, 126
ADP, 40
adrenal gland, 18
adrenaline, 130
adult obesity, 114
adulthood, 114, 116, 123
adults, 12, 33, 36, 46, 53, 55, 84, 87, 96, 114, 119, 136, 176
adverse conditions, 121
adverse effects, 143
aerobic exercise, 54
agar, 176, 177
age, 34, 39, 92, 93, 95, 97, 115, 117, 118, 125, 174, 184
aggregation, 7, 46
agonist, 78, 131
alanine, 65, 78, 143
alanine aminotransferase, 143
albumin, 84
alcohol consumption, viii, 33
aldolase, 106
aldosterone, xii, 173, 180, 181
allele, 4, 13
ALT, 143
alters, xi, 5, 92, 158
amino, 2, 4, 13, 47, 62, 64, 65, 66, 70, 71, 72, 75, 77, 78, 80, 81, 86, 112, 142, 167, 168, 169
amino acid(s), 2, 13, 62, 64, 65, 66, 70, 71, 72, 77, 112, 142, 168, 169
amplitude, xi, 10, 157, 160, 162, 166, 184
amyloid beta, 12, 13
amyloid deposits, 7
anabolism, 135
androgen(s), 85, 92, 93, 96, 97, 103, 107
angiogenesis, x, 34, 35, 36, 62, 80, 113, 141, 142, 145, 147, 148, 149, 150, 151, 152, 153, 154, 155
angiotensin II, 125
anorexia, 2, 10, 104, 118, 130
anorexia nervosa, 10, 130
ANOVA, 160, 162
antagonism, 137
antibody, 23, 86, 142, 144, 147
anti-cancer, 40
anticonvulsant, 9
antidepressant, 8, 15

antigen, 154
antioxidant, 66
antitumor, 40
APA, 107
apnea, 158
apoptosis, 3, 11, 40, 41, 43, 85, 90, 95, 108, 113, 122, 126, 138
apoptotic mechanisms, 7
appetite, ix, 18, 28, 47, 54, 55, 59, 61, 73, 104, 112, 114, 122, 131, 158, 175
ARC, 113, 116
arginine, 185
arrest, 40
arterial hypertension, 27, 127
artery, 28, 119
aspartate, 4, 143
assessment, 40, 105
astrocytes, 4
atherosclerosis, 46, 53, 119, 120, 121, 126
ATP, 6, 11, 64, 167, 171
atrophy, 7, 120
Austria, 176, 177
axons, 168

B

barriers, 47, 49, 51
base, 158
basement membrane, 35
BBB, 49, 51
beneficial effect, vii, 1, 4, 6, 7
benefits, vii, 1
bias, 12, 176
binding globulin, 84, 97, 107, 109
bioavailability, 2, 47, 63, 85
biochemistry, 42, 137, 138, 139
biosynthesis, vii, 6
birth weight, 114, 115
bisphenol, 139
blood, viii, xi, 2, 4, 11, 18, 19, 22, 27, 28, 29, 33, 34, 35, 47, 49, 51, 56, 58, 62, 63, 65, 69, 78, 85, 89, 94, 98, 99, 102, 105, 116, 118, 121, 125, 127, 131, 133, 142, 143, 144, 146, 147, 150, 174, 175, 178, 183
blood monocytes, 11
blood pressure, 19, 22, 27, 28, 29, 34, 121, 127
blood vessels, xi, 35, 142, 144, 146, 147, 150
blood-brain barrier, 49, 58, 62, 63, 78, 89, 102, 131
bloodstream, 94, 174, 175
body composition, viii, 30, 33, 36, 97, 105, 114
body fat, 2, 25, 30, 46, 57, 84, 93, 97, 112, 113, 116, 117, 118, 174, 183, 186
body fluid, 27
body mass index (BMI), viii, 2, 6, 7, 9, 33, 53, 84, 92, 96, 114, 118
body weight, x, 8, 15, 18, 36, 46, 47, 48, 49, 50, 51, 52, 57, 58, 73, 80, 85, 100, 104, 112, 113, 115, 116, 117, 122, 125, 131, 132, 137, 141, 142, 143, 153, 168, 185
bone, x, 31, 34, 62, 77, 112, 120, 122, 126, 129, 130, 131, 132, 133, 134, 135, 136, 137, 138, 139, 142, 154
bone biology, 77
bone cells, x, 129
bone form, x, 62, 129, 131, 132, 133, 134, 135, 136, 138, 139, 142, 154
bone growth, 137
bone marrow, 120, 126, 131, 133, 134, 138
bone mass, x, 34, 112, 122, 129, 130, 131, 132, 133, 136, 137, 139, 154
bone resorption, 131, 133, 136
bone volume, 132, 133, 135
bones, 130, 136
brain, vii, viii, ix, x, 1, 2, 3, 4, 5, 6, 7, 8, 9, 10, 11, 12, 13, 14, 18, 34, 45, 47, 49, 51, 56, 57, 58, 75, 76, 77, 89, 92, 101, 102, 104, 111, 112, 113, 115, 118, 121, 123, 124, 129, 130, 131, 136, 142, 153, 154, 159, 167, 169, 170, 185
brain stem, 159, 167
brain structure, 12
brainstem, 160, 167, 168, 171
branching, 151
breast cancer, vii, viii, 35, 37, 39, 40, 41, 42, 43
breast carcinoma, 42
breast milk, 112
breathing, xi, 157, 158, 160, 162, 169, 170
breeding, 176, 185
bulimia, 118
burn, x, 141, 143, 146

C

Ca^{2+}, 4, 107, 167, 170
cachexia, 26, 29, 31
calcification, 117, 119
calcium, 3
caloric restriction, 21, 92, 119
calorie, 19, 31, 114, 132
cancer, viii, 8, 34, 35, 36, 37, 39, 40, 41, 42, 43, 106
cancer care, 43
cancer cells, 37, 40
cancer death, 34
candidates, 92
carbohydrate, 119, 124
carcinogen, 34
carcinogenesis, 34, 37

cardiomyopathy, 119
cardiovascular, vii, viii, ix, 17, 26, 28, 31, 45, 53, 54, 57, 58, 59, 84, 96, 111, 119, 120, 121, 126, 186
cardiovascular disease, viii, ix, 45, 53, 54, 59, 84, 96, 111, 119, 120, 121, 126
cardiovascular function, 54, 57
cardiovascular physiology, 28
cardiovascular risk, x, 53, 112
cardiovascular system, 31, 120
carotene, viii, 33
cartilage, 65
cascades, 3
caspases, 3
C-C, 98
CD8+, 52
cDNA, 52, 178, 179
cell biology, 139
cell culture, 135
cell cycle, 29, 40
cell death, 13, 15, 95, 103
cell differentiation, 95, 120
cell division, 93, 99
cell line(s), 11, 13, 34, 36, 71, 76, 77, 79, 80, 97, 103, 144
cell proliferation, 20, 29, 34, 63, 80, 117, 133, 138, 144, 147, 153
cell signaling, 13, 42, 85
cell size, 119, 120
cell surface, 4
central nervous system, xii, 2, 10, 11, 46, 56, 62, 116, 168, 173
cerebellum, 159
cerebral cortex, 11
cerebrospinal fluid, 6, 15, 47, 51, 89, 159, 160
chemical, x, 64, 121, 130, 141, 143, 146, 168, 171, 178
chemoreceptors, 159
chemotherapy, 40, 153
childhood, 85, 119
children, 105, 115, 116, 117, 119, 125, 135, 136
cholesterol, 4, 5, 12, 13, 93
cholesterol-lowering drugs, 4
choroid, 47, 89
chronic diseases, 54, 119
chronic renal failure, 30
cigarette smoking, viii, 33
circadian rhythm, 117
circulation, viii, 2, 4, 18, 30, 45, 63, 64, 117, 118
classes, 72
classification, 2
cleavage, 93
climate, 175
clinical application, 58
clinical significance, vii, viii, 39
clinical symptoms, 7
clinical trials, 22
cloning, 9, 27, 56, 79, 80, 81, 112, 122, 136, 153, 155, 184, 187
clustering, 11
CNS, 6, 46, 52, 54, 55, 87, 118, 169
CO2, 158, 159
cocaine, 90, 105, 131
coding, 167, 169
coffee, 36
cognition, vii, 1, 2, 4, 5, 6, 9, 10, 12, 102, 115
cognitive development, 10, 123
cognitive function, 3, 5, 123
cognitive impairment, vii, 1, 5, 6, 7, 14, 15
cognitive performance, 114
cognitive profile, 7
collagen, 24, 25, 65, 138, 143, 144, 147
colon, 34, 36
colon cancer, 36
colorectal cancer, 35, 37
commercial, 178
common symptoms, 7
community, 12
comparative analysis, 30
competition, 178
complex interactions, x, 129
complexity, x, 41, 129, 135
complications, 46, 112
composition, 4, 5, 12, 13, 67, 97
compounds, 41
computer, 160
conditioning, 6
conflict, 96
conflict of interest, 96
connective tissue, x, 65, 141, 142, 143, 145, 146, 147, 148, 153
consensus, 75, 167
consolidation, 113
constant rate, 160
consumption, 51, 52, 63, 85, 119, 158
contradiction, 34
control group, xii, 143, 144, 145, 146, 147, 148, 174, 177, 179
controversial, 134
cooperation, 136
coordination, 137
copper, 8
coronary artery disease, 127
coronary heart disease, 117, 118
correlation(s), 46, 53, 95, 96, 107, 118, 158
cortex, 2, 123
cortical bone, x, 129, 130, 132, 133, 135, 136, 137

cortical neurons, 3
corticobasal degeneration, 7
cortisol, 90, 126
counseling, 54
craniotomy, 159
creatinine, 20
Creutzfeldt-Jakob disease, 8
critical period, 114, 115, 121
crown, 150
CRP, 20
CSF, 6, 118
cues, xi, 173, 176, 185
cure, 14
cycles, 118, 175
cycling, 183
cysteine, 65, 76
cystine, 66
cytochrome, 93
cytokines, ix, 2, 3, 11, 27, 34, 35, 46, 52, 53, 111, 118, 120, 121, 126
cytoplasm, 64, 75
cytoskeleton, 11, 13
cytotoxicity, 40, 120

D

database, 6, 179
Dead Sea, 176
deep brain stimulation, 14
defects, 3, 51, 58, 98, 102
deficiency(ies), 2, 3, 4, 5, 6, 9, 10, 20, 34, 35, 59, 62, 85, 95, 98, 101, 106, 107, 108, 123, 131, 132, 136, 139, 183
degradation, 22, 68, 89
dementia, vii, 1, 2, 6, 7, 8, 12, 14, 15
dentin, xi, 142, 149, 150
deposition, 7, 18, 25, 119
deposits, 6, 174
depression, vii, 1, 3, 8, 15, 170
deprivation, 132, 154, 183
depth, 159
desensitization, 74, 118
destruction, 53
detection, 86, 143, 178, 179
developed countries, 96
diabetes, 2, 8, 10, 18, 26, 27, 34, 57, 73, 76, 112, 114, 115, 117, 119, 123, 126
diabetic patients, 115
dialysis, 25, 26, 30, 31
diaphragm, xi, 157, 160, 161, 162, 163, 165
diet, viii, 19, 20, 21, 22, 23, 24, 28, 29, 30, 33, 36, 49, 51, 52, 58, 64, 65, 73, 78, 100, 101, 102, 119, 183
diet composition, 29
dietary intake, viii, 33
diffusion, 64
dimerization, 87
dipeptides, 72, 76, 78
direct action, xi, 70, 84, 90, 133, 158, 175
disease progression, 4, 8, 15
diseases, vii, viii, ix, x, 1, 4, 8, 15, 45, 54, 83, 84, 112, 114, 121, 123, 139
disorder, 2, 7, 8, 9
distribution, 3, 14, 96, 97, 105, 107, 116, 142, 150, 167
diuretic, 20
diversity, 47
DNA, 95, 108
DOI, 77
donors, 138
dopamine, 7, 131
dopaminergic, 7, 15
dosage, 41
down-regulation, 41, 43, 78
drugs, 7, 40, 41, 42, 43
duodenum, 64, 76

E

eating disorders, 5, 118, 126
ecosystem, xi, 173
electrodes, 160
ELISA, 178
EMG, 160, 161, 162, 163, 165
enamel, xi, 142, 149, 150
encephalopathy, 7, 8
encoding, 144
end stage renal disease (ESRD), 31
endocrine, ix, xii, 2, 36, 46, 55, 63, 74, 76, 83, 84, 86, 96, 98, 106, 117, 122, 130, 173, 174, 175, 183, 184, 185
endocrine disorders, 84
endocrine system, 175
endocrinology, 18, 126, 137, 138, 173
endothelial cells, xi, 20, 24, 25, 28, 29, 35, 47, 52, 81, 117, 121, 122, 142, 143, 144, 146, 148, 150, 151
endothelial dysfunction, ix, 111, 121
endothelium, 154
end-stage renal disease, 26, 27
energy conservation, 135
energy density, 174
energy expenditure, vii, xii, 17, 47, 48, 54, 62, 73, 79, 113, 115, 122, 158, 173, 174, 175
England, 77, 78
environment, ix, xii, 67, 111, 114, 121, 125, 173

environmental change, 175, 181
environmental conditions, 92, 182
environmental influences, 114
environmental stimuli, 121
environments, xii, 124, 173, 176
enzyme(s), 64, 69, 93, 178
enzyme immunoassay, 178
epidemic, 97, 114
epidemiology, 168
epididymis, 87, 99
epilepsy, 8, 15
epileptogenesis, 4, 12
epinephrine, 131
epithelia, 65, 76
epithelial cells, x, 69, 76, 77, 141, 142, 149
epithelial transport, 76
epithelium, 81, 144, 147, 149
equilibrium, 50
ESRD, 31
estrogen, 39, 92, 100, 105, 107, 139
ethnicity, 118
etiology, 115
European Regional Development Fund, 75
evidence, vii, viii, 17, 18, 20, 28, 34, 35, 39, 41, 51, 78, 97, 99, 100, 105, 114, 115, 116, 127, 150, 153, 154, 158, 167, 175, 185
evolution, 102, 116
excitatory synapses, 113
excitotoxicity, 15
excretion, 4, 20, 21, 22, 23, 26, 29
exercise, 54, 59
exposure, viii, 34, 45, 50, 51, 52, 68, 134, 139, 186
extracellular domain, 18
extracellular matrix, 25, 35, 120
extracellular signal-related kinases, 3, 86
extraction, 178

F

families, 85
family history, 120
family members, 89
fasting, 51, 73, 77, 92, 103, 106, 115, 118, 122, 126, 184
fasting glucose, 115, 126
fat, ix, x, 18, 22, 23, 30, 31, 46, 51, 52, 57, 81, 84, 94, 105, 107, 111, 112, 115, 117, 118, 126, 129, 130, 131, 133, 135, 136, 139, 153, 154, 174, 185
fatty acids, 4, 72
fear, 6
feedback inhibition, 100
female rat, 104, 184
femur, 130
fertility, 62, 84, 85, 86, 87, 89, 95, 97, 98, 101, 108, 183
fertilization, 95
fetal development, 114, 115
fetal growth, 115, 123
fetal growth retardation, 115
fetus, 116
fiber, 119
fibroblasts, 65, 117, 146, 147
fibrosis, 24, 30
filtration, 24
fluid, 10, 57, 58, 102, 159
follicle,(s) 90, 175
food, vii, viii, ix, xi, xii, 10, 14, 15, 17, 33, 34, 46, 51, 52, 57, 58, 61, 62, 66, 76, 79, 85, 90, 92, 104, 111, 113, 115, 116, 120, 122, 125, 132, 154, 158, 168, 170, 173, 175, 176, 177, 180, 182, 183, 186
food intake, vii, viii, ix, xii, 14, 15, 17, 33, 34, 46, 51, 57, 61, 62, 76, 79, 85, 104, 111, 113, 115, 116, 120, 122, 125, 132, 158, 168, 170, 173, 175, 177, 186
formaldehyde, 160
formation, 7, 40, 115, 132, 133, 143, 146, 149, 150
fragility, 137
fragments, 161, 163, 165
France, 58
fructose, ix, 61, 63, 64, 65, 69, 70, 75, 115
functional activation, 126, 153
functional analysis, 137
functional changes, 30

G

GABA, 48
gastric mucosa, 63, 76
gastrointestinal tract, 57, 63, 74, 81
gel, 176, 177
gene expression, xii, 8, 10, 25, 30, 50, 70, 81, 88, 92, 94, 99, 106, 116, 119, 123, 133, 153, 174, 178, 179, 180, 183, 184, 186
gene promoter, 78, 90, 106, 107
gene regulation, 88
genes, xii, 3, 13, 88, 93, 95, 103, 104, 108, 133, 139, 147, 174, 176
genetic background, 87
genetic defect, 51
genetics, 14, 105, 114
genome, 114
genotype, 13, 114
germ cells, 85, 86, 94, 95
Germany, 176, 177, 178
gestation, 116
gestational age, 116

gingival, x, 141, 143, 144
gingival epithelium, x, 141
gland, 40
glial cells, 4, 115
glucagon, 43, 75, 80
glucocorticoids, 63, 118
gluconeogenesis, 66, 69
glucose, ix, 6, 11, 13, 25, 56, 61, 64, 65, 68, 69, 70, 73, 77, 78, 79, 80, 81, 92, 94, 107, 114, 115, 118, 122, 125, 126, 127, 153, 170
glucose tolerance, 94, 107, 114, 115, 126
glucoside, 69
GLUT, 64, 69
GLUT4, 13, 57
glutamate, 8, 9, 65, 66, 67, 71, 76, 78, 79
glutamine, ix, 61, 65, 66, 70, 77
glutathione, 66
glycogen, 13, 138
gonadotropin-releasing hormone (GnRH), 90, 175
gonads, ix, xii, 83, 86, 87, 93, 113, 174, 175, 178, 182, 183
Gori, 138
grants, 74
granules, 63, 76
gray matter, 3
grouping, 87
growth, viii, ix, xi, 33, 34, 35, 36, 37, 39, 40, 42, 43, 56, 80, 81, 85, 88, 90, 101, 105, 111, 113, 114, 115, 120, 122, 123, 124, 125, 126, 139, 142, 149, 151, 152, 153, 155, 175, 184
growth factor, xi, 36, 39, 40, 113, 120, 122, 139, 142, 149, 151, 152, 153, 155, 184
growth hormone, 80, 85, 105, 126, 149
guanine, 89
gymnasts, 139

H

habitat, xi, 173, 182
head and neck cancer, 153
healing, x, 141, 143, 145, 146, 153
health, vii, 17, 27, 81, 84, 96, 114, 121
heart disease, 18
height, viii, 33, 36
hematopoiesis, x, 34, 62, 77, 117, 141, 142
hemodialysis, 25, 30, 31, 139
hepatic stellate cells, 120, 126
hepatocytes, 142
hepatoma, 97
heritability, 158, 169
heterogeneity, 9, 41, 118
high fat, 24, 28, 36, 49, 51, 58, 75
hippocampus, vii, 1, 2, 3, 4, 7, 8, 12
histology, 149, 155
homeostasis, vii, ix, x, 1, 2, 4, 6, 9, 15, 26, 34, 46, 47, 56, 57, 90, 94, 103, 104, 111, 112, 113, 115, 120, 121, 122, 126, 129, 130, 135, 141, 142, 158, 170, 175, 184
hormonal control, 122
hormone levels, 97, 107, 108
HSB, 147
human brain, 12, 78, 168
human experience, 123
human skin, 147, 148
human subjects, 75, 106, 184
hybridization, 107
hydrolysis, 64
hydrophobicity, 46
hyperactivity, 123
hyperglycemia, 35, 119, 126
hyperinsulinemia, 10, 25, 35, 84, 117, 119
hyperplasia, 67, 119, 120
hypertension, viii, ix, 17, 18, 19, 20, 22, 26, 27, 28, 29, 30, 75, 111, 114, 120, 121, 123, 125
hypertriglyceridemia, 51
hypertrophy, 18, 67, 119, 120, 121
hypogonadism, ix, 83, 85, 90, 92, 97, 98, 102, 107
hypothalamus, vii, viii, ix, x, xii, 1, 2, 3, 12, 17, 18, 19, 20, 33, 45, 47, 48, 51, 57, 58, 62, 79, 83, 85, 89, 90, 91, 92, 93, 96, 100, 103, 104, 105, 111, 112, 113, 115, 116, 124, 129, 131, 132, 134, 137, 142, 154, 169, 170, 171, 174, 175, 184
hypothesis, 22, 34, 35, 51, 53, 114, 115, 123, 159
hypoxia, 37, 94, 106, 121, 170
hypoxia-inducible factor, 37, 94, 106

I

identification, 27, 74, 76, 80, 112
IFN, 53
ileum, 79
immune function, 13, 62, 112, 117
immune response, 56, 79
immune system, 2, 46, 52, 62, 79, 98, 112, 120
immunity, 77, 90, 122
immunofluorescence, 87
immunoglobulin, 155
immunohistochemistry, 86, 87, 99, 147
immunolocalization, 56
immunoreactivity, 103, 104, 155, 168, 187
immunosuppression, 56
impairments, 4, 12
in situ hybridization, 27, 86, 87, 154, 169
in utero, 114, 116, 117
in vitro, xi, 4, 7, 11, 15, 34, 41, 52, 56, 69, 74, 80, 92, 101, 104, 106, 137, 157, 159, 167, 168, 169

in vivo, xi, 6, 28, 41, 47, 56, 68, 70, 71, 72, 74, 76, 78, 80, 105, 106, 133, 137, 157, 159, 167, 169, 170, 171
incidence, 14, 18, 25, 34, 39, 84
incisors, 149, 150
income, 43
India, 29
indirect effect, 112, 175, 182
individuals, ix, xii, 3, 5, 6, 46, 51, 62, 73, 83, 85, 89, 112, 113, 114, 118, 119, 134, 158, 174, 176, 177, 180
inducer, 11
induction, 18, 40, 51, 121
inevitability, 14
infants, 114, 115
infertility, ix, 34, 83, 85, 89, 92, 95, 96, 108, 112, 186
inflammation, 26, 29, 30, 31, 34, 35, 46, 52, 53, 54, 55, 58, 59, 77, 81, 112, 117, 119, 120, 121, 125, 126
inflammatory disease, 52
inflammatory mediators, 117
inflammatory responses, 117, 118, 120
inflation, 158
ingestion, 94
inhibition, vii, 12, 18, 35, 41, 43, 68, 69, 70, 77, 85, 88, 89, 93, 99, 102, 113, 125, 131, 132, 158, 175
inhibitor, 41, 70, 86, 87, 91, 120
injury, 9, 120, 121
inositol, 11, 123
insertion, ix, 61, 68, 69, 70, 75
insulation, xii, 173, 174
insulin, viii, 11, 19, 20, 25, 29, 30, 33, 36, 45, 48, 52, 54, 56, 63, 68, 73, 75, 79, 80, 84, 92, 93, 94, 95, 97, 100, 102, 106, 107, 115, 117, 118, 119, 122, 123, 125, 126, 139, 184, 186
insulin resistance, viii, 20, 29, 45, 54, 73, 84, 94, 115, 117, 118, 119, 125, 126
insulin sensitivity, 48, 52, 79, 119
insulinoma, 11
integrated EMG, xi, 157, 160, 161, 162, 163, 165
integration, 41, 105
integrin, 41
integrity, 5, 108
interface, 26, 131
interneurons, 169
intervention, 41, 54
intestine, 63, 65, 67, 69, 70, 73, 74, 75, 79
intima, 55, 119
intraocular, 36
intrauterine growth retardation, 125
intravenously, 28
ion transport, 76
ischemia, 121
ischemia reperfusion injury, 121
Israel, 103, 176, 177, 178, 179, 185
issues, 135
Italy, 36, 39, 80

J

Japan, 143, 144, 146, 147
jejunum, 68, 72, 74, 75, 76
joints, 65

K

K^+, 28, 29, 64, 67, 74
keratinocyte, 147, 154
keratinocytes, x, 141, 146, 147, 148
kidney(s), 18, 19, 20, 24, 28, 29, 30, 31, 62, 66, 76, 79, 115, 118, 139
kinase activity, 125

L

labeling, 3
lactate dehydrogenase, 106
lactation, ix, 100, 111, 115, 124, 175
large intestine, 76
L-arginine, 91
latency, 36
later life, 114, 121
lean body mass, 30
learning, 3, 4, 12
learning behavior, 3
leptin receptors, vii, xi, 1, 2, 3, 9, 19, 29, 40, 42, 46, 47, 52, 62, 68, 69, 73, 76, 79, 86, 90, 94, 99, 101, 103, 104, 112, 113, 116, 131, 132, 133, 135, 136, 138, 154, 158, 167, 175, 182, 187
lesions, 75, 90
leukemia, 2, 46
leukocytes, 121
libido, 175
lichen planus, 153
life expectancy, 84, 96, 114
ligand, 47, 113, 134
light, 136, 175, 177
lipid metabolism, x, 11, 57, 78, 117, 124, 141, 142, 153
lipids, 4, 6, 14, 72, 119
lipodystrophy, 2, 10
lipolysis, 48, 84, 94, 97, 185
lipoproteins, 14, 72
liver, 2, 3, 9, 18, 48, 66, 69, 84, 104, 115, 119, 154

liver disease, 9
localization, 29, 79, 95, 107, 136, 143, 147, 149, 152, 154
LTD, 3, 12, 24
lumen, 63, 74
luteinizing hormone, 90, 104, 105, 175, 184, 186
lymph node, 35
lymphocytes, 65
lymphoid, 34

M

macromolecules, 2
macrophages, 11, 35, 53, 59, 79, 120, 121
magnitude, 23, 54, 55, 115, 136, 158
majority, 7, 13, 118, 135
malignant melanoma, 36
malnutrition, 30, 77, 86, 99, 114, 115, 124
mammals, ix, 85, 111, 118, 122, 153, 159, 171, 174, 175, 185
man, 27, 108
management, 30, 40, 170
mandible, 149
manipulation, 114
mapping, 103
marrow, 130, 134, 138
mass, viii, ix, xii, 2, 6, 20, 24, 25, 29, 31, 33, 36, 45, 46, 53, 54, 57, 84, 92, 96, 97, 108, 111, 112, 114, 117, 118, 119, 125, 126, 130, 131, 132, 133, 135, 136, 137, 139, 174, 183
materials, 149
matrix, 35, 80, 149
matrix metalloproteinase, 35, 80
mean arterial pressure, 19, 119
measurement(s), 6, 79, 160, 184
meat, 8
media, 55, 119, 134
median, 6
mediation, 167
medical, 42
medication, 8, 9
medicine, xi, 139, 141
Mediterranean, 185
medulla, 159, 169
megakaryocyte, 100
melanoma, vii, viii, 33, 34, 35, 36
melanoma development, viii, 33
melatonin, 149, 155, 180, 181, 185, 186, 187
mellitus, 119
melting, 179
membranes, 75, 159, 175
memory, vii, 1, 2, 3, 4, 7, 12, 14, 115
memory function, 4
menarche, 184, 186
menopause, 2
menstruation, 105, 174
mesangial cells, 25
mesenchymal stem cells, 138, 139, 140
messenger ribonucleic acid, 99, 106, 124, 137, 169
messenger RNA, 124
metabolic, 27, 42, 53, 111, 185
metabolic changes, 114
metabolic disorder(s), 122
metabolic disturbances, 7, 136
metabolic dysfunction, 59, 114
metabolic pathways, 34
metabolic responses, 47, 186
metabolic syndrome, viii, ix, 24, 28, 30, 45, 46, 53, 54, 55, 59, 94, 104, 107, 108, 109, 111, 114, 115, 117, 119, 120, 125
metabolism, vii, ix, x, xii, 4, 20, 23, 24, 49, 62, 76, 85, 111, 112, 114, 115, 117, 119, 120, 125, 126, 127, 129, 130, 131, 135, 138, 154, 158, 171, 173, 185
metalloproteinase, 121
metastasis, viii, 35, 39, 40
Mexico, 111
microcirculation, 126
microclimate, 67
microinjection, xi, 157, 159, 160, 161, 162, 163, 165, 169
migration, viii, x, 34, 35, 39, 41, 117, 141, 144, 145, 147, 148, 153
mineralization, 137, 138, 139
miniature, 160
mitogen, 3, 7, 15, 18, 40, 86, 100, 154
mitogen activated protein kinase (MAPK), 18
mitogen activated protein kinase cascade (MAPK), 3
mitogens, 36
MLT, 175, 177, 178, 179, 180, 181, 182, 183
MMA, 91
models, x, 3, 4, 5, 8, 9, 10, 15, 20, 40, 51, 85, 87, 89, 93, 96, 98, 102, 103, 114, 115, 117, 123, 129, 130, 133, 135
modifications, ix, x, 68, 73, 111, 112
molecular mass, 174
molecules, 18, 47, 49, 52, 64, 68, 74, 155
monoclonal antibody, 40, 154
monocyte chemoattractant protein, 81, 121
monosodium glutamate, 75
morbidity, ix, 83, 123
morphogenesis, 149
morphology, 12, 84, 108
morphometric, 12
mortality, 36
MRI, 3, 10

mRNA, xii, 10, 15, 27, 69, 73, 80, 86, 92, 93, 99, 103, 104, 116, 124, 133, 137, 139, 144, 147, 154, 167, 169, 174, 178, 180, 182, 185, 187
mucosa, x, xi, 63, 68, 75, 76, 141, 142, 143, 144, 145, 147, 148, 153
mucus, 63
muscle mass, 139
muscle strength, 93
muscles, xi, 157, 158, 160, 161, 162, 163, 165
musculoskeletal, 137
mutagenesis, 14
mutant, 8
mutation(s), 7, 8, 27, 34, 76, 85, 86, 98, 112, 158, 169
mutational analysis, 100
myocardial infarction, x, 59, 112, 121
myocardium, 120

N

Na^+, ix, 28, 29, 61, 64, 65, 66, 67, 70, 71, 74, 78, 79, 80, 81
NaCl, 177, 178
National Academy of Sciences, 75, 186
National Health Service, 41
natural killer cell, 120
necrosis, 40, 120
negative effects, 175
neocortex, 2
neonates, 114
nerve, 27, 28, 166, 168
nervous system, xii, 19, 22, 116, 170, 173, 175
neural network, 169, 171
neurodegeneration, 4
neurodegenerative diseases, 5, 13
neurodegenerative disorders, 4, 8, 9
neurokinin, 170
neuronal cells, 13, 52
neuronal circuits, 113
neurons, 3, 4, 5, 6, 7, 10, 15, 48, 51, 56, 87, 88, 89, 90, 91, 92, 100, 101, 102, 103, 104, 113, 116, 123, 125, 130, 132, 159, 167, 168, 170, 171, 175
neuropeptides, 55, 62, 113, 116, 124, 130
neurotransmission, 7
neurotransmitters, 63, 114
neutral, 19, 65, 70, 78, 80, 81
nitric oxide, 19, 22, 28, 91, 95, 100, 108, 121
nitric oxide synthase, 91
NK cells, 120, 126
NMDA receptors, 4, 5, 12
norepinephrine, 131
normal distribution, 160
Norway, 36, 169
nuclear receptors, 102
nuclei, 116, 130, 168
nucleus, vii, xi, 1, 14, 19, 28, 47, 52, 80, 90, 92, 104, 113, 116, 123, 124, 130, 131, 132, 135, 157, 158, 166, 167, 169, 171
nutrient(s), vii, ix, 61, 63, 64, 67, 74,75, 79, 81, 92, 114, 149, 153, 181
nutrition, ix, 10, 111, 112, 116, 123, 125, 184
nutritional imbalance, 114
nutritional status, 63, 79, 104, 130, 175

O

obstructive sleep apnea, 158
old age, 123
oligomerization, 100
oligomers, 13
omega-3, 4
oocyte, 80
opioids, 159, 167
oral cavity, x, 141, 142, 153
organ(s), viii, 2, 18, 19, 34, 45, 55, 61, 112, 113, 115, 117, 118, 135, 153, 174, 175, 183, 184
organism, 62, 114, 181
osmotic stress, xii, 173, 176
ossification, 133, 138, 154
osteoclastogenesis, 131, 134
ovaries, xii, 112, 174, 180, 181, 183
overweight, 26, 84, 96, 114, 120, 174
ovulation, 175, 186
oxidation, 6, 81, 100, 119
oxidative stress, 22, 29, 30, 52, 79, 117
oxygen, 94

P

pachytene, 95
pancreas, 56, 115
parallel, 48, 68, 74, 78, 115
parkinsonism, 7, 14
participants, 7
pathogenesis, 6, 29, 57, 78, 100, 117
pathology, vii, 1, 5, 6, 7, 8, 13, 14
pathophysiological, 23, 26, 54
pathophysiology, 24, 97, 105, 115, 168
pathways, x, xii, 3, 4, 9, 10, 11, 41, 43, 48, 56, 68, 77, 86, 88, 93, 100, 103, 113, 116, 120, 121, 122, 125, 129, 130, 132, 133, 134, 135, 136, 170, 174, 175
PCR, xii, 27, 87, 133, 144, 147, 174, 178, 182, 185

peptide(s), vii, ix, xii, 11, 14, 17, 43, 61, 63, 64, 66, 72, 73, 75, 78, 79, 90, 92, 95, 105, 113, 132, 137, 159, 167, 173
perfusion, 68, 70
perinatal, ix, x, 86, 111, 112, 116, 124, 168
permission, 21, 22, 23, 24, 25
pH, 63, 65, 70, 71, 78, 79
phagocytosis, 52
pharmaceuticals, 7
pharmacological approaches, viii, 39, 40, 41
pharmacological treatment, 76
pharmacology, 78
phenocopy, 132
phenotype, viii, x, 39, 40, 41, 85, 86, 87, 98, 112, 114, 123, 129, 130, 131, 132, 133, 136, 139
phenotypes, 40, 85, 87, 130, 136
phenylalanine, 65
phosphate, 143, 178
phospholipids, 4
phosphorylation, vii, 1, 3, 6, 11, 13, 19, 41, 47, 49, 50, 52, 70, 78, 87, 89, 95, 124
physiological, vi, 21, 62, 111, 141, 173
physiology, ix, 24, 57, 58, 83, 95, 100, 105, 122, 125, 138, 140, 158, 183, 186
PI3K, 3, 18, 77, 86
pigs, 86, 99
pilot study, 14, 138
pineal gland, 183
pineal hormone melatonin, 175
pituitary gland, viii, 61, 104, 112, 113, 142, 153, 175
placenta, viii, 40, 61, 62, 79, 112, 113, 116, 124, 142, 153
plaque, 6
plasma levels, 58, 62, 69, 73, 183
plasma membrane, 5, 13, 67, 69, 72
plasminogen, 120
plasticity, vii, 1, 113, 115, 122, 123
platelet aggregation, ix, 111, 117
plexus, 47, 89
point mutation, 112
polarity, 12
polarization, 115
polymerase, 40
polymerase chain reaction, xii, 174, 178, 182
polymorphisms, 15
polypeptide, viii, 45, 100, 132, 142, 174
polyunsaturated fatty acids, 13
population, 18, 53, 73, 84, 92, 95, 96, 120, 126, 150, 151, 152, 160, 176
positive correlation, 33, 46, 53, 121, 174
potassium, 3, 167, 171
precursor cells, 97
pregnancy, ix, 89, 100, 102, 111, 114, 116, 124, 175
prejudice, 96
prematurity, 125
prevention, 42, 153
pro-atherogenic, 120
progenitor cells, 3, 13, 131, 138
progesterone, 11, 39, 94, 116, 178
prognosis, viii, 35, 39, 40, 41
programming, 112, 114, 115, 116, 123
progressive supranuclear palsy, 7
pro-inflammatory, 46, 52, 53, 57, 118
prolactin, 14, 89, 97, 116, 124
proliferation, viii, 3, 11, 20, 24, 29, 34, 35, 39, 40, 63, 80, 95, 102, 113, 115, 117, 120, 121, 122, 126, 133, 138, 144, 147, 153, 184
proline, 65, 66, 78, 79
promoter, 47, 49, 102
propagation, 15
propranolol, 131
prostate cancer, 36
prostate gland, 95, 108
proteasome, 89
protection, 53, 54
protein kinase C, 69, 79
protein kinases, 68
protein misfolding, 8
protein synthesis, 12
protein tyrosine phosphatase, 18, 101, 102
proteins, 3, 5, 8, 11, 13, 15, 34, 41, 47, 50, 51, 52, 64, 66, 86, 89, 117, 118, 149
proteinuria, 24, 25
psychosis, 14
PTEN, 12
pubertal development, 93, 103, 117
puberty, 85, 90, 92, 104, 105, 139, 184
public health, viii, 45
pulp, 151
purification, 178

Q

quality of life, ix, 83
quantification, 178, 179, 181, 182

R

radiotherapy, 153
reactions, 47, 52, 178
reactive oxygen, 95, 108
real time, 179
recognition, 6
recovery, 92, 93, 162
recruiting, xi, 121, 142, 151

rectal temperature, 159
recycling, 5
regulator gene, 79
regulatory systems, 26
relevance, vii, 17, 23, 99, 135
renal cell carcinoma, 34, 35
renal dysfunction, 26
renal medulla, 20, 21, 29
renal osteodystrophy, 26, 31
renal regulation, vii, 17, 26
renin, 30
repair, 77, 144, 147, 154
repression, 93, 101, 113, 134
reproduction, ix, xii, 9, 34, 62, 76, 83, 84, 85, 86, 87, 89, 90, 91, 92, 93, 98, 99, 100, 103, 105, 111, 173, 174, 176, 183, 184, 185, 186
reproductive age, 96
reproductive organs, 2
reproductive state, 104
requirements, xi, 14, 158, 167
reserves, ix, 111, 181
residues, 46, 47, 49, 50, 86
resistance, viii, ix, 2, 6, 10, 19, 20, 21, 22, 27, 28, 34, 45, 50, 51, 52, 53, 54, 55, 57, 58, 59, 73, 74, 83, 85, 88, 89, 90, 95, 96, 98, 101, 102, 113, 116, 117, 118, 119, 124, 127, 138, 139, 158, 170, 175, 183, 184, 186
resources, xii, 174
respiration, xi, 157, 159, 160, 162, 167, 168
respiratory disorders, 84
respiratory rate, xi, 157, 158, 162
response, ix, 5, 11, 19, 23, 28, 29, 31, 34, 39, 41, 53, 54, 58, 72, 73, 76, 77, 89, 90, 92, 93, 94, 101, 106, 111, 117, 120, 122, 131, 132, 133, 136, 158, 159, 161, 162, 163, 165, 179, 180, 181, 183
responsiveness, 23, 124
restoration, 21, 74, 105
restrictions, 86
reticulum, 11, 89, 102, 150
retinol, viii, 33, 120
reverse transcriptase, xii, 87, 174, 179, 182
rhythm, xi, 157, 159, 167, 168, 169, 170, 171, 187
rhythmicity, 14
ribose, 40
rings, 19, 68, 70
risk(s), viii, x, 4, 5, 6, 12, 13, 18, 29, 33, 35, 36, 37, 40, 46, 53, 59, 94, 96, 112, 114, 117, 118, 119, 120, 124
risk factors, 53, 59, 114, 119, 120
RNA, 42, 79, 178, 179, 184
rodents, ix, xii, 3, 5, 9, 12, 15, 61, 69, 80, 85, 86, 94, 95, 116, 118, 158, 173, 174, 175, 176, 183, 185, 187
Russia, 159

S

safety, 29
salinity, xii, 173, 174, 176, 178, 183, 185, 186
saliva, x, 141, 142, 154
Sartorius, 176, 177, 178
saturation, 2
Saudi Arabia, 139
seasonal changes, 175
seasonality, 185
secrete, xii, 35, 63, 73, 149, 173, 174
secretin, 63
secretion, 6, 11, 14, 15, 49, 53, 63, 76, 78, 79, 80, 84, 85, 89, 90, 91, 92, 95, 96, 99, 102, 103, 104, 105, 106, 115, 117, 118, 119, 120, 122, 133, 134, 174, 175, 182, 183, 186
seizure, 9
selectivity, 19, 80
semen, 96, 102, 108
seminal vesicle, 95, 108
seminiferous tubules, 85, 86, 94, 95
sensing, 81, 113, 153
sensitivity, 59, 70, 73, 94, 101, 121, 122, 126, 175, 182, 185
serine, 19
serotonin, 122
Sertoli cells, 86, 87, 95
serum, ix, xii, 2, 6, 10, 15, 24, 25, 30, 31, 35, 36, 37, 57, 59, 84, 85, 86, 92, 93, 94, 95, 98, 102, 106, 107, 108, 111, 112, 116, 120, 121, 124, 125, 135, 139, 174, 178, 179, 180, 181, 183, 184, 187
sex, viii, 33, 36, 84, 85, 90, 92, 97, 103, 105, 106, 107, 109, 174, 178
sex differences, 92
sex hormones, 85, 92, 97, 174, 178
sex steroid, 36, 92, 97, 106
shape, 167
sheep, 10, 104, 175, 183, 185
short splice variant, 18
showing, ix, 46, 92, 96, 111, 115, 118, 119, 143, 159
signal transduction, 18, 34, 47, 56, 63, 81, 86, 88, 89, 93, 100, 101, 113, 117, 118, 122
signaling pathway, ix, 3, 11, 19, 47, 57, 61, 86, 87, 88, 93, 94, 100, 101, 118, 120, 123
signalling, 9, 40, 41, 43, 47, 77, 80, 100, 102, 130, 131, 132, 133, 134, 135
signals, viii, ix, xii, 27, 33, 46, 47, 55, 64, 80, 89, 100, 101, 105, 111, 120, 131, 134, 135, 149, 167, 173, 174
siRNA, 133
skeletal muscle, viii, 40, 48, 61, 76, 102, 142, 154

skeleton, 130, 132, 135, 137
skin, x, 65, 77, 141, 142, 146, 147, 148, 153, 154, 155
small intestine, 64, 70, 73, 76, 77, 78, 79, 80
smoking, 36, 120
smooth muscle, 20, 29, 117
smooth muscle cells, 121, 138
SNS, 25, 131, 132
society, 136, 184
sodium, 20, 21, 22, 23, 24, 26, 29, 30, 64, 65, 67, 77, 81, 146, 183
software, 160
solution, 143, 146, 159, 162, 177
Spain, 61
spatial memory, 3, 12
species, xi, 86, 87, 94, 95, 108, 173, 174, 175, 176, 183
sperm, 84, 86, 95, 97, 99, 107, 108
sperm function, 96
spermatogenesis, ix, 83, 85, 90, 93, 95, 99
spine, 136
spleen, 18
stability, 178
stabilization, 15
standard error, 160
starvation, 51, 56, 106, 120, 132, 133, 135
state(s), viii, xii, 2, 9, 23, 35, 45, 46, 51, 52, 53, 54, 55, 64, 67, 69, 73, 92, 115, 116, 121, 133, 134, 163, 165, 170, 173, 175, 183
status epilepticus, 9, 15
steel, 160
stem cell differentiation, x, 129
stem cells, 42, 134
sterile, 177
steroids, 104, 105
stimulant, 158, 159, 162, 166, 167
stimulation, xi, 4, 14, 18, 19, 20, 22, 42, 70, 80, 89, 93, 104, 113, 136, 158, 160, 162, 166, 168, 171
stimulus, 56, 63
stomach, viii, 40, 61, 63, 64, 75, 76, 80, 85, 112, 113, 142, 153
stomatitis, 153
storage, xii, 116, 119, 173, 174, 183
stress, xii, 11, 89, 102, 173
stroke, x, 8, 112, 121
stroma, 35, 134
stromal cells, 138
structural changes, 24
structural characteristics, 46
structure, viii, 2, 9, 12, 45, 46, 55, 67, 78, 112, 114, 118
style, 175
subgroups, 7, 9
substrate(s), 19, 47, 49, 58, 65, 69, 70, 77, 80, 116, 174
suicide, 5
supplementation, 31, 114, 131
suppression, 9, 18, 102, 116, 131, 138
suprachiasmatic nucleus, 169
surface area, 36
survival, xi, 7, 11, 15, 35, 40, 99, 103, 115, 173
survival rate, 7
susceptibility, 77, 84, 121
sympathetic denervation, 22, 29
sympathetic nervous system, x, 18, 19, 20, 22, 25, 26, 57, 121, 129, 130, 131, 136
symptoms, 85, 93
synaptic plasticity, 3, 7, 12
synaptic strength, 3
synaptic transmission, 12, 15
synaptogenesis, 3, 4
syndrome, viii, 12, 42, 45, 94, 103, 123, 158, 167, 168, 170
synthesis, 4, 24, 25, 62, 66, 68, 73, 80, 84, 85, 118, 120, 134, 138, 174, 186
systemic vasculature, 18
systolic blood pressure, 20

T

T cell, 47, 53, 120
T lymphocytes, 126
tangles, 6
target, viii, 2, 3, 20, 39, 40, 42, 51, 87, 88, 103, 112, 113, 121, 142, 168, 179
tau, vii, 1, 5, 6, 7, 8, 13, 14
technical assistance, 26
technology, 179
teeth, 155
temperature, vii, 17, 176, 177, 186
tendons, 65
testing, 6, 35
testis, ix, xii, 83, 85, 86, 88, 89, 93, 94, 95, 97, 98, 99, 103, 106, 108, 174, 178, 180, 182, 183
testosterone, ix, 83, 84, 85, 86, 88, 89, 92, 93, 94, 96, 97, 98, 106, 107, 108, 109, 178
TGF, 24
therapeutic applications, viii, 39
therapeutic approaches, 14
therapeutic use, 122
therapeutics, 135
therapy, vii, 1, 7, 8, 9, 10, 13, 39, 40, 53, 54, 55, 105, 106, 112, 118, 139
third molar(s), 150
threonine, 65
threshold level, 93

thrombosis, ix, 111
thymus, 120
tissue, xii, 5, 8, 15, 18, 26, 27, 34, 35, 40, 48, 50, 54, 55, 57, 58, 79, 85, 113, 116, 117, 118, 127, 130, 142, 143, 146, 148, 151, 152, 153, 154, 158, 173, 174, 184
TNF, 125
TNF-alpha (TNF-α), 12, 46, 53
tobacco, 36
tooth, x, xi, 141, 142, 149, 150, 151, 152, 153, 155
toxicity, 8, 13, 41
trachea, 159
tracks, 15
trafficking, ix, 4, 5, 12, 61, 81, 123
training, 54, 59, 123
transcription, 3, 18, 47, 49, 59, 72, 86, 87, 89, 94, 100, 101, 118, 123, 124, 126, 167, 178, 179, 185
transcription factors, 86, 89
transducer, 59, 86, 100, 118, 120, 123, 124, 167
transduction, 18, 47, 113
transforming growth factor, 133
translocation, 13, 72, 87, 89, 101, 168
transmission, 8, 168
transplantation, 131, 139
transport, ix, 2, 4, 5, 13, 18, 47, 51, 58, 61, 63, 64, 65, 66, 68, 69, 70, 71, 72, 73, 75, 76, 77, 78, 79, 81, 89, 92, 118, 123
treatment, viii, 3, 5, 6, 7, 11, 14, 15, 22, 27, 39, 40, 41, 42, 57, 58, 62, 69, 70, 85, 90, 92, 98, 118, 120, 124, 126, 127, 134, 138, 153, 178, 179, 180, 183, 186
tremor, 7
triggers, 50, 52, 69, 90
triglycerides, 4, 51, 72, 89
tumor, viii, 33, 34, 35, 36, 37, 46, 120, 125
tumor development, 37
tumor growth, viii, 33, 34, 35
tumor necrosis factor, 46, 120, 125
tumo(u)rs, 34, 35, 36, 37, 39, 40, 41
turnover, 81, 132
type 2 diabetes, ix, 53, 84, 94, 111, 114, 115, 117, 119, 124, 126
tyrosine, 18, 47, 49, 50, 52, 58, 86, 87, 101, 102, 125, 167

U

UK, 160, 178
ulcer, x, 141, 143, 144, 145, 146, 148
undernutrition, 114, 115, 116
uniform, 115
United States (USA), 13, 17, 18, 26, 33, 40, 75, 77, 78, 114, 136, 153, 154, 159, 160, 168, 178, 179, 186
urea, 66
urethane, xi, 157, 159

V

vagus nerve, 63
validation, 19
variations, 174, 183
vascular diseases, 26
vascular endothelial growth factor (VEGF), 37
vascular system, 120, 121
vasculature, 18, 121
vasoconstriction, 19
vasodilation, 28, 121
vasodilator, 127
vasopressin, xii, 173, 185, 186
VEGF expression, 35
ventilation, xi, 158, 159, 162, 164, 166, 167, 168
vertebrae, 130
vessels, 146, 151
villus, 77
visceral adiposity, 186
vision, ix, 61, 74
vitamin A, 36
vitamin E, viii, 33

W

water, xi, xii, 20, 23, 24, 173, 174, 176, 177, 182, 183, 185
weight gain, 14, 35, 46, 115, 119
weight loss, viii, 8, 13, 14, 21, 26, 31, 45, 46, 51, 53, 54, 55, 88, 96, 109, 119, 158
western blot, 70, 87
wild type, 132
World Health Organization, 84
worldwide, viii, 39, 45, 84, 96, 114, 120
wound healing, x, xi, 62, 141, 142, 143, 144, 145, 146, 147, 148, 153, 154

Y

yang, 104
yin, 104
young adults, 27